Governors State University
Library
Hours:
Monday thru Thursday 8:30 to 10:30
Friday and Saturday 8:30 to 5:00
Sunday 1:00 to 5:00 (Fall and Winter Trimester Only)

DEMCO

PHYSICIAN RECRUITMENT AND EMPLOYMENT

A Complete Reference Guide

Second Edition

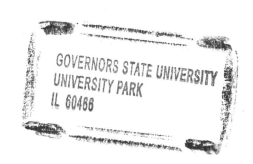
By
The Coker Group
Atlanta, GA

Eugene Nelson   **Kay B. Stanley, FACME**

JONES AND BARTLETT PUBLISHERS
Sudbury, Massachusetts
BOSTON   TORONTO   LONDON   SINGAPORE

World Headquarters
Jones and Bartlett Publishers
40 Tall Pine Drive
Sudbury, MA 01776
978-443-5000
info@jbpub.com
www.jbpub.com

Jones and Bartlett Publishers
Canada
6339 Ormindale Way
Mississauga, Ontario L5V 1J2
CANADA

Jones and Bartlett Publishers
International
Barb House, Barb Mews
London W6 7PA
UK

Jones and Bartlett's books and products are available through most bookstores and online booksellers. To contact Jones and Bartlett Publishers directly, call 800-832-0034, fax 978-443-8000, or visit our website, www.jbpub.com.

Substantial discounts on bulk quantities of Jones and Bartlett's publications are available to corporations, professional associations, and other qualified organizations. For details and specific discount information, contact the special sales department at Jones and Bartlett via the above contact information or send an email to specialsales@jbpub.com.

Production Credits
Executive Editor: David Cella
Associate Production Editor: Daniel Stone
Editorial Assistant: Lisa Gordon
Production Director: Amy Rose
Associate Marketing Manager: Laura Kavigian
Manufacturing Buyer: Amy Bacus
Cover Design: Timothy Dziewit
Printing and Binding: Courier Westford
Cover Printing: Courier Stoughton

This publication is designed to provide accurate and authoritative information in regard to the Subject Matter covered. It is sold with the understanding that the publisher is not engaged in rendering legal, accounting, or other professional service. If legal advice or other expert assistance is required, the service of a competent professional person should be sought.

Library of Congress Cataloging-in-Publication Data
Stanley, Kay, 1944–
    Physican recruitment and employment / The Coker Group ; Kay Stanley. — 2nd ed.
       p. ; cm.
    Rev. ed. of: Physician recruitment and employment / Eugene E. Olson, Kay B. Stanley ; the Coker Group. © 2004.
    Includes index.
    ISBN-13: 978-0-7637-3867-9
    ISBN-10: 0-7637-3867-0
    1. Physicians—Recruiting.   2. Physicians—Employment.   I. Olson, Eugene E., 1943– Physician recruitment and employment.   II. Coker Group.   III. Title.
    [DNLM: 1. Personnel Selection—legislation & jurisprudence—United States—Guideline.   2. Personnel Selection—standards—United States—Guideline.   3. Physicians—United States—Guideline.   W 76 S788p 2007]
    R729.5.R87O448 2007
    362.11068'3—dc22

                                    2006015679

Printed in the United States of America
10 09 08 07 06   10 9 8 7 6 5 4 3 2 1

PHYSICIAN RECRUITMENT AND EMPLOYMENT

A Complete Reference Guide

Second Edition

By
The Coker Group
Atlanta, GA

Eugene Nelson   **Kay B. Stanley, FACME**

JONES AND BARTLETT PUBLISHERS
Sudbury, Massachusetts
BOSTON   TORONTO   LONDON   SINGAPORE

World Headquarters
Jones and Bartlett Publishers
40 Tall Pine Drive
Sudbury, MA 01776
978-443-5000
info@jbpub.com
www.jbpub.com

Jones and Bartlett Publishers
Canada
6339 Ormindale Way
Mississauga, Ontario L5V 1J2
CANADA

Jones and Bartlett Publishers
International
Barb House, Barb Mews
London W6 7PA
UK

Jones and Bartlett's books and products are available through most bookstores and online booksellers. To contact Jones and Bartlett Publishers directly, call 800-832-0034, fax 978-443-8000, or visit our website, www.jbpub.com.

Substantial discounts on bulk quantities of Jones and Bartlett's publications are available to corporations, professional associations, and other qualified organizations. For details and specific discount information, contact the special sales department at Jones and Bartlett via the above contact information or send an email to specialsales@jbpub.com.

Production Credits
Executive Editor: David Cella
Associate Production Editor: Daniel Stone
Editorial Assistant: Lisa Gordon
Production Director: Amy Rose
Associate Marketing Manager: Laura Kavigian
Manufacturing Buyer: Amy Bacus
Cover Design: Timothy Dziewit
Printing and Binding: Courier Westford
Cover Printing: Courier Stoughton

This publication is designed to provide accurate and authoritative information in regard to the Subject Matter covered. It is sold with the understanding that the publisher is not engaged in rendering legal, accounting, or other professional service. If legal advice or other expert assistance is required, the service of a competent professional person should be sought.

Library of Congress Cataloging-in-Publication Data
Stanley, Kay, 1944–
    Physican recruitment and employment / The Coker Group ; Kay Stanley. — 2nd ed.
        p. ; cm.
    Rev. ed. of: Physician recruitment and employment / Eugene E. Olson, Kay B. Stanley ; the Coker Group. © 2004.
    Includes index.
    ISBN-13: 978-0-7637-3867-9
    ISBN-10: 0-7637-3867-0
    1. Physicians—Recruiting. 2. Physicians—Employment. I. Olson, Eugene E., 1943– Physician recruitment and employment. II. Coker Group. III. Title.
    [DNLM: 1. Personnel Selection—legislation & jurisprudence—United States—Guideline. 2. Personnel Selection—standards—United States—Guideline. 3. Physicians—United States—Guideline. W 76 S788p 2007]
    R729.5.R87O448 2007
    362.11068'3—dc22

                                2006015679

Printed in the United States of America
10 09 08 07 06   10 9 8 7 6 5 4 3 2 1

Contents

ENCLOSED CD-ROM

The CD-ROM included in this book contains PDFs of all exhibits displayed throughout the text. In addition, all Templates and Tools from Part IV are included.

Preface

Is the government taking a meaner and tougher approach to healthcare fraud? In its budget justification for Fiscal Year (FY) 2007, the US Department of Health and Human Services Office of Inspector General noted:

> FY 2005 expected recoveries from audit disallowances and investigative receivables was $2.88 billion—$657 million more than the $2.23 billion target. Audit disallowances in FY 2005 were almost double the amount experienced in FY 2004, and nearly four times the amount in FY 2003 . . . OIG average annual return on investment during the FY 2003 to 2005 period was $11.6:1—seven percent higher than the 10.8:1 target. This continues the well-established pattern of effective and efficient conduct of the OIG mission.[1]

Meanwhile, in April 2006, a federal prosecution in San Diego based on alleged federal anti-kickback statute violations involving physician recruitment, ended in a second mistrial. Six months earlier, a large nonprofit health system agreed to pay $40 million to settle civil false claims allegations that it entered into a series of transactions, including recruiting agreements, through which it paid remuneration intended to induce physicians to refer patients to its facilities. Clearly, physician recruitment arrangements have become a target of increasing government scrutiny.

Physician Recruitment and Employment: A Complete Reference Guide is a comprehensive orientation and instruction manual for physician recruitment and employment policies and contracts. The federal government has instituted a number of broad-ranging laws and statutes over the years that seriously affect healthcare providers and physicians. The relevant laws and regulations include the Medicare Fraud and Abuse Statute (sometimes called the "anti-kickback statute"), the Ethics in Patient Referral Act of 1989 (sometimes called the "Stark amendment" or "Stark I"), the Comprehensive Physician Ownership and Referral Act of 1993 (sometimes called "Stark II") (Stark I and Stark II are called collectively the "Stark law"), and the False Claims Act. Regulations promulgated pursuant to the Stark law have been published in stages, with the most recent revisions published in March, 2004.

Why was this important?

Virtually every aspect of health care is affected by some form of government control at both the federal and state level. That control extends to hiring practices, business relationships and how they are established, patient referrals, what services are provided, how much is charged for those services, how those services are recorded, and how payment for those services is accomplished. This book focuses on those controls applying to physician recruitment and hiring.

Taking a tougher and meaner approach, the federal government has made known its intentions toward full-force investigations of any evidence of fraud and abuse in government-funded programs, and its resolve to prosecute violators. Any breach of regulations, whether intentional or not, could bring the Office of Inspector General (OIG), Department of Justice (DOJ), Internal Revenue Service (IRS), or state agencies knocking on the door, not to mention the possibility of a "whistle blower" or Qui Tam lawsuit by a private citizen who could share in any money damages awarded by a court in connection with a violation of federal regulations.

Enforcement actions have clearly increased, with the number of federal criminal prosecutions of healthcare companies and workers increasing in 2004 to 395 involving 646 defendants, and with convictions of 459 defendants for healthcare fraud-related crimes. In addition, in FY 2004, the Department of Justice opened 868 new civil healthcare fraud investigations, and filed complaints or intervened in 269 civil healthcare cases.

Between 1996 and 2003, Congress more than tripled the budget for Medicare and Medicaid fraud enforcement for the OIG and more than doubled the budget for the same type of work by the FBI. Under the Health Insurance Portability and Accountability Act of 1996, civil and criminal penalties collected in health fraud probes help fund enforcement of antifraud laws.

The purpose of this book is an attempt to answer many of the questions about the government regulations pertaining to physicians and health systems in the area of physician recruitment and employment practices. The government regulations have a broad influence and are sometimes vague and even contradictory at times. This book attempts to make hospitals and healthcare providers aware of these far-reaching regulations and to encourage consultation with an attorney in any transaction touching any of the regulated areas described in this book.

The initiatives that are designed to prevent healthcare fraud and abuse are pervasive and widespread. Providers, institutions, and companies cannot afford to be uninformed about and must adhere to the myriad statutes affecting every aspect of the industry. The potential pitfalls are plentiful, and the consequences are great for those in health care who violate federal and state laws. This book introduces many of the pitfalls and presents some suggested ways to help keep away from infringements and ensure legal compliance. In all matters of legal responsibility, however, it is essential to consult an attorney for specific legal advice. A qualified attorney should be engaged to review all activities, correspondence, and documentation regarding physician recruitment to ensure compliance with federal and state laws.

REFERENCES

1. Department of Health and Human Services, Office of Inspector General. Fiscal year 2007 justification of estimates for appropriation committees. Available at: http://oig.hhs.gov/publications.html. Accessed April, 27, 2006.

About the Authors

Eugene E. Olson, attorney at law, is a partner in the law firm of Connolly, O'Malley, Lillis, Hansen & Olson, LLP, located in Des Moines, Iowa. He received his juris doctorate in 1968, and then served as assistant city attorney and later as city solicitor in Des Moines.

Practicing in the areas of healthcare law, hospital law, real estate, and zoning, Mr. Olson personally has been involved in hospital and health law for 20 years. Although his primary activity has been in connection with hospitals, he has also been involved with physicians in private practice, as well as licensed nursing facilities.

Kay B. Stanley is an associate partner of The Coker Group, a national healthcare services firm headquartered in Atlanta, Georgia. She heads the company's publishing and training initiative. Major projects include *Practice Success!*, a medical practice management guidebook, and the *Practice Success!* series, 10 publications on medical practice management published by the American Medical Association. Under Ms. Stanley's purview, Coker has over 40 published books on various aspects of the business of health care. With The Coker Group since 1988, Ms. Stanley has more than 20 years of experience in administration and personnel management. She is a member of the Medical Group Management Association at the local, state, and national levels and a Fellow in the American College of Medical Practice Executives.

As a recognized leader in practice management consulting, The Coker Group serves its clients by providing independent appraisals of physician practices; development and administration of management services organizations (MSOs); primary care network establishment and administration;

physician services such as independent group formation and practice sale brokering; physician compensation plan design; physician and hospital integration; and managed care strategic planning.

CONTRIBUTORS

Craig W. Hunter, an associate partner with The Coker Group, has over 15 years experience in health care. Since joining the firm in 1989, he has worked extensively with health systems, hospital-based networks, multispecialty and single-specialty groups, and independent private practices to achieve performance improvement. Mr. Hunter has facilitated many phases of integration and practice development for Coker clients. Working in the area of practice mergers, strategic planning, management reviews, negotiations, and disengagements are among his major strengths.

Mr. Hunter's focus includes physician network development, physician manpower plans, practice brokerage, appraisals and operational assessments, physician compensation plans, and medical staff surveys. Mr. Hunter provides integrated network services to hospitals and independent practices.

Mr. Hunter frequently conducts physician need and feasibility analyses for hospitals and private practices, which specifically involve staff planning and market analysis. Assignments involve physician contracts preparation, analysis, and negotiations.

Mr. Hunter is a frequent program speaker at conferences and workshops sponsored by pharmaceutical companies, medical associations, and healthcare organizations. His audiences comprise health system executives, physician executives, senior administrators, and other healthcare personnel. Recent publishing accomplishments include *Beyond Disengagement: Recreating the Physician Practice* and articles in *Managed Care Quarterly* and the American Osteopathic Association's *Practice Pointers*. Hunter's article on expanding market share was featured recently in the *Journal of Medical Practice Management*. Hunter is a contributor to the second edition of *Integration Strategies*, and the second edition of *Physician Compensation Strategies*.

Mr. Hunter is a graduate of David Lipscomb University in Nashville, Tennessee.

Gabriel L. Imperato, JD, has practiced healthcare law in both the public and private sectors for more than 20 years and is board certified as a specialist in health law by the Florida bar. Mr. Imperato presently represents individuals and organizations accused of criminal and civil healthcare fraud in jurisdictions throughout the United States. Prior to joining Broad and Cassel, Mr. Imperato was the deputy chief counsel, Office of the General Counsel, US Department of Health and Human Services, where he advised and represented various agencies of the Department of Health and Human Services, including the Health Care Financing Administration (Medicare and Medicaid), the Public Health Service, the Social Security Administration, and the Office of the Inspector General. Mr. Imperato has extensive criminal and civil trial and appellate experience in administrative, state, and federal courts and has personally handled leading national cases concerning criminal and civil care fraud and abuse and healthcare law and policy. He has also handled numerous matters involving the formation of integrated delivery systems and managed care organizations. He is considered a national expert on fraud and abuse, reimbursement, and antitrust and has published numerous articles on such issues as medical staff proceedings, antitrust in the healthcare field, handling a healthcare fraud investigation, and administrative and judicial procedural rights and the fraud and abuse laws under Medicare, Medicaid, and private health insurance programs. He is a member of the Illinois, Florida, and District of Columbia Bars; the American Health Lawyers Association; the Health Law Section of the Florida Bar; the American Bar Association Antitrust Health Care Committee, White Collar Crime Committee, and the Subcommittee on Health Care Fraud, where he has been a member of the Planning Committee of the American Bar Association Health Care Fraud Institution. Mr. Imperato was a long-time member of the now dissolved American Academy of Hospital Attorneys, where he was chair of the Reimbursement and Payment Committee and the Health Care Reform Task Force.

Lester J. Perling, JD, MHA, is a board-certified health law attorney and holds a Masters degree in health care administration. He has significant experience with Medicare and Medicaid reimbursement and fraud and abuse issues, privacy of healthcare information (HIPAA), federal and state administrative proceedings, provider operations issues, corporate compliance programs, managed care and integrated delivery systems, and various administrative and corporate matters for healthcare providers. Prior to becoming an attorney, Mr. Perling had more than 10 years experience as a healthcare executive and held various administrative positions, including chief executive officer with investor-owned and community hospitals. Mr. Perling is a partner at the Ft. Lauderdale office of Broad and Cassel, on the executive counsel of the health law section of the Florida bar, vice chair of the American Health Lawyers Association Regulation, Accreditation and Payment practice groups, member of the health law section of the American and Florida bar, author of numerous published works in the healthcare field, and is a frequent speaker on health law topics.

Mike Segal, JD, LL.M, attended the University of Florida, receiving his Bachelor of Arts in political science in 1967 and his juris doctorate in law in 1969. In 1971, he received an LL.M. in taxation from New York University. Thereafter, he was an attorney advisor for the US Tax Court in Washington, DC. He has been associated with Broad and Cassel for 25 years. Mr. Segal is a partner of the Miami office of Broad and Cassel, serves on the firm's executive committee, and is the chair of the firm's healthcare practice group. Mr. Segal's practice is primarily devoted to healthcare transactional matters, which includes structuring medical group practices throughout the United States, forming integrated delivery systems between physicians and hospitals, and representing buyers and sellers in complex purchase and sale of healthcare-related businesses. He is a member of AHLA, the healthcare sections of the American and Florida.

Edward J. Hopkins, Esq., is a partner in the West Palm Beach office of Broad and Cassel, and a member of the Firm's Health Law and White Collar and Civil Fraud Defense Practice Groups. He has limited his practice exclusively to the representation of healthcare providers and companies for the last 30 years. Much of Mr. Hopkins' practice is devoted to counseling clients regarding the regulatory healthcare fraud and false claims implications of corporate and financial transactions; advising them regarding various aspects of compliance plan development, implementation, training, and operation; and defending clients in healthcare fraud and false claims-related voluntary disclosures, investigations, and litigation. He has also represented a significant number of public and private hospitals, healthcare systems, hospices, physician group practices, practice management companies, and other healthcare companies in facility and system reorganizations, acquisitions and divestitures, joint ventures, third-party reimbursement appeals, and issues relating to tax exemption, as well as general corporate, regulatory, financial, and operational issues confronting the healthcare industry.

Mr. Hopkins is a regular speaker at regional and national seminars and at officer and trustee training programs on corporate governance and the implications for officers and trustees of fraud and abuse and compliance issues. He is a recipient of the Healthcare Financial Management Association's Follmer Bronze and Reeves Silver Merit Awards for Outstanding Service, and is listed in *The Best Lawyers in America (Health Care Law),* and in *Law and Leading Attorneys*.

Mr. Hopkins is licensed to practice law in both Florida and Texas, and is board certified in health Law by the Florida Bar. He is a member of the American Health Lawyers Association, Florida Association of Healthcare Attorneys, and the Health Law Section of the Florida Bar, the Healthcare Financial Management Association, and the Health Care Compliance Association. Mr. Hopkins received his AG, magna cum laude, from Xavier University in 1970, and his JD from Duke University School of Law in 1973.

Part I

General Guiding Principles

The primary regulatory considerations applicable to physician recruitment emanate from the rules governing the tax-exempt status of hospitals and the prohibitions under the federal anti-kickback statute. The principles of "community benefit" as a factual matter and "community need" are important to establish as a factual matter to preserve global tax-exempt status and to reflect that the "intent" under the federal anti-kickback statute in the physician recruitment program was to procure a physician to fulfill a community and hospital need instead of paying remuneration in return for the referral of the physician's patients. The following discussion of the law governing tax-exempt status and the application of the federal anti-kickback statute frames the necessity for justification of "community benefit" and "community need."

TAX-EXEMPT STATUS

A § 501(c)(3) not-for-profit (i.e., nonprofit) organization is an entity that has been determined to be exempt from federal income taxation pursuant to § 501(c)(3) of the Internal Revenue Code. While § 501(c) lists 28 different types of exempt status, 501(c)(3) status is the most advantageous status. Advantages of § 501(c)(3) status include the following:

1. Avoidance of federal (and generally, state) income taxes on net income
2. Ability to receive contributions that are deductible to donors for their own income tax purposes

3. Qualification for grants from governmental and other charitable sources
4. Ability to utilize tax-exempt bond financing
5. Ability to use certain employee benefit programs (e.g., tax-deferred annuities)
6. Exemption from federal (not state) unemployment taxes
7. Qualification for preferential postal rates
8. Depending on local law, exemption from state and local real and personal property taxes
9. Depending on local law, exemption from state and local sales and use taxes on purchases of goods and services

Section 501(c)(3) applies to a broad range of organizations, including those that are charitable, religious, educational, or scientific in nature. The "promotion of health" has been determined to constitute a charitable purpose.[1]

Section 501(c)(3) regulations established the "community benefit" standard for exemption of healthcare organizations. Key criteria include the following:

1. An emergency room open to all, regardless of ability to pay.[2]
2. Provision of hospital care for all who can afford to pay, including through Medicare and Medicaid
3. Use of surplus funds to further exempt purposes
4. Open medical staff
5. Community board (i.e., majority of board are independent community or civic leaders)
6. Charity care, while not explicitly required by Rev. Rul. 69-545, often serves as a key indicator of community benefit.[3]

An organization may qualify for (c)(3) status either on a "stand-alone" basis (i.e., on the basis of its own purposes and activities) or on the theory that it constitutes an "integral part" of the exempt activities of another (c)(3) organization.[4] An organization must be organized exclusively for one or more exempt purposes, and generally it must be formed as a nonprofit or nonstick entity under applicable state laws. The organization must be organized as a corporation, association, trust, foundation, or community chest. In recent years, the IRS has recognized that limited liability companies may obtain (c)(3) status, if they elect to be treated as corporations (rather than as pass-through entities).

The operational test an organization must meet is whether it is to be operated exclusively for one or more exempt purposes, meaning it must engage "primarily" in activities that further its exempt purpose or purposes.

If an organization engages in activities that are not in furtherance of any exempt purpose, it must do so only to an insubstantial degree. Moreover, it may have to pay taxes on income derived from such activities.[5] If an activity is not in furtherance of an exempt purpose, the organization must be prepared to show that it is merely "incidental" to its primary (exempt) activities. The IRS looks at: (1) the amount of income derived from the activity in comparison to total income; (2) the amount of expenditures for the activity in comparison to total expenditures; and (3) the amount of time the organization's employees devote to the activity in comparison to total hours worked.

The operational test is not met if either private inurement or substantial private benefit is present. An organization must serve a public, rather than a private, interest. The class of persons served by the organization's activities must be so broad as to be deemed the "public." Any private benefit (such as to physicians) that results from the organization's activities must be incidental, both quantitatively and qualitatively, to the public benefit resulting there from.[6]

A subset of private benefit is private inurnment. An organization's earnings must not inure in whole or in part to the benefit of "insiders," meanings persons having a personal and private interest in the activities of the organization (founders, directors, officers, key employees, or relatives thereof; or in the case of hospitals, to physicians). This prohibition is absolute, meaning as an organization it cannot have even a de minimis amount of inurement (in contrast to private benefit).[7] For several years, the IRS indicated that all physicians on a hospital's medical staff would be considered "insiders."[8] In recent years, however, they have taken a different view.[9]

The practical application of these restrictions means that (c)(3) organizations must do the following:

- Pay not more than reasonable compensation for services rendered to the organization.
- Pay not more than fair market value for property being purchased by the organization.
- Receive not less than fair market value for services being rendered by the organization.
- Receive not less than fair market value for property being sold by the organization.

Up until 1995, the IRS's only remedy for cases of private benefit or inurement was to revoke the tax exemption for the offending organization. Today, in inurement cases, the IRS can impose immediate sanctions (i.e., penalty excise taxes) on persons who received improper benefit and on the organization's managers. The IRS also may revoke the organization's tax-exempt status, but likely will do so only in rare circumstances.[10]

ANTI-KICKBACK STATUTE

The federal anti-kickback statute states in pertinent part:

   A. Whoever knowingly and willfully solicits or receives any remuneration (including any kickback, bribe, or rebate) directly or indirectly, overtly or covertly, in cash or in kind
      1. in return for referring an individual to a person for the furnishing or arranging for the furnishing of any item or service

for which payment may be made in whole or in part under a Federal health care program, or

2. in return for purchasing, leasing, ordering, or arranging for or recommending purchasing, leasing, or ordering any good, facility, service, or item for which payment may be made in whole or in part under a Federal health care program shall be guilty of a felony and upon conviction thereof, shall be fined not more than $25,000 or imprisoned for not more than five years, or both.

B. Whoever knowingly and willfully offers or pays any remuneration (including any kickback, bribe, or rebate) directly or indirectly, overtly or covertly, in cash or in kind to any person to induce such person

1. to refer an individual to a person for the furnishing or arranging for the furnishing of any item or service for which payment may be made in whole or in part under a Federal health care program, or

2. to purchase, lease, order, or arrange for or recommend purchasing, leasing, or ordering any good, facility, service, or item for which payment may be made in whole or in part under a Federal health care program, shall be guilty of a felony and upon conviction thereof, shall be fined not more than $25,000 or imprisoned for not more than five years, or both.[11]

The case law is instructive regarding the application of the law to physician recruitment activities. The decision in *United States v. Greber*[12] also established the "one purpose" test for interpreting the application of the statute. Over defendant's objections, the court held that the anti-kickback statute covers any arrangement where *one purpose* of the remuneration was to obtain money for the referral of services or to induce further referrals. The court stated that even in cases in which a physician performs some service for the money received, "the potential for unnecessary drains on the Medicare system remains. The statute is aimed at the inducement factor."

The scienter requirement of *knowingly* and *willfully* is also an important aspect in the application of the statute and is reflected in a number of cases. In *United States v. Baystate Ambulance*[13] the court approved the following jury instruction: "*Knowingly* simply means to do something voluntarily, to do it deliberately, not to do something by mistake or by accident or even negligently. *Willfully* means to do something purposely, with the intent to violate the law, to do something purposely that [the] law forbids." The court stated that the scienter requirement mitigated any due process vagueness challenge, especially with respect to the adequacy of notice to the defendant that his conduct is proscribed. The Ninth Circuit Court of Appeals in *Hanlester Network v. Shalala*[14] later found that the anti-kickback statute requirement of "knowingly" and "willfully" requires individuals to "know that Section 1128B prohibits offering or paying remuneration to induce referrals, and engage in prohibited conduct with the specific intent to disobey the law." The court states in a footnote that "[t]he legislative history demonstrates that Congress, by use of the phrase 'knowingly and willfully' to describe the type of conduct prohibited under the anti-kickback laws, intended to shield from prosecution only those whose conduct 'while improper, was inadvertent.' "[15]

The decision in *United States v. Starks*[16] rejected many of the arguments for imposing a heightened scienter requirement, but this case did not involve an innocent business practice or a misunderstanding of a technicality. There was evidence in *Starks* that the defendants tried to conceal payments to government employees for referrals to a drug-treatment program. Such a classic bribery case may have been the wrong vehicle for defining the outer contours of the anti-kickback statute, since the defendants' conduct would likely have satisfied any standard of criminal intent.[17]

This part sets forth the general principles and concepts that serve to guide hospitals and health systems in lawfully recruiting physicians. The following areas are covered:

- Justification of community need and benefit
- Policies concerning the categories of practice as they relate to existing medical practices
- Other guiding principles, such as the overall reasonableness of recruitment activities

The objective of this part is to draw attention to the areas most likely to be scrutinized carefully. Because of the potential for extreme penalties and retributions, it is essential to work closely with legal counsel in all areas of physician recruitment.

PRINCIPLES OF COMMUNITY NEED AND COMMUNITY BENEFIT

As a general rule, any physician recruitment transaction should be able to identify actual community need or community benefit. The concepts of community need and community benefit, within the context of physician recruitment, are evolving standards. Moreover, in November 1999, the Office of Inspector General (OIG) stated that while a "demonstrated community need" standard is appealing, it presents too many difficulties in application to warrant safe harbor protection. Despite this lack of safe harbor protection, every hospital should require that each recruitment transaction specifically delineate that the community need be met and document any community benefits imparted by each physician the hospital is recruiting.

The community need and benefit preconditions generally should conform to identified standards set forth in this section. If a transaction cannot be supported by either of these two articulated standards, the transaction should not proceed without approval of the board of trustees.

Community Need: Acceptable Justifications

Evidence of community need for a particular physician and that physician's specialty can be demonstrated by a variety of factors and documented by a number of sources. These include but are not limited to the following:

- Absence of physicians in the recruited physician's specialty
- Government studies of health manpower needs or other related development plans
- Patient travel patterns
- Physician and patient survey results
- Comments and data from private and governmental insurers, employers, and managed care payers
- Medical staff development plans, long-range strategic plans, and other similar hospital studies
- Newspaper and periodical articles
- Demand for a particular medical service, coupled with a documented lack of such service, or long waiting periods for the service.

Other determining factors include waiting times for appointments, office waiting times, physician referral patterns, current physicians' willingness to treat, and Medicaid/Medicare/indigent patients (see the next section, "Community Benefit: Acceptable Justifications"). These sources of data can help demonstrate that physician manpower is needed to provide new services or procedures that are unavailable in the community, improve access to medical care, and improve patient convenience. The best sources for this information are a statistically valid community survey and a medical staff survey.

For a discussion of one method of quantitatively documenting community need, see Exhibit 1-1, "Community Need Analysis," at the end of this chapter.

Community Benefit: Acceptable Justifications

In addition to, or in lieu of, a documented quantitative need for a particular physician in a community (i.e., "community need"), there may be evidence of other significant benefits to the community through hospital recruitment of a specific physician. Community benefit can be demonstrated by, but not limited to, any of the following:

- A new service or procedure in the community
- A new physician in the community
- Improved patient accessibility
- Increased physician accessibility

- Each physician's willingness to treat Medicare/Medicaid and indigent patients
- Each physician's participation in managed care programs
- Additional educational and research activities
- Expansion of health care resources
- Improvement in treatment modalities
- Increased efficiency
- Enhanced quality
- Reduction in costs
- Promotion of a hospital's charitable mission.

Unacceptable Justifications

The following criteria cannot be used to support a physician recruitment arrangement under any circumstances:

- Obtaining patient referrals
- Avoiding new competition.

While criteria focusing on "improvement or maintenance of a hospital's financial viability" may not be used as the sole basis for supporting a physician recruitment arrangement, such criteria may be used in conjunction with any of the acceptable justifications to support recruitment of a particular physician.

Absence of Community Need or Community Benefit

In the absence of significant community need or benefit, all physician recruitment contracts should require full repayment of all funds extended to any physician, consistent with commercially reasonable market rates, terms, and conditions. In all recruitment contracts, it is strongly advised that, at a minimum, each recruited physician convey some degree of documentable community benefit. Recruitment that does not result in some community benefit is undoubtedly of questionable validity.

POLICIES CONCERNING CATEGORIES OF PRACTICE

The safe harbors to the anti-kickback statute issued in November 1999 did not include any protection for retaining existing physicians or assisting existing medical practices. The safe harbors provide protection from sanctions under the anti-kickback statute for certain relationships that meet specific criteria. Although there is a safe harbor for newly recruited physicians, the OIG specifically declined to consider a safe harbor for recruitment into existing practices. Accordingly, there presently are no safe harbor protections for physician retention and assistance to existing medical practices. There is a Stark law exception for physician recruitment activities, including support for existing practices. The following is a discussion, however, of some practices that have occurred historically between hospitals and physicians. In any of these examples, consultation with legal counsel is appropriate to make certain that there is no violation of the anti-kickback statute or the Stark law.

Policies Applying to All Categories of Physicians

All recruitment and retention policies and procedures must be evaluated under both the anti-kickback statute and the Stark law as well as relevant state laws to ensure that they are compliant with these statutes. Most all activities of this nature implicate these statutes. Even free educational courses can be considered a financial relationship under the Stark law. There is a specific exception to the Stark law for compliance training provided by entities, including hospitals, to physicians; however, there is not a specific exception for other types of training. Consequently, there is a risk that such training could be considered a compensation arrangement for which there is potentially no exception. The outcome of this is not clear but both hospitals and medical practices should be aware of this potential.

All recruitment policies should be applied consistently across various categories of the medical staff. Exceptions to such policies need to be approved by the board of trustees.

Except for medical practices that are being started or expanded as a result of clearly demonstrated community need or benefit, established physicians in a particular community should pay for or reimburse a hospital for practice support services when such support is provided directly by a hospital. This support includes services such as physician recruitment expenses, practice management services, consulting services, and marketing services. Payment or reimbursement for services should be at commercially reasonable rates.

The preceding provision does not prohibit a hospital from conducting studies of specific practices as part of the development process for a new service or product line to address an existing community need or to convey additional health care benefits to the community.

With respect to existing medical practices and physician recruitment activities, where community need or benefit is clearly established, a hospital may incur certain expenses as long as those expenses are clearly associated with establishing either a new community service or expanding an existing service. In all cases, community need must be clearly demonstrated.

From time to time, a hospital should be able to conduct seminars for physicians and their office staffs as a courtesy and to assist its medical staff in complying with Medicare/Medicaid program requirements, Occupational Safety and Health Administration (OSHA) requirements, Medicare's Resource-Based Relative Value System (RBRVS) requirements, managed care requirements, and other requirements relating to the benefit of its community at large. However, seminars and educational programs should be offered consistently and evenhandedly to all physicians in the medical community, not just to that hospital's medical staff. Note that the content of training and educational programs is also a factor. In minutes from a November 4, 1992, meeting between a coalition of health care providers and OIG officials and in a December 23, 1992, memo, the OIG indicated that it considers problematic any training or educational program offered by hospitals to physicians that "solely and primarily" benefits the physician "in his or her private practice and does not relate directly to his or her duties in the hospital." Note that the value of free seminars must fit within a Stark law exception such as the de minimus exception. Any hospital may provide certain informational services as a courtesy to all physicians.

Directly or indirectly, the hospital may provide loans, arrange for lines of credit, or make other financial support available to physicians for various purposes, as long as those purposes are related to the business aspects of their medical practices and some degree of benefit to the community can be documented. Such loans carry risk under the anti-kickback statue, and care should be taken to fit within an exception to the Stark law. The preferred and first method of financing the preceding should be through banks and other lending institutions. In all instances, the interest rate on loans, as well as the terms and conditions of such loans, should be based upon the prevailing market. Loans should relate only to the business aspects of the medical practice and must be authorized by the hospital's chief executive officer or his or her designee. The board of trustees must directly approve any exceptions to the preceding.

No loan to any physician should be made or guaranteed by a hospital without a component of personal risk and a personal guarantee by the physician.

Lease of facilities (including lease assignments), space, or equipment, or assistance with "build-out" should be provided under fair market terms and conditions. A hospital may provide deferrals of lease payments and other beneficial provisions under certain conditions where there is a clear community need or benefit, or where it can be documented that the beneficial provisions are consistent with local fair market value terms and conditions.

The purchase of any physician practice or real estate assets should require, at a minimum, an appropriate business plan and pro forma submitted prior to formalizing the purchase and a fair market value purchase price.

Policies Applying to Existing Medical Practices

Existing medical practices should pay for all management support services, loans, rentals, leases, and other services based upon prevailing market rates and "arms-length" transactions (defined as transactions negotiated by unrelated parties, each acting in his or her own self-interest).

Existing medical practices should pay prevailing market rates for any recruiting services provided by or through a hospital where there is no documented community need or significant community benefit. If an existing medical practice is recruiting a physician or providing a service for which there is a demonstrated community need, then a hospital may elect to provide certain practice services. Each hospital should evaluate such a provision on a case-by-case basis.

In the case of a physician who announces the intent to retire, relocate, or otherwise cease practicing in a service area, and who has been providing a service, the loss of which would be detrimental to the community, a hospital may elect to provide certain recruiting and practice support services. Each hospital should evaluate these on a case-by-case basis.

A hospital may provide loans to existing medical practices for the purpose of expanding, relocating, making management or marketing enhancements, or acquiring real estate, furnishings, or equipment. Such loans should be fully repayable and maintain an interest rate and other terms and conditions that are consistent with those of the commercial market. Physicians receiving such financial support should be expected to take some degree of financial risk and provide a personal guarantee. As with financial support from any hospital, community need or some degree of documented community benefit should be present in all such transactions.

Where it is demonstrated or contemplated that a hospital will be involved in a transaction, that hospital may elect to provide and pay for a medical practice valuation, a practice assessment, and certain reasonable legal work relating to the transaction. However, when a transaction occurs strictly between two or more physicians without the involvement of a hospital, those physicians should be expected to contract and pay for these services independently.

Care should be taken not to violate the anti-kickback statute to comply with an exception to the Stark law (see preceding discussion).

Policies Applying to New or Significantly Expanding Medical Practices

With respect to new and expanding medical practices that do not meet community need and benefit criteria, the policies should apply as if these practices were existing medical practices (see the section on unacceptable justifications). Any deviation from the policies applying to existing medical practices should be justified only by documentation of community need or benefit. This documentation should be prepared by hospital personnel and reviewed by an independent outside party.

In circumstances in which community need or benefit is clearly justified, a hospital may provide and pay for recruiting physicians in each specific specialty and be able to provide the specific level of incentives justified by community need and benefit analyses. In circumstances in which new physicians are recruited based upon justified community need or benefit, a hospital may provide practice support services, management services, and marketing services as long as it can clearly demonstrate that the services it provides are not simply to enhance an existing medical practice but to establish a new or needed practice.

Following the start-up phase of a practice or new service (with *start-up* defined as that phase ending with the achievement of financial self-sufficiency, but in no case exceeding 24 months after initiation of the practice), the physician or physicians should pay for management or marketing services provided by any hospital, either directly or through loan arrangements.

To establish a newly needed specialty, hospitals may provide loans, lines of credit, or other financial support incentives. Regardless of the form of the financial support itself, any and all amounts advanced by a hospital, directly or indirectly, should be considered a loan fully repayable either in cash or through legitimate "work-off" provisions.

Care should be taken not to violate the anti-kickback statute and to comply with an exception to the Stark law (see "Community Need: Acceptable Justifications").

OTHER GUIDING PRINCIPLES

Other guiding principles relate to the areas discussed in the following sections.

Overall Reasonableness of Recruitment Incentives

When viewed together as a package, all recruitment incentives must not exceed a reasonable amount. Thus, it is not sufficient that individual components of a recruitment package be reasonable when viewed separately.

In determining reasonableness, a hospital should consider the following:

- A physician's benefit and value to a hospital (e.g., a new service, enhanced productivity)
- A physician's benefit and value to a community (e.g., a needed specialty)
- Additional independent sources for determining the reasonableness of physician incentives (e.g., national studies or fair market valuations)
- The type of practice (e.g., specific specialty, practicing in specialty for less than a year, relocating to establish a new practice)
- A physician's experience
- Comparative incomes of similar physicians in a physician's specialty
- Cap on incentives provided

In addition to or as a component of the overall reasonableness considerations mentioned in the preceding section, each incentive or benefit must have a financial or volume cap on the amount of incentive offered. The following sample contract language gives an example:

Financial Cap

Following a review of receipts by the Chief Financial Officer, Hospital shall reimburse physician for reasonable costs of a professional mover to move Physician's personal goods from [City and State of Present Residence] to [Hospital's City and State]. The amount of this reimbursement shall not exceed [Amount of Financial Cap]. Physician shall submit to Hospital copies of all invoices prior to reimbursement.

Volume Cap

Physician shall be entitled to a maximum of [Volume Cap in Days] days per calendar year for continuing medical education and professional conferences.

Type of Physician to Whom Recruitment Incentives Can Be Extended

Subject to exceptions set forth in each physician recruitment policies document, recruitment incentives should be extended only to physicians who have the following:

- Practiced their specialties for less than one year
- Relocated their residences and practices to the communities served by a hospital (i.e., communities within each hospital's service area).

Requirement for Written Agreement

All recruitment incentives must be documented by a written agreement. Additionally, the identified community need and benefit should be documented throughout each agreement, particularly in the recitals section of the agreement.

Duration of Recruitment Incentives

The incentives provided under any physician recruitment arrangement should be for a period not to exceed 3 years.

Prohibition Against Renegotiation

The terms of the agreement or agreements should not be renegotiated during the duration of the benefit period.

Requirement for Reporting to the IRS

The Internal Revenue Service has begun to increase its audit activity dramatically with regard to physician payment of income tax on certain "free" recruitment incentives provided by hospitals. Examples of such incentives include relocation expenses, free or discounted office rent, and "forgiven" start-up loans.

Although certain recruitment incentives can become a tax issue for physicians, providing these incentives can also become significant reporting and tax-exemption (private inurement) issues for any hospital.

For these reasons, every hospital must be careful to not only inform physicians in writing of the taxable income potential of certain incentives provided in advance of executing any agreement, but also file appropriate IRS income reporting forms in a timely manner (e.g., IRS Form 1099).

Exceptions to Guidelines

There may be some isolated or unique instances in which some reasonable deviation by a hospital from established recruitment policies may be necessary to meet community needs or to provide community benefits. Examples of such unique circumstances include the following:

- Recruited physicians whose practices do not develop as quickly as anticipated. An existing incentive may have to be extended beyond the usual period of time or otherwise modified to avoid losing a needed physician from a community. (Please note that the community need or significant benefit established at the initiation of the original agreement must still prevail at the time the incentive is extended.)
- An existing incentive may have to be extended or modified for recruited physicians who are unexpectedly called to active duty in the armed forces of the United States.
- Reasonable deviations may be necessary to recruit or retain a physician in a rural community with a definite acute shortage of physicians.
- If deviations from specific recruitment policies are proposed, it is critical that both hospital legal counsel and the governing board be consulted and that there is documented justification for the deviation.

REFERENCES

1. *See* Rev. Rul. 69-545, 1969-2 C.B. 117.
2. *But see* Rev. Rul 83-157. 1983-C.B. 157 (emergency room not required for exemption, as where such would duplicate services already available in the community).
3. *See,* e.g. FSA 200110030.
4. *See* Treas. Reg. 1.502-1(b); GCMs 39830 and 39508; *Geisinger Health Plan v. Commissioner,* 100 TC 394 (1993), *aff'd* 30 F.3d 494 (3d Cir. 1994).
5. *See* § 1.50(c)(3)-1(c)(1).
6. *See* § 501(c)(3) and Treas. Reg. 1.501(c)(3)-1(d)(1)(ii); *See also* Rev. Rul. 76-206, 1976-1 C.B. 154; Rev. Rul. 75-384, 1975-2 C.B. 204; GCMs 39862, 39598, 39498, and 37789; PLRs 9233037 and 9231047.
7. *See* Treas. Reg. 1.501(c)(3)-1(c)(2) and Treas. Reg. 1.501(a)- 1(c).
8. *See* GCMS 39862 and 39498.

9. *See* Rev. Rul. 97-21, 1997-18 IRB 8; Final Regulations regarding intermediate sanctions, TC 8978, 67 Fed. Reg. 3076 (January 23, 2002).

10. *See* § 4958 and Final Regulations, TD 8978, 67 Fed. Reg. 3076 (January 23, 2002).

11. 42 U.S.C. § 1320a-7b(b).

12. 760 F.2d 68 (3d Cir.), cert. denied, 474 U.S. 988 (1985).

13. 874 F.2d 20, 33 (1st Cir. 1989).

14. 53 F.3d 1390 (9th Cir. 1995).

15. *Id.* at n. 16 (citing H.R. No. 96-1167, 96th Cong., 2d Sess. 59 (1980)), *but see United States v. Neufeld*, 908 F. Supp. 491 (S.D. Ohio 1995) and *United States v. Davis*, 132 F.3d 1092 (5th Cir. 1998).

16. 157 F.3d 833 (11th Cir. 1998).

17. *But see United States v. Butcher*, 1998 U.S. Dist. LEXIS 22137 (N.D. Fla. Dec. 7, 1998) (distinguishing *Starks* as a case in which the defendants could "reasonably anticipate that [their] conduct [was] wrongful").

EXHIBIT 1-1 COMMUNITY NEED ANALYSIS

How to Create a Quantitative Community Need Analysis for Your Hospital

Definitions

Community. When referring to a community need analysis, the term *community* is the geographic area containing a defined patient population. Another common term used to describe the geographic community served by a hospital is *service area.* For the sake of this discussion, *community* and *service area* are indistinguishable.

A hospital may have one or several defined communities or service areas, depending on how detailed the hospital wishes to segment its drawing area. For most community hospitals, it is only necessary to define a *primary* and a *secondary* service area. Depending on the expected drawing range of each clinical specialty (e.g., cardiovascular surgery versus family practice) in determining need, both the primary and secondary service areas may be combined to define that specialty's primary service area.

It is important to remember that how one chooses to define the patient population determines the geographic boundaries of the hospital's community or service area, not the converse. Thus, service areas do not always properly match political or geographic boundaries, such as rivers or county lines.

A hospital's community usually changes over time. As competition, service lines, and patient populations change, so does the geographic composition of the community that each hospital serves.

Primary Service Area. One widely used definition of a hospital's primary service area is "[t]hat contiguous geographic area surrounding the hospital from which it receives 75% of its total admissions volume."

To be meaningful, this should represent the majority of a hospital's total admissions and should be greater than 60%. In most cases, looking at a list of admissions arranged in descending frequency by zip code of patient origin aids in establishing a reasonable definition.

Secondary Service Area. A hospital's secondary service area is defined as that geographic region beyond the hospital's primary service area that generates an important, but smaller, percentage of the hospital's admissions. As with the primary service area, any meaningful percentage of contribution to its admissions level can be selected.

Data Sources

Physician-to-Population Ratios. Any of several standardized physician-to-population ratios can be used as the established guideline for projecting the demand for physician services. The physician-to-population ratio estimates the number of persons that a physician in a particular specialty can satisfactorily serve and still afford those persons adequate access.

By convention, these ratios are expressed as "1 physician per 4000 units of population." For example, if the physician-to-population ratio for family practitioners is 1:4000, this signifies that each family practitioner can serve 4000 patients and still afford adequate access to those persons.

The most widely recognized physician-to-population ratios are those determined by the Graduate Medical Education National Advisory Committee and are conventionally termed the *GMENAC ratios.* The latest revision of these ratios has been updated to 1990 practice standards.[1]

It is well known, however, that GMENAC ratios tend to overstate the demand for physician services. Thus, relying exclusively on these ratios may provide analyses that tend to overestimate required physician numbers. Other nationally recognized ratios have their own biases and shortcomings as well.[2]

---

[1]*1990 Update: Report of the Graduate Medical Education National Advisory Committee.* U.S. Department of Health and Human Services.

[2]Other recognized sources include ratios provided by *Medical Economics*, the Medical Group Management Association, and the American Medical Association.

Regardless of the ratio you choose, it must be nationally acceptable and established by a well-known outside source if your community need analysis is to be legally defensible.

Population Data. Population data by zip code for your community can be obtained from a variety of sources. One of the most accurate and readily available data sources is the National Planning Data Corporation (NPDC), with offices in Ithaca, New York, and other cities. In addition to NPDC, numerous other firms sell population data by zip code. Also, the United States Census Office in Washington, D.C., is an additional source for inexpensive population data.

These are all national population data resources; local chambers of commerce or state planning agencies may have equally accurate population data for your community.

Physician Data. The most difficult data to obtain in completing a community need analysis concerns the number of physicians by practice location within a service area. Although while the NPDC and other firms have estimates that you may purchase, the most accurate way to determine current physician numbers is to create a database on your own.

Several sources are available for creating your own physician database. The local telephone Yellow Pages Directory (electronic or otherwise) is an excellent source for current, accurate physician data. Also, local and state medical societies have lists of members. In addition, the state board of medical examiners retains a complete listing of physicians by location.

Office Visit Data. Many prefer to calculate physician demand on the basis of office practice statistics. Using such statistics has the advantage over physician-to-population ratios in that most office visit data can be fine-tuned to population demographics (e.g., age, sex) rather easily. The data are also very applicable as we see medical care shift more to office-based practice and preventive and primary care. Some sources of data to help develop office visits per population statistics are the following:

- Socioeconomic Characteristics of Medical Practice, AMA Center for Health Policy Research
- National Ambulatory Medical Care Survey, National Center for Health Statistics
- U.S. Bureau of Census data.[3]

The primary purpose for these quantitative data is to provide documentation and justification of community need. Use as many sources of data as possible in documenting community need. Although any one source can be questioned, corroborating evidence lends strength and credence to justifying community need.

Completing the Community Need Analysis

The analytical method employed in this exhibit calculates current and projected community need through the following five steps:

1. A current and projected population for the primary service area is determined.
2. The current *supply* of practicing physicians, by specialty, is determined for the primary service area.
3. The number of physicians, by specialty, required to care for patients residing within the primary service area is calculated from nationally accepted physician-to-population ratios.
4. The projected *demand* for each specialty within the primary service area is calculated by dividing the service area population by that specialty's physician-to-population ratio.
5. The estimated *demand* is compared with the current *supply* of physicians, and the result expressed as current and projected physician manpower *surpluses* and *deficits*.

Note that all steps in this process should be well documented.

The following table is only for illustration purposes. A market-specific study should be completed before utilizing any numbers.

---

[3]Medical Search Institute. 1995. "Documenting Community Need." Available at: http://worldmall.com/msi/secure/lib/docneed.htm. Accessed July 11, 2001.

Community Need Analysis, Anytown, USA

2005 Population   163,078
2010 Population   180,823

Specialty	Current Supply	2005 Ratio	2005 Demand	2005 Surplus Deficit	2010 Ratio	2010 Demand	2010 Surplus Deficit
Primary Care							
Family Medicine	50.2	4,000	40.8	9.4	4,000	45.2	5.0
Internal Medicine	16.0	4,000	40.8	−24.8	4,000	45.2	−29.2
Obstetrics/Gynecology	18.6	10,000	16.3	2.3	10,000	18.1	0.5
Pediatrics	9.6	8,500	19.2	−9.6	8,500	21.3	−11.7
Medical Specialties							
Allergy & Immunology	1.0	85,000	1.9	−0.9	85,000	2.1	−1.1
Cardiology	7.7	30,000	5.4	2.3	30,000	6.0	1.7
Dermatology	1.4	40,000	4.1	−2.7	40,000	4.5	−3.1
Endocrinology	0.3	120,000	1.4	−1.1	120,000	1.5	−1.2
Gastroenterology	5.1	30,000	5.4	−0.3	30,000	6.0	−0.9
Geriatrics	0.5	35,715	4.6	−4.1	35,715	5.1	−4.6
Hematology/Oncology	4.0	50,000	3.3	0.7	50,000	3.6	0.4
Infectious Disease	0.2	120,000	1.4	−1.2	120,000	1.5	−1.3
Nephrology	0.4	95,000	1.7	−1.3	95,000	1.9	−1.5
Neurology	2.0	40,000	4.1	−2.1	40,000	4.5	−2.5
Phys. Med./Rehab	1.0	50,000	3.3	−2.3	50,000	3.6	−2.6
Psychiatry	1.3	13,000	12.5	−11.2	13,000	13.9	−12.6
Pulmonology	1.4	70,000	2.3	−0.9	70,000	2.6	−1.2
Rheumatology	0.0	130,000	1.3	−1.3	130,000	1.4	−1.4
Surgical Specialties							
Cardiothoracic Surgery	0.1	90,000	1.8	−1.7	90,000	2.0	−1.9
Colon & Rectal	0.0	300,000	0.5	−0.5	300,000	0.6	−0.6
General Surgery	2.1	15,000	10.9	−8.8	15,000	12.1	−10.0
Neurosurgery	0.5	80,000	2.0	−1.5	80,000	2.3	−1.8
Ophthalmology	3.8	20,500	8.0	−4.2	20,500	8.8	−5.0
Orthopedic	8.0	16,000	10.2	−2.2	16,000	11.3	−3.3
Otorhinolaryngology	2.3	32,000	5.1	−2.8	32,000	5.7	−3.4
Plastic	0.2	45,000	3.6	−3.4	45,000	4.0	−3.8
Urology	3.0	31,000	5.3	−2.3	31,000	5.8	−2.8
Vascular	1.0	100,000	1.6	−0.6	100,000	1.8	−0.8

Part II

Current Legal Environment

Health care in the United States continues to evolve at a revolutionary pace. Entrepreneurs and strategic not-for-profit institutions alike are restructuring the delivery of health care. Government regulation at the federal, state, and local levels continues to accelerate in scope and complexity, with new rulings occurring frequently. Litigation threatens to engulf many institutions and companies in liability as they seek to understand and embrace changes in rules and rulings.

Medicare and Medicaid fraud and abuse laws, the Stark laws, and state laws prohibiting kickbacks and physician self-referrals, loom heavily over healthcare organizations. Health care provider activities that fall within these fraud and abuse prohibitions include submission of false claims or fraudulent billing, kickbacks and illegal remuneration, and violations of physician self-referral restrictions. These laws are to be considered in structuring health care business arrangements, such as joint ventures, physician recruitment, purchases of physician practices, personal services and management contracts, leases, physician employment arrangements, group purchasing, and managed care activities.

The information in the next section provides some background around the current legal environment of health care and how the rules apply to provider activities.

FRAUD AND ABUSE

Anti-Kickback Statute

The anti-kickback statute was designed to impose criminal, civil monetary penalties, and/or exclusion on providers of health care services who give or receive kickbacks related to referrals for services paid for by any federal health care program, including Medicare or Medicaid. Under the statute, it is illegal to knowingly and willfully offer, pay, solicit, or receive any remuneration, directly or indirectly, in return for referring a patient for the furnishing, recommending the furnishing, or arranging for the furnishing of any services for which payment may be made by a federal health care program. Violation of this statute is all of the following:

- A felony offense
- Punishable by a fine of up to $25,000
- Punishable by imprisonment for up to 5 years
- Grounds for exclusion from federal health care programs by the Office of the Inspector General (OIG)
- Grounds for imposition of a civil money penalty.

Each act may be considered a separate offense under this statute; therefore, the offending party or parties may be subject to maximum penalties for each violation.

On a different front, the Internal Revenue Service (IRS) has stated that tax-exempt hospitals that violate the anti-kickback statute are acting inconsistently with their § 501(c)(3) tax-exempt charitable purposes, and thus their tax-exempt status could be jeopardized in addition to other penalties.

Legal precedent suggests that any violation of the law must be substantial to warrant revocation of a hospital's tax exemption. In addition, there appears to be some push by some members of Congress to impose "intermediate penalties" (monetary penalties) for hospitals as an alternative to revocation of tax-exempt status. This is an area that is currently evolving from a legal and regulatory standpoint and should be monitored closely. It is important to emphasize that the anti-kickback statute will certainly continue to have important implications for the tax-exempt status of a hospital.

Safe Harbors to the Anti-Kickback Statute

In 1987 Congress authorized the OIG in the Department of Health and Human Services (DHHS) to impose civil monetary penalties and to exclude a person or entity from participation in the Medicare and Medicaid programs to the extent that the party has engaged in a prohibited remuneration scheme. Congress also required the OIG to promulgate "safe harbor" regulations specifying those payment practices that would not be subject to criminal prosecution or civil sanctions, assuming *all* requirements are met. Falling outside of a safe harbor does not mean that a relationship violates the anti-kickback statute.

The safe harbors apply to the following activities, assuming all of their specific requirements are met:

- Certain investment interests
- Space rentals
- Equipment rentals
- Personal services and management contracts
- Sale of physician practices to other physicians
- Payment for referral services
- Warranties
- Discounts
- Bona fide employment
- Group purchasing organizations
- Waiver of beneficiary coinsurance and deductible amounts
- Remuneration between providers and managed care plans
- Wavier or reduction by pharmacies of cost sharing imposed under Medicare Part D
- Remuneration between a federally qualified health center and a Medicare Advantage organization
- Remuneration between a federally qualified health center and certain individuals or entities' provision of items or services, financial arrangements related to health plans
- Physician recruitment and relocation
- Obstetrical malpractice insurance subsidies
- Investment by providers in their practices
- Payments between a cooperative hospital services organization and a participating hospital
- Ambulatory surgery center and joint ventures
- Certain agreements to refer patients for specialty services
- Ambulance restocking arrangements

(See Exhibit 2-1, 1991 Fraud and Abuse Safe Harbors, U.S. Department of Justice, for additional information and related correspondence.)

Here are three safe harbors that apply most directly to physician recruitment and employment activities:

- The agreement must be in writing and signed by the parties, specifying the benefits to be provided, the terms under which the benefits will be provided, and the obligations of the parties.
- If the practitioner is leaving an established practice, at least 75% of the new practice's revenues must come from new patients, not patients from the former practice.
- The agreement can neither exceed 3 years nor be renegotiated during the 3-year term in any substantial aspect; however, if during the term of the agreement, the area to which the physician was recruited ceases to qualify as a Health Professional Shortage Area, the safe harbor will continue to be satisfied through the term of the agreement.
- Benefits must not be contingent on referrals or generating business, although the entity can require the practitioner to maintain staff privileges.

- The practitioner's ability to establish staff privileges at or refer business to another entity must not be restricted.
- The amount or value of benefits must not vary based on the volume or value of referrals or business otherwise generated for which payment may be made in whole or in part by Medicare, Medicaid, or other federal health care programs.
- The practitioner must agree to treat all federal health care program beneficiaries in a nondiscriminatory manner.
- A minimum of 75% of revenues from the new practice must come from patients living in a HPSA, Medically Underserved Area, or Medically Underserved Population.
- Other than the recruited practitioner, no payment or exchange of anything of value may be given to a person or entity in a position to make or influence referrals.
- The OIG will look to whether there is documented evidence of an objective need for the practitioner's services. A hospital's determination of need must be based on what is necessary to provide adequate access to medically necessary care for patients in the community as opposed to its own competitive interests.
- The degree of risk is heightened when the recruited practitioner has an existing stream of referrals within the hospital's service area. Hospitals should consider recruiting a new practitioner or one that is relocating from a substantial distance.
- The OIG will consider whether the benefits exceed that which is reasonably necessary to attract qualified physicians.
- A recruiting arrangement will be subject to heightened scrutiny if the total benefit payout period exceeds 3 years from the initial agreement.

The OIG intends these points to clarify the anti-kickback statute. Because the statute is so broad, concern had been expressed that it would technically cover some relatively innocuous commercial arrangements and, therefore, be subject to criminal prosecution.

Keep in mind the following several important points concerning the safe harbor for physician recruitment:

- The fact that a recruitment arrangement does not fall clearly within the safe harbors does not necessarily make it illegal. The safe harbors are fairly narrow in scope. Hospitals should be cautious, however, in considering any arrangement for physician recruitment that does not fall within the safe harbors.
- There are conflicts between the safe harbors and the Stark law. For example, the exception for physician recruitment, as set forth in the Stark regulations, permits payment by a hospital to an existing medical group to recruit physicians, even though these payments are specifically excluded from the new anti-kickback safe harbors.
- Although the safe harbors permit those in practice for less than 1 year to be recruited without having to relocate, Stark requires a physician to relocate to qualify for the recruitment exception, even if he or she has been in practice for less than 1 year.

- Any physician recruitment package has to be evaluated under both the Stark law and the physician recruitment safe harbors. Compliance with one does not necessarily ensure compliance with the other. State law must be considered also.

Other OIG Pronouncements

As of yet, no court cases or administrative decisions discuss the effect of the safe harbors on physician recruitment and support incentives. Furthermore, despite the urging of commentators that the OIG issue advisory opinions regarding specific transactions and generic criteria that could be considered in evaluating business arrangements, the preamble to the safe harbor regulations holds to the OIG's long-standing policy not to provide such guidance other than by creating new safe harbors through the rule-making process.

The preamble to the safe harbor regulations, however, also states that they do not expand the scope of activities that the anti-kickback statute prohibits and that the statutory language continues to describe the scope of illegal activities. In other words, the failure of a particular transaction or arrangement to fall within a safe harbor will not necessarily subject it to investigation or enforcement action. The conduct may be legal, it may be in a gray area, or it may be subject to immediate enforcement action.

Some examples of the OIG's interpretive stance also merit discussion. The first is a management advisory report (MAR) issued by the OIG on January 31, 1991. (See Exhibit 2-2 at the end of this chapter.) This MAR is aimed at arrangements that require physicians to pay less than fair market value for services provided by hospitals or that compensate physicians for more than the fair market value of goods and services that they provide the hospitals.

This MAR states that arrangements requiring physicians to split portions of their income with hospitals are highly suspect, although not technically in violation of the anti-kickback statute. Although this MAR focuses on income-splitting agreements, it also includes recommendations for all arrangements between hospitals and hospital-based physicians. Specifically:

- The arrangement should be based on fair market value.
- The nature and value of all services performed should be stated separately, and the fair market value should be documented.
- The arrangement should be unrelated to physician income or billings.
- The arrangement should be limited to goods and services necessary for the provision of medical services by the hospital-based physicians.
- The arrangement should be typical of what most other hospitals provide hospital-based physicians.

A second, more relevant, interpretation appears in an OIG Special Fraud Alert issued on May 5, 1992, addressing hospital incentives to physicians. (See Exhibit 2-3 at the end of this chapter.) This alert identifies the following 10 commonly used physician recruitment and retention practices as suspect incentive arrangements that are indicators of potentially unlawful activity:

- Payment of any sort of incentive by the hospital each time a physician refers a patient to the hospital
- Use of free or significantly discounted office space or equipment (in facilities usually located close to the hospital)
- Provision of free or significantly discounted billing, nursing, or other staff services
- Free training for a physician's office staff in areas such as management techniques, CPT coding, and laboratory techniques
- Guarantees that provide that if the physician's income fails to reach a level, the hospital will supplement the remainder up to a certain amount
- Low-interest or interest-free loans, or loans that may be "forgiven" if a physician refers patients (or some number of patients) to the hospital
- Payment of the cost of a physician's travel and expenses for conferences
- Payment for a physician's continuing education courses
- Coverage on the hospital's group health insurance plans at an inappropriately low cost to the physician
- Payment for services (which may include consultations at the hospital) that require few, if any, substantive duties by the physician, or payment for services in excess of the fair market value of services rendered.

Although these suspect activities are not illegal, they will be subject to even greater scrutiny by the OIG. Hospitals are advised to be careful with all future physician incentive arrangements and to review all current contracts containing any of the above incentive arrangements.

At the same time, however, the following criticism has been leveled against the alert:

- It fails to clearly distinguish illegal kickback arrangements from bona fide recruitment arrangements in which the benefits conferred upon the physician are not linked to the volume of referrals or even a requirement to refer.
- Classification of all listed incentives as suspect fails to recognize that there may be factors such as the structure of the arrangement, the need for physicians, the benefit to the community, and other related factors that would make the arrangement legal.

Frequently, issuance of a Special Fraud Alert precedes filing of one or more test cases on a particular aspect of the anti-kickback statute. It is interesting to note that shortly after the issuance of the May 1992 Special Fraud Alert, the Inspector General began an investigation in Cobb County, Georgia, concerning Kennestone Hospital's recruitment activities. (The settlement of this case will be discussed in detail later in this section.)

A third relevant insight into contemporary OIG thinking appeared in the form of a letter from the OIG's Associate General Counsel, D. McCarty Thornton, to Mr. T. J. Sullivan of the IRS on December 22, 1992. In this letter (see Exhibit 2-4 following this chapter), Thornton describes the IRS's stance on anti-kickback implications when a tax-exempt organization acquires a private physician's practice assets and subsequently employs that physician. Thornton clearly pierces the statutory exemption for payments made to employees where these payments can be shown to be compensation to the physician for referrals to the tax-exempt organization. Specifically, Thornton states:

> The statute exempts only payments to employees which are for the provision of covered items or services. Accordingly, since referrals do not represent covered items or services, payments to employees which are for the purpose of compensating such employees for the referral of patients would likely not be covered by the employee exemption.

In this letter, Mr. Thornton reaffirms that the safe harbor regulations do not cover "purchases of physicians' practices by hospitals" or situations where the seller "remains in a continuing position to make referrals or influence referrals" to the purchasing hospital.

Thornton goes on to specify that payment for the following items "would raise a question as to whether payment was being made for the value of a referral stream":

- Payment for goodwill (Note that statements made in January 1994 by Thornton appear to modify this blanket prohibition against all types of goodwill. Thornton appears to distinguish between goodwill that is attributable to the perpetual or going-concern value of a practice (i.e., institutional goodwill) and the goodwill that merely represents the "value of future business from that practice to the hospital." He has indicated that the former would be permissible, while the latter form of goodwill value clearly would not be allowable.)
  - Payment for the value of the ongoing business unit
  - Payment for covenants not to compete
  - Payment for exclusive dealing arrangements
  - Payment for patient lists
  - Payment for patient records

Finally, Thornton provided some additional guidance as to how the IRS might determine that practice acquisition payments might constitute payments for future referrals. The two tests stipulated by Thornton were:

- To compare the financial welfare of the physicians involved beforehand after the acquisition.
- To compare referral patterns before and after the acquisition.

Clearly, this letter provides critical insight into contemporary OIG thinking regarding enforcement of the anti-kickback statute and another demonstration of the IRS's increasing coordination and cooperation with the OIG concerning anti-kickback compliance.

In 2001 the OIG issued an Advisory Opinion (No. 01-4) addressing a physician recruitment arrangement that did not fit within the applicable safe harbor because the hospital was not located in an HPSA, but was located in a medically underserved area. The OIG found that the reviewed arrangement not be subject to sanction. Essentially, the relationship complied with all of the safe harbor requirements other than the location. In the opinion the OIG looked to more key factors:

- Whether there is documented evidence of an objective need for the practitioner's services
- Whether the practitioner has an existing stream of referrals within the recruiting entity's service area (which would indicate a greater risk of a potential kickback arrangement)
- Whether the benefit is narrowly tailored so that it does not exceed that which is reasonably necessary to recruit a practitioner
- Whether the remuneration directly or indirectly benefits other referral sources

Additionally, the OIG has addressed the issue of physician relationships with hospitals in both its model compliance programs for individual and small-group physicians as well as its compliance guidance for hospitals.

Anti-Kickback Case Law

As a general matter, the anti-kickback statute has been interpreted very broadly in court cases and administrative decisions. In *United States v. Greber* (1985), the court held that the anti-kickback statute is violated if only one purpose of a payment is to induce referrals, even if the transaction reflected reasonable compensation for services rendered.

Subsequent cases have affirmed the broad interpretation taken in *Greber*. For example, in *United States v. Kats* (1989), the court agreed with *Greber* and additionally approved of jury instructions, which stated that the term *kickback* extends not only to the secret return of a sum of money received but also to the *payment or granting of assistance to one in a position to control a source of income*, unless such payment is wholly attributable to the delivery of goods or services.

In *United States v. Bay State Ambulance and Hospital Service* (1989), the court reiterated that the main focus of the anti-kickback statute is inducement, not whether the practice increases costs to the Medicare and Medicaid programs. The *Bay State* court also made clear that actual Medicare or Medicaid funds need not be used for the illegal remuneration and that *simply giving an individual an opportunity to earn money* may well be an inducement.

Kats and *Bay State* fail to clarify whether the illegal purpose of any arrangement must be the *primary purpose*. Nevertheless, they contain stringent language that could prohibit many legitimate business practices if applied literally.

A more recent case employing civil sanctions under the anti-kickback statute also saw the OIG adopt a broad interpretation. In *Inspector General v. Hanlester Network* (1991), the OIG alleged that dividends paid to physician investors in clinical laboratories were payments for referrals. Originally, the administrative law judge found insufficient grounds to exclude the physicians from the Medicaid and Medicare programs because the physicians *made no explicit agreement to refer* in connection with obtaining their investment interest.

On reconsideration, however, the physicians were excluded. It was held that a party could be found to have unlawfully received remuneration for referrals if that party received a benefit in return for the referral, consisting of *anything of value*, in any form or manner whatsoever. In other words, *an actual agreement to refer is not necessary* to establish a violation of the anti-kickback statute.

Finally, in the first case of its kind, a federal magistrate judge ruled that a physician recruitment agreement violated the anti-kickback statute and was therefore void and unenforceable. The case, *Polk County v. Peters* (1992), involved a rural hospital in eastern Texas that had provided various incentives to a surgeon to commence private practice in the area. The incentives extended to the physician by the hospital included an interest-free loan, free office space, rent and utility subsidies, and reimbursement for malpractice insurance. (See Exhibit 2-5, analysis section of *Polk County v. Peters* decision.)

The hospital never sought repayment on the loan until years later, when it brought suit against the physician, who was then using another hospital. It is important to note that the hospital and the physician were also embroiled in other litigation relating to the termination of the physician's privileges at the hospital.

The court took judicial notice from this other litigation that the hospital's stated reason for terminating the physician's medical staff privileges was his failure to use the hospital as his "primary hospital." The court held that "while the Hospital may well have been motivated to a greater or lesser degree by a legitimate desire to make better medical services available in the community, there can be no doubt that *the benefits extended to [the physician] were, in part, an inducement to refer patients to the Hospital.*"

Polk County is important for a number of reasons. The court cites the Special Fraud Alert almost as having the force of law. It does not mention that the alert only represents the OIG's opinion on what arrangements are suspect. Additionally, the court does not clarify that under the right circumstances, even suspect recruitment arrangements can be legal. Further, the case is unusual because by claiming that the contract was void as an illegal arrangement, the physician risked federal criminal and civil prosecution for both himself and the hospital.

As demonstrated by its plain language, the anti-kickback statute is extremely broad. Although the statute requires that the government establish scienter, meaning criminal intent, under a "knowingly and willfully" standard, these terms are not defined. Thus, the courts have had to address the exact scope of the requisite intent, resulting in different standards. Furthermore, because the statute is aimed at preventing intentional inducements, another interpretive question for the courts became what standard to apply in determining whether the purpose of the payments was to induce referrals.

Many courts as well as the OIG have adopted the "one-purpose test," which states that if one purpose of the payment is to induce referrals, then the statute is violated regardless of any other legitimate purposes for the payment. Therefore, in order for a transaction to fall outside the ambit of the statute, *no purpose* of the payment can be to induce referrals. Some courts have slightly modified the one purpose test, while still keeping within its framework. For example, remuneration designed entirely for legitimate purposes may not violate the statute if the individual merely hoped, expected, or believed that referrals may result from the arrangement. Some jurisdictions apply a slightly less expansive standard, by looking to whether the payments were made *primarily* for the purpose of inducing referrals.

Standards applied to the statute's scienter requirement are even more varied. In some jurisdictions, *knowingly* simply means to do something voluntarily and deliberately, while *willfully* means to do something purposely, with the intent to violate the law. Under this standard, the government can prove the requisite intent by showing that the individual voluntarily made payments in violation of the statute, and did so with the intent of violating the law. Other jurisdictions apply a slightly heightened scienter requirement by requiring knowledge that the conduct was unlawful. Under this standard, the government must prove that the individual knew the anti-kickback statute prohibited paying or offering remuneration to induce referrals, and that the defendant engaged in the prohibited conduct with the specific intent to disobey the law.

In view of the current political climate and in light of the increased governmental scrutiny in the area of fraud and abuse, hospitals should increase their awareness of applicable federal and state laws to avoid even an appearance of impropriety. This increased government scrutiny also underscores the absolute necessity of consulting with legal counsel having expertise in the area of health law before beginning the physician recruitment process, during negotiations, and at all times during preparation of the recruitment contract.

Furthermore, it would be prudent for hospitals to have legal counsel periodically audit recruitment contracts after execution for compliance with federal and state law. It is important to note that numerous proposals regarding antifraud and abuse restrictions and sanctions were common threads throughout all of the health care and budgetary reform proposals raised in Congress in 1995, and they continue to be important issues in the ongoing consideration of health care legislation.

TAX EXEMPTION AND PRIVATE INUREMENT

Private Inurement and Private Benefit

A §501(c)(3) tax-exempt hospital is subject to prohibitions against private benefit and inurement. A §501(c)(3) organization must be organized and operated exclusively—which has been interpreted as *primarily*—for charitable purposes. An organization is not organized or operated exclusively for charitable purposes unless it serves public rather than private interests.

It is generally recognized, however, that a charitable organization must often confer benefits upon private persons as an incidental part of carrying out its larger exempt purposes. For example, the fact that a hospital makes its facilities available to private physicians does not threaten its tax-exempt status.

Violation of the private benefit prohibition generally can be avoided by showing that the private benefit conferred is "incidental" in both a qualitative and a quantitative sense:

- In a qualitative sense, it must be shown that the public benefit cannot be achieved without necessarily benefiting certain private individuals.
- In a quantitative sense, the private benefit must not be substantial when measured in the context of the overall public benefit.

As to the private inurement prohibition, an organization is not operated exclusively for one or more exempt purposes if its net earnings inure in whole or in part to the benefit of private individuals. Several important definitions of this statement include the following:

- *Private individual* refers to a person having a personal and private interest in the activities of the organization.
- A *person* is defined as "an individual, trust, estate, partnership, association, company, or corporation."
- The word *private* is intended to limit the scope of those persons who personally benefit from the net earnings of the charitable organization to the interested beneficiaries of the organization's exempt activities.

The IRS's Position on "Insiders"

Case law and IRS rulings historically have applied the private inurement prohibition only to "insiders," defined as persons receiving a benefit as a result of their control or influence over the tax-exempt entity, such as shareholders, founders, directors, officers, or major contributors. The IRS concern is that a financial arrangement between an exempt organization and insiders cannot be negotiated on an arm's-length basis because of the control that the insiders exercise over the exempt organization.

The IRS now takes the position, which is not completely supported by case law, that *any member of a tax-exempt hospital's medical staff is an insider.* The IRS reasons that the physician has a unique role in relation to the hospital and controls patient flow to the hospital—and thus is able to affect the hospital's revenue materially.

Violation of the private inurement prohibition can be avoided by showing that there has been no inurement of the hospital's net earnings to private persons. In practical application, inurement is frequently analyzed in terms of reasonable compensation. The reasonableness of compensation is judged against what would be paid for like services from a like organization in like circumstances.

Applying this reasonableness standard, an inurement challenge could be defended against by showing that *the entire compensation is reasonable* relative to the services rendered to, or the benefits conferred upon, the hospital and the community.

At a theoretical level, the framework for analyzing tax exemption is straightforward. The private benefit prohibition must be considered in all arrangements involving a tax-exempt hospital. The private inurement provision applies only to insiders.

In reality, IRS rulings, and even some cases, occasionally blur the distinction. The practical result is that arrangements involving physicians who are insiders will be subjected to much greater scrutiny than would otherwise be the case. Because of this, *the risk to exempt status is much greater where an insider relationship is involved.*

To allow the IRS to be able to impose penalties on insiders receiving impermissible private benefits from tax-exempt organizations without having to pursue revocations of §501(c)(3) tax-exempt status on the organization itself as the only possible relief, in 1996 Congress enacted, as part of its Taxpayer Bill of Rights 2, Section 4958 of the Internal Revenue Code—the "intermediate sanctions" penalty. Section 4958 permits the IRS to impose significant excise taxes upon certain persons (but not the tax-exempt organization itself) who improperly benefit from transactions with exempt organizations. Specifically, intermediate sanctions may be imposed upon any "disqualified person" who receives an "excess benefit" from a "covered organization," and on each "organization manager" who approves the excess benefit.

A "covered organization" is, essentially, any organization that is tax-exempt under §§501(c)(3) or (4).

A "disqualified person" is a person who was in a position to exercise substantial influence over the affairs of an exempt organization. The person need not be only an individual; it may also be an organization, partnership, or unincorporated entity. Section 4958 identified certain persons, such as family members of disqualified persons, organizations at least 35% owned by a disqualified person, as being disqualified as a matter of law. Others are determined to have substantial influence and are considered to be presumptively disqualified. Examples of those persons are the organization's executive officers, treasurer, and chief financial officer. On the other hand, an employee who does not fit into those above categories and who is both not highly compensated and is not a substantial contributor to organization is conclusively *not* a disqualified person.

In all other cases, a fact and circumstances test applies. The U.S. Treasury regulations interpreting §4958 contain two lists of facts and circumstances. The first includes facts and circumstances that tend to show that the person *does* have substantial influence. Some (but not all) of those facts and circumstances are: the person is a substantial contributor (as that term is defined in §507); the person is the founder of the exempt organization; the person has or shares authority to control or determine a substantial portion of the organization's operating budget; or the person's compensation is primarily based on revenues derived from an activity of the organization that the person controls. The second list tends to show that the person *does not* have substantial influence. Some examples (not inclusive) include a religious organization where the person has taken a vow of poverty and when the person's direct supervisor is not a disqualified person.

An "organization manager" is an officer, director, trustee, or person having similar powers or duties of such person, regardless of title. An organization manager who participates in an excess benefit transaction with knowledge that it is such a transaction is liable for penalties unless his or her participation was not willful and was due to reasonable cause.

An "excess benefit transaction" occurs when a disqualified person receives an economic benefit from an exempt organization that exceeds the value of the benefit provided to the organization by the disqualified person. For example, unreasonable compensation paid to a disqualified person is subject to penalties.

A "reasoned written opinion" from an appropriate professional can protect a person from penalties for an otherwise excess benefit transaction.

Penalties that may be imposed on a disqualified person who has entered into an excess benefit transaction include return of the benefit to the organization, plus interest, and an excise tax of 25% of the excess benefit, which can increase to 200% of the excess benefit if the monies are not returned within the statutory period.

An excise tax of 10% of the excess benefit may also be imposed on each liable organization manager, up to $10,000 per transaction.

The Current IRS Concept of Community Benefit

On December 4, 1991, the IRS issued a major pronouncement in the form of a general counsel memorandum (GCM 39862) focusing on joint ventures between tax-exempt hospitals and their staff physicians. This GCM is important because the IRS makes broad statements about what would constitute "acceptable" community benefit.

In particular, the IRS states that when determining whether any private benefit of the joint venture arrangement is incidental in light of the public benefit derived therefrom, the public benefit must be a benefit to the "community," as distinguished from a benefit to the hospital and its continued financial viability.

The following are examples of acceptable community benefits:

- Providing a new service or new physician for the community
- Pooling diverse and distinct areas of expertise
- Improving patient convenience
- Increasing physician accessibility to patients

Examples of "unacceptable" justifications include the following:

- Obtaining patient referrals
- Avoiding new competition

(For additional information on completing a community need analysis, see Exhibit 1-1 in Part 1.)

Expanded Hospital Audit Guidelines

Efforts by tax-exempt hospitals and other organizations to implement physician–hospital integration generally involve incentives to recruit and retain physicians. These recruitment and retention incentives implicate federal tax-exempt laws, fraud and abuse statutes, federal and state antireferral prohibitions, and other miscellaneous federal and state laws. Recruitment and retention incentives involve varying degrees of risk to an institution's tax-exempt status.

On April 1, 1992, the IRS published expanded hospital audit guidelines to be used by IRS examiners in reviewing a tax-exempt hospital's compliance with §501(c)(3). Under the 1992 guidelines, the IRS audit agents are instructed to look for certain incentives extended by hospitals to physicians that are not reasonable compensation for services rendered, such as the following:

- Physicians being charged no rent or below-market rent for space in hospital-owned office buildings or being charged less than fair market value for practice management services
- Hospitals providing physicians with private practice income guaranties
- Hospitals providing financial assistance to physicians for home purchases or the purchase of office equipment
- Outright cash payments by hospitals to physicians for home purchases to secure or retain their services
- Hospitals purchasing the practice of a physician and then employing the physician (in many cases to operate the same practice)

In addition, the new audit guidelines establish a dual test for reasonableness and community need/benefit, emphasizing that:

> To establish that any loans, income guaranties, or other subsidies used as recruiting incentive or further charitable purposes are reasonable, the specialist must be able to determine that there is a need for the physician in the community served by the hospital. Absent evidence of a compelling community need or a significant other benefit to the community, the recruitment contract should require full payment (at prevailing interest rates). Evidence of need may include the previous absence of practitioners in a given specialty, governmental studies of health manpower, patient travel patterns, and so on.

Last, the audit guidelines indicate that to determine that a recruiting incentive is reasonable, it should be linked to the physician's value to the hospital (i.e., a new service or enhanced productivity) or community (i.e., a specialty that is lacking in the community), and that all incentives should be considered together and may not exceed a reasonable amount. In addition, the type of practice, the physician's experience, and the relative incomes must be considered.

A second expansion of guidelines for its auditors occurred when the IRS published the *1994 Exempt Organizations Technical Instruction Book*. In Chapter N (pp. 212–243) of the instruction book, the IRS sets forth its position on integrated organizations, especially issues involving medical practice acquisition and physician compensation within these organizations as they relate to private inurement concerns.

The IRS reaffirms that it will not consider a situation as constituting private inurement if the organization can prove that all of its relationships with a physician in question are"truly at arm's length," and "the physician has no chance to employ inside influence."

The IRS lists the following five critical facts that would point away from private inurement in this area:

- Fair market value was paid for all assets conveyed to the applicant.
- Independent negotiations took place between unrelated parties to determine the value of the assets conveyed.
- Certified appraisals were obtained from independent third parties when the medical group's assets were being purchased, licensed, or leased.
- The fee schedule and physician compensation are determined by an independent community board and are comparable to what other physicians receive in fees and compensation in the same geographic area, taking into consideration the transfer of capital assets.
- None of the other arrangements suggests any dividend-like sharing of charitable assets or other expenditures for the benefit of private interest.

Finally, the 1994 book lists several key issues or documents that the auditors should review during an examination, including the following:

- The integrated organization's governing board should represent a broad cross-section of the community, with physicians constituting no more than 20% of the board. (This has since been liberalized so that it may be possible to increase physician participation to constitute up to 50% of the board.)
- Independent appraisals were used in the purchase of medical practice assets and the lease or purchase of equipment and real estate, and fair market value was paid.
- There is a commitment to provide charity care and nondiscriminatory treatment of Medicare and Medicaid patients.
- For any intangible assets to be included in the purchase price, they should "contribute directly and substantially to the accomplishment of the purchaser's exempt purposes."
- There should be a disclosure policy for potential conflicts of interest.
- If the fees to be charged to the exempt organization or patients are determined prospectively by a fee committee, that committee should be independent, with physicians constituting a minority of its membership.

- Physician compensation should be reasonable, negotiated at arm's length, and comparable to the prevailing compensation for physicians in that specialty in the local marketplace.
- Any extended (i.e., multiyear) payout for purchase or lease of practice assets is discouraged.

In its technical instruction text for the 1996 fiscal year (titled *Continuing Professional Education (CPE), Exempt Organizations, Technical Instruction Program for FY 1996*), released on August 24, 1995, the IRS updated and supplemented Chapter N. Chapter P ("Integrated Delivery Systems and Health Care Update") of the CPE textbook reviews such key topics as integrated delivery system governance (including a refinement of the 20% safe harbor exemption), implications of the sale of a tax-exempt hospital and the creation of a tax-exempt foundation to distribute the proceeds from the sale, PHO tax status and capitalization, and problems associated with stock liquidations of medical practice when acquired by exempt hospitals and IDSs. The level of detail and analysis in Chapter P exceeds that of Chapter N of the 1994 CPE textbook.

Hermann Hospital Closing Agreement

The closing agreement reached on October 14, 1994, between the commissioner of internal revenue and the Hermann Hospital in the state of Texas also provides guidance for tax-exempt hospitals in recruiting physicians. Care should be taken, however, in evaluating the closing agreement because it was unique to Hermann Hospital circumstances and also, in part, may have been more aggressive than might be expected under existing law.

In the Hermann case, the hospital voluntarily disclosed to the IRS certain physician recruitment and retention activities engaged in by the hospital from 1989 through 1992. In the agreement, the IRS agreed that the hospital's tax-exempt status would not be revoked. In return, the hospital agreed to certain conditions regarding physician recruitment and retention. The agreement provided, in part, that the hospital agree to adopt verbatim the hospital physician recruitment guidelines set forth as an exhibit to the closing agreement. (Physician Recruitment Guidelines, Exhibit 1 to Closing Agreement with the Hermann Hospital Estate, are presented as Exhibit 2-6.)

IRS Announcement 95-25

On March 15, 1995, the IRS announced that it was considering issuing a revenue ruling addressing the question of whether a hospital violates the requirements for exemption from federal income tax when it provides incentives to recruit private-practice physicians. Proposed Revenue Ruling 9525 (Announcement 95-25) provides four examples of situations in which a physician recruitment program does not violate the exemption rules of Internal Revenue Code Section 501(c)(3) and provides one example of a situation in which a hospital's recruitment policies would threaten its exempt status. This proposed revenue ruling ultimately became final in Revenue Ruling 97-21.

In the announcement, the IRS addressed standards for review of recruitment arrangements generally and applied that analysis to specific fact situations. The IRS outlined the following four basic standards for analyzing physician recruitment incentives:

1. **Further exempt purposes:** The hospital may not engage in substantial activities that do not further its exempt purposes. All recruitment incentives must be reasonably related to the accomplishment of those purposes.
2. **Inurement:** The hospital must not engage in activities that result in inurement of its net earnings to a private shareholder or individual ("insiders"). *Net earnings* in this context include providing insiders with an "advantage, profit, fruit, privilege, gain, or interest" derived from the hospital.
3. **Private Benefit:** The hospital may not engage in substantial activities that cause it to be operated for the benefit of a private rather than a public interest so that it has a substantial nonexempt purpose. Private benefit issues are not limited to transactions with insiders.
4. **Legality:** The hospital may not engage in substantial unlawful activities. For example, a minor violation of the law (such as an unlawful disclosure of medical records, which in many states is a misdemeanor) would not trigger loss of tax exemption, but a massive, intentional coding violation under Medicare could.

Several aspects of the announcement represent new IRS positions, including the following:

1. The hypothetical examples include 3-year limits on the incentive, but the ruling does not suggest that there is an inherent cap.
2. Recruitment in the same city as the hospital may be permissible.
3. Hospitals may pay physicians to take on charity care and Medicaid patients.
4. Income guarantees are expressly recognized as permissible. Further, there is no requirement that a physician pay back the guaranteed amounts or that paybacks be forgiven under a formula requiring a physician to remain in a community for a long time.
5. Reasonable compensation is examined in terms of the physician's specialty without regard to the locality, recognizing that hospitals are competing in a national market.
6. Reasonable compensation is examined in light of whether there are charitable, community-oriented reasons for the physician's entire package.

Finally, the announcement also provides information on the basic documentation requirements and process for approving recruitment arrangements. Each recruitment arrangement should be set forth in a written agreement, negotiated at arm's length, approved by the hospital's governing board or its designees, limited so that all incentives provided are described in the agreement (i.e., no "off agreement" incentives provided), and supported by documented community need and benefit related to the particular specialty, with a higher degree of community benefits required for cross-town recruitment.

It is important to note that it remains unclear just how the fraud and abuse and antireferral considerations fit into the IRS proposal, especially in light of the November 19, 1999, safe harbors. The announcement outlined a situation in which the hospital's recruiting activities were held as not exempt because the hospital received a criminal conviction for anti-kickback violations. However, the example is not particularly helpful, as it provided no details about the illegal activities. In addition, while the proposed rule explicitly states that an anti-kickback statute violation will end an organization's qualification for tax exemption, it does not address the issue of Stark violations.

Although the proposed revenue ruling is encouraging in that the IRS is willing to attempt a clarification in the area of physician recruitment, the proposed ruling applies to areas that are not very questionable—for example, a rural hospital located in an economically depressed inner city with a shortage of obstetricians, and a hospital convicted of knowingly and willfully violating the Medicare and Medicaid anti-kickback statute for providing recruitment incentives that constituted payments for referrals. Nevertheless, this proposed revenue ruling should be carefully monitored and reviewed upon final issuance by IRS. (See Exhibit 2-7 for the full text of Announcement 95-25.)

In view of the current political climate and in light of the increased governmental scrutiny in the area of fraud and abuse, hospitals should increase their awareness of applicable federal and state laws and avoid even an appearance of impropriety. This increased governmental scrutiny also underscores the absolute necessity of consulting with legal counsel having expertise in the area of health law prior to beginning the physician recruitment process, during negotiations, and at all times during preparation of the recruitment contract.

Furthermore, it would be prudent for hospitals to have legal counsel periodically audit the recruitment contracts after execution for compliance with federal and state law. It is important to note that increased antifraud and abuse restrictions and sanctions were common threads throughout all of the current health care reform proposals proposed in Congress in 1994, and they continue to be important issues in the ongoing discussion of health care legislation.

ANTITRUST CONSIDERATIONS

In the course of physician recruitment, hospitals may increasingly be involved in collaboration or joint ventures among physicians, other health care providers, and health plans. As in other aspects of physician recruitment, legal counsel must be consulted to make certain there is no violation of state anti-competition laws or federal antitrust statutes. The importance of this is underscored by the 1994 jury verdict (which was later reversed) awarding nearly $50 million in antitrust damages against a Marshfield, Wisconsin, clinic.[1]

In the *Marshfield* case, Blue Cross & Blue Shield United of Wisconsin (Blue Cross) and its subsidiary, Compcare Health Services Insurance Company, an HMO, brought suit under sections 1 and 2 of the Sherman Act (discussed below) against the Marshfield Clinic and its IIMO subsidiary, Security Health Plan of Wisconsin, Inc. Compcare, Blue Cross' HMO, claimed that the Marshfield Clinic (a nonprofit corporation owned by the 400 physicians it employed) had a monopoly that it acquired and maintained by alleged improper practices that excluded Compcare from the HMO market in which the Marshfield Clinic and its HMO subsidiary (Security) operated. Blue Cross claimed that Marshfield, partly through its own alleged monopoly power and partly by alleged collusion with other providers of medical services, charged supracompetitive prices to patients insured by Blue Cross. After a 2-week trial, the jury returned a verdict for both plaintiffs that, after remittitur, trebling, and addition of attorneys' fees, produced a judgment just short of $50 million.

On September 18, 1995, the U.S. Court of Appeals for the Seventh Circuit reversed virtually all of the district court's ruling and, in doing so, made observations that could mean that providers can deal with the insurance industry on their own terms, even when they are the only providers in the market. On January 11, 1999, the U.S. Supreme Court denied Blue Cross and Blue Shield's petition for writ of certiorari.

The decision in the Marshfield Clinic case provides some guidance for physician groups, hospitals, clinics, and payers organizing physician networks. However, the case also serves as a warning that, while "natural monopolists" such as sole community providers may be able to act without violating antitrust laws under certain circumstances, care must be taken in the structure of the activity and the intent so as to avoid an antitrust claim.

The following federal acts are sometimes referred to collectively as the federal antitrust laws: the Sherman Act, the Clayton Act, the Federal Trade Commission Act, and the Robinson-Patman Act. Only the Sherman Act and the Clayton Act are pertinent to this review.

The Sherman Act

Section 1 of this act prohibits concerted or collusive activity by two or more persons resulting in a restraint on competition. The following elements must be proved:

- A contract, combination, or conspiracy
- Restraint of trade
- An effect on interstate commerce.

Section 2 of the act also prohibits monopolies and describes them as follows:

- Monopoly power consists of the power to control prices or exclude competition.

- An attempted monopolization occurs when a competitor with a dangerous probability of success engages in anticompetitive practices, the specific designs of which are to build a monopoly or exclude or destroy competition.

The Clayton Act

This act prohibits any exclusive dealing and tying arrangements involving sales of commodities if the arrangements lessen competition or tend to create a monopoly. It allows individuals to sue to enforce the Sherman Act and to seek treble damages and injunctive relief.

Examples of "Per Se" Antitrust Violations

Shortly after the Sherman Act was adopted, the U.S. Supreme Court established special categories of conduct that became known as "per se offenses" under that act. If certain conduct is illegal per se, the person seeking to enforce the Sherman Act (whether it be the government or an individual) need only prove that the conduct in question actually occurred. The defendant is permitted to justify the conduct or explain why the parties involved in the practice did what they did or that the actual effects of the acts were not anticompetitive.

Per se offenses include the following:

- **Price fixing among competitors:** This includes any practice or agreement with the purpose of raising, lowering, or stabilizing prices or terms of a sale. This also includes any agreement among competitors to fix employee salaries or fringe benefits.
- **Resale price maintenance:** This includes any agreement that controls the price at which a product is resold or distributed.
- **Agreements among competitors not to compete:** This includes, for example, agreements not to remain open at night, agreements not to bid against each other, or agreements not to offer a particular product or services.
- **Agreements to allocate markets or customers:** This includes establishing exclusive districts or agreements as to a division of the market or customers among competitors.
- **Group boycotts:** This includes agreements among competitors not to deal with certain third parties.
- **Tie-in agreements:** A tie-in is a sale or lease, for example, of a product with which the seller has "economic power" and with terms dictating that the customer must take another product, thus giving the customer little or no choice.

Examples of "Rule of Reason" Antitrust Violations

Practices under the antitrust laws that are not illegal per se are subject to court analysis under the "rule of reason." The courts weigh the business purposes and the actual anticompetitive and procompetitive effects to determine whether or not there has been a violation of the antitrust laws. Many of the collaborative efforts between hospitals and physicians, as well as hospital mergers throughout the United States, are being evaluated on a "rule of reason" basis. The U.S. Department of Justice (DOJ) and the Federal Trade Commission (FTC) (or the courts) carefully evaluate each set of circumstances to determine if the acts in question (assuming they are not illegal per se) have an anticompetitive or procompetitive effect.

Role of the "Expedited Business Review"

The DOJ has established an expedited business review procedure (58 Fed. Reg. 6132, 1993) pursuant to 28 C.F.R. 50.6 that allows health care providers to request preapproval for any collaborative activities that might involve potential antitrust risk. (See Exhibit 2-8 at the end of this chapter for an example of an expedited review request and response.)

If a hospital elects to use the expedited business review procedure, it is mandatory that the business venture not be commenced until after the DOJ has issued its response. In addition to consulting the federal regulations, hospitals (through their legal counsel) may want to contact the DOJ at the following address for more details:

Assistant Attorney General
Antitrust Division
United States Department of Justice
10th St. and Constitution Avenue, N.W.
Washington, D.C. 20530
Telephone: (202) 514-2000

Furthermore, the DOJ and the FTC have jointly issued statements concerning antitrust.[2]

Six policy statements were issued that identify antitrust safety zones in an attempt to provide greater certainty to the health care community and to encourage cost-cutting arrangements through cooperative activities. The six antitrust safety zones address the following:

1. Hospital mergers
2. Hospital joint ventures involving high technology or expensive equipment
3. Physician's provision of information to purchasers of health care services
4. Hospital participation in price and cost information exchanges
5. Joint purchasing arrangements
6. Physician network joint ventures.

In the area of physician network joint ventures, for example, an antitrust safety zone has been created for any group comprising 20% or less of the physicians in the relevant geographic market. A greater percentage may be permitted if, applying the rule of reason analysis, the group would enhance competition, reduce costs, and improve the delivery of health care.

Concerned that antitrust laws discourage the formation of procompetitive health care provider networks, House Judiciary Committee chairman Henry J. Hyde (R-Ill.) introduced a bill on February 1, 1996, that would have permitted more information sharing among network members. Congressman Hyde stated that the formation of procompetitive health care provider networks is being discouraged by the "arbitrarily narrow definition" of permissible integration contained in the DOJ and FTC policy statements. Congressman Hyde's bill would have required that as long as certain conditions are met, the information sharing among members of such networks is judged under antitrust laws pursuant to the "rule of reason" rather than treated as per se violations.

Physician-Hospital Organizations: Antitrust and PHO Contracting Activities

Physician-hospital organizations (PHOs) are proliferating in the United States today. Because PHOs provide a mechanism for hospitals and physicians to join together in networks of sufficient scope and coverage to attract contracts from insurers and employers, hospitals and practitioners are viewing them as one of many steps toward integration for more effective delivery of health care. Because most PHOs are associations of independent and competing providers, their organization and operation may raise significant antitrust concerns.

Two separate recent lawsuits for alleged antitrust violations mark the first enforcement actions brought by either of the federal antitrust enforcement agencies (the DOJ and the FTC) against PHOs and their constituent members. The enforcement actions address the managed care contracting activities of PHOs and likely signal the beginning of continued governmental antitrust scrutiny.

All health care providers participating in physician–hospital collaborations, or planning to do so in the future, should be aware of the background of these recent lawsuits and their implications for other PHOs.

The lawsuits involve PHOs and their participating providers in Danbury, Connecticut, and St. Joseph, Missouri. The DOJ alleged that the defendants in both cases had entered into agreements, the purpose and effect of which were to unlawfully reduce or eliminate the development of managed care and otherwise limit competition in the area.

Although both cases have been tentatively settled, subject to local federal district court approval, the proposed settlements offer a number of lessons on how a PHO may and may not conduct its managed care activities.[3]

BONA FIDE EMPLOYEE STATUS

In light of the rather narrow safe harbor regulations issued on November 19, 1999, regarding physician recruitment, and in view of the existing statutory exception for payments to employees (as also incorporated in Stark II), hospitals may wish to give more consideration to recruiting physicians and establishing them as bona fide employees of the hospital until they can enter private practice, assuming that doing so would be otherwise permitted by state law. (See Exhibit 2-9 for 20 key factors that the IRS looks at to determine independent contractor versus bona fide employee status.)

Again, it is extremely important that the hospital consult legal counsel to make certain that the hospital fully complies with the bona fide exception to the statute and applicable state law. Some states prohibit the corporate practice of medicine. This prohibition also may be changing in some states, such as Michigan, where the attorney general on September 17, 1993, opined that the corporate practice of medicine prohibition would not apply to a nonprofit corporation such as a § 501(c)(3) hospital.

See also the opinion of the Iowa attorney general dated July 12, 1992, reversing, in part, a 1954 opinion and finding that the corporate practice of medicine regarding a nonprofit organization may not be unlawful if on a case-by-case basis it can be demonstrated that the corporate entity does not exercise undue dominion and control over the licensed professional.

In 1995 the Illinois Circuit Court (Fifth Circuit) in Charleston, Illinois, ruled that a physician contract with a hospital was unenforceable because direct employment of physicians by a corporation violated the Illinois Medical Practice Act of 1987. The case was eventually appealed to the Illinois Supreme Court.[4] In the *Berlin* case, the Illinois Supreme Court reversed the decisions of both the circuit court and the appellate court and held that a licensed hospital, whether a for-profit or nonprofit organization, is exempt from the prohibition of corporate practice of medicine, and, therefore, such hospital may employ licensed physicians to provide medical services.[5]

The area of physician employment also points out the sometimes divergent views of the OIG, the IRS, and the state laws prohibiting the corporate practice of medicine. Some hospitals have retained physicians as independent contractors and not as employees to avoid violating their state's prohibition. Accordingly, the hospital does not withhold any taxes from amounts paid to the physician. The IRS has recently increased its scrutiny of such arrangements, and upon an audit may take the position that the physician is really an employee. Consequently, the hospital may be subject to penalty for not withholding taxes even though it has designated the physician as an independent contractor.

THE KENNESTONE SETTLEMENT

In 1993, a settlement was reached with the OIG in the Kennestone Hospital at Windy Hill, Inc., investigation in Cobb County, Georgia. This settlement may offer some guidance to hospitals regarding physician recruitment. Following an extensive criminal investigation by the OIG, a settlement was reached in connection with certain income guarantees that had been offered as part of a physician recruitment agreement.

- The settlement, as reported, suggests that income guarantees, under limited conditions, may be permissible as long as certain standards are met, including the following: Payments in cash and kind must be based on a written agreement for a term of at least 1 year and must set forth all of the services to be provided by the physician.
- Aggregate payments consistent with fair market value must be set in advance in an arm's-length transaction and must not be determined by the volume and value of referrals.
- Although a hospital may require a physician to practice within the hospital's service area, it cannot restrict referrals within that area.

The Kennestone settlement further provides the following:

- Payments for moving expenses were acceptable under the circumstances.
- Future physician recruitment activities and agreements must be given a review by independent legal counsel.

Although the Kennestone settlement is not a binding precedent for hospitals, it does provide some guidance concerning enforcement of the antifraud and abuse statute by the OIG. This is especially helpful in view of the narrow scope of the proposed physician recruitment safe harbor regulations (i.e., safe harbor only for hospitals located in rural areas).

FELDSTEIN, M.D., V. NASH COMMUNITY HEALTH SERVICES, INC.

Court decisions regarding physician recruitment are rare. On March 16, 1999, the U.S. district court in North Carolina rendered a decision in the case of *Feldstein, M.D., v. Nash Community Health Services, Inc.* (51 F. Supp. 2d 673 1999) that provides some insights into how the federal courts view physician recruitment arrangements.

In *Feldstein*, the Community Hospital of Rocky Mount entered into a physician recruitment arrangement with Dr. Feldstein. The hospital was later acquired by Nash Community Health Services, Inc. ("Nash"). Feldstein sued for an alleged breach of contract. The agreement provided, among other things, that the physician was not required to admit patients to the hospital and that his compensation was not conditional upon the use of any item or service offered by the hospital:

> We, of course, hope that the quality and cost-effective nature of our Hospital's services will commend themselves to your patients. However, we clearly understand that the choice of services and the choice of service suppliers which you make on behalf of your patients must be, and will be, made *only* with regard to the best interests of the patients themselves. Therefore, so there will be no misunderstanding, the compensation that you are to receive is not conditional on the use of any item or service offered by this Hospital.

The central issue in *Feldstein* was whether or not this statement violates the federal anti-kickback statute. Nash contended that the provisions of the agreement violated the anti-kickback statute (as well as Stark), and, therefore, the hospital was entitled to a summary judgment from the court that the recruitment arrangement was unenforceable under state law.

The *Feldstein* case contains an extensive discussion of the federal regulatory structure. The court also noted that it had been able to locate only one published case involving physician agreements and the anti-kickback statute [*Polk County v. Peters,* 800 F.Supp. 1451, 1455 (Ed. Tex. 1992)]. In *Polk*, a hospital brought suit against a physician in an attempt to recover money advanced to the physician pursuant to a recruiting contract that the physician allegedly breached. The court in *Feldstein* found that the *Polk* case was not dispositive of the issue because in *Polk*, the physician was explicitly required to refer patients to the hospital. In *Polk*, the court found that the agreement violated the anti-kickback statute, and, consequently, the contract was illegal and unenforceable under Texas law.

In *Feldstein*, Feldstein argued that summary judgment should be granted in his favor because the language of the recruitment agreement expressly disavowed any connection between the compensation provided to the physician and the physician's use of the hospital. Nash requested summary in its favor, and because of ambiguity in the agreement asked the court to look beyond the explicit language of the recruitment agreement and to infer such intent from the agreement read as a whole. The court concluded by stating that the language in the recruitment agreement was ambiguous. When the language is ambiguous, the parties' intent is a question for the jury. Consequently, the court did not grant summary judgment to either party on the anti-kickback issue. One possible lesson to be learned from *Feldstein* is to draft recruitment agreements carefully and not make any gratuitous or affirmative statements that could lead to potential ambiguity or claim.

There are some encouraging points in the Feldstein case despite the fact that the court held that a jury should decide the issue regarding the anti-kickback statute. For example, the court declined the defendants' invitation to issue a ruling so broad that it would render almost every physician recruitment contract illegal. The court stated:

> Such a determination would set dangerous precedent in light of the fact that any recruitment contract, particularly one involving the relocation of a physician, will involve the extension of significant monetary benefits to that physician.

The court went on to note:

> All physician recruitment contracts involving relocation are going to contain the extension of significant monetary benefits to physicians to entice them to relocate and to make them believe that starting a medical practice in a new location will be a viable enterprise. Similarly, every physician recruitment contract is, by definition, a hospital giving a physician an opportunity to earn money. While such an opportunity "may well be" an inducement to refer

patients, [citation omitted], it may well not be intended as such an inducement.

The court also concluded that it could not find, as a matter of law pursuant to a motion for summary judgment, that the recruitment agreement violated Stark. It noted that Stark contains a specific exception under which a physician recruitment agreement would not be a prohibited compensation arrangement.[6]

ALVARADO HOSPITAL MEDICAL CENTER, INC.

In 2003 Alvarado Hospital Medical Center, a Tenet health care hospital, and its CEO, Barry Weinbaum, were indicted for criminal violations relating to payments to physicians based on numerous physician relocation agreements entered into between the hospital and physicians. The government alleged that established physicians, rather than newly recruited physicians, received the substantial portion of the benefit and that these payments were made in exchange for referrals. This case was tried and in early 2005 ended in a hung jury. Nonetheless, it indicates the government's concern with regard to recruitment payments being made that benefit existing physicians rather than newly recruited physicians.

Following a 4-year hiatus in advisory opinion activity, and in the same breath as a MEDPAC recommendation to Congress, the OIG issued four favorable advisory opinions in 2006 on what have come to be known as "gainsharing" arrangements. Two more favorable opinions are also to be issued in 2006, and it does appear that the regulatory door is opening to such arrangements that meet the strict criteria described in the opinions.

Gainsharing and Its Regulatory History

Gainsharing is an arrangement between a hospital and physicians on its medical staff who refer patients to the hospital and provide services to the hospital's patients, under which the hospital pays the physicians a portion of a hospital's savings in exchange for the physicians implementing certain cost-saving strategies. It is intended to align incentives between physicians who bear none of the burdens of such costs, and the hospital, which bears them all.

Although variations of gainsharing arrangements have been discussed since before the enactment of the hospital inpatient prospective payment system, the present generation of such arrangements can be traced back to the late 1990s. It was in response to these proposals that the OIG, almost regrettably, issued a Special Advisory Bulletin in July 1999, in which it advised existing and prospective gainsharing participants that they would be subject to civil monetary penalties under 42 U.S.C. §1320a-7a(b)(1) if they knowingly made a payment directly or indirectly to a physician as an inducement to reduce or limit services to Medicare or Medicaid beneficiaries in the physician's care.

Despite rather harsh commentary at the time from several advisers to the health care industry, the OIG did not relent in its position; however, in January 2001, the OIG issued its first advisory opinion (No. 01-01), in which it declined to impose sanctions on a gainsharing arrangement structured much like the arrangements described in the 2005 advisory opinions. Other than occasional commentary, such as in its recommended compliance guidance for hospitals, that was the last formal communication from the OIG on the subject.

At its January 12, 2005, meeting, MEDPAC issued a recommendation to Congress that it enact legislation permitting CMS to authorize gainsharing arrangements under strict rules CMS would adopt. At the same time, the OIG was finalizing the six new gainsharing opinions, each submitted by an Atlanta-based consulting firm, for programs it designed for client hospitals seeking to achieve cost savings either from their cardiac surgery programs or cardiac catheterization laboratories. Some of these opinion applications had been under OIG scrutiny for as long as 2 1/2 years; the programs had already been completed, and the gainsharing payments placed in escrow pending favorable OIG opinions.

The programs before the OIG had the following major elements in common:

- Each program included a hospital and one or more physician groups already on the hospital's medical staff, whose physicians provided all of the hospital's cardiac surgery or cardiac catheterization services.
- The consultant was hired as a program administrator to manage the program for a fixed fee. Among the program administrator's responsibilities were to prepare a "practice pattern report" examining both historic practices at the applicable hospital department and among the participating physicians, and then to present cost-saving recommendations based on these findings. These recommendations typically fell into the categories of "open as needed" supplies savings, blood cross-matching as needed, substitution of less costly items, and product standardization.
- The program administrator also established a base line for costs and utilization and set controls to ensure that participating physicians were not rewarded for reducing costs, increasing referrals, or "cherry picking" patients for the program.
- Participating physician groups were to be paid 50% of the documented cost savings resulting from adoption of the recommendations in the practice pattern report for the first year of the program only. No provision was made for sharing in savings in subsequent years. Physician groups receiving gainsharing payments also agreed to distribute such funds per capita among group members.
- The arrangement was to be disclosed to patients prior to admission, unless emergency circumstances did not permit, in which case disclosure had to be made at least prior to the subject procedure. The parties were expected to document the patients' authorizations in writing.

The OIG's Analysis

As it did in its previous Special Advisory Bulletin and Advisory Opinion No. 01-01, the OIG noted that the present arrangements could be subject to civil monetary penalties, and if unlawful intent was present, could violate 42 U.S.C §1320a-7b(b), the federal anti-kickback statute. The OIG also noted that the arrangements could implicate federal Stark II referral prohibitions (42 U.S.C. §1395nn), but declined to opine regarding Stark II, that falling within CMS's jurisdiction. The OIG also declined to opine on the implications of the arrangements for the tax-exempt status of any of the applicant tax-exempt hospitals.

Despite the potential in the OIG's opinion for the proposed gainsharing arrangements to violate one or more of these authorities, the OIG declined to impose civil monetary penalties or to commence an enforcement action under the federal anti-kickback statute. The OIG noted that each arrangement before it had built-in program safeguards, leading the OIG to conclude that these particular gainsharing programs posed little prospect for Medicare or Medicaid program abuse. The safeguards included the following:

- Cost-saving actions and the savings resulting from them were clearly and separately identified, allowing for public scrutiny and individual physician accountability for any adverse effects of the arrangements.
- Credible medical support existed indicating that patient care would not suffer.
- Payments were to be based on all procedures regardless of the patient's insurance so that procedures were not disproportionately performed on Medicare/Medicaid beneficiaries; savings were based on actual hospital out-of-pocket expenses.
- Baseline thresholds for cost and utilization protected against inappropriate reductions in services.
- Even after adopting product standardization recommendations, physicians would still have the same devices available to them, should patient care considerations dictate one product or another in the physician's judgment.
- The arrangements would be transparent to the patient, who could make an informed decision before undergoing the particular procedure.
- Financial incentives were reasonably limited in duration and amount, and were mitigated vis-à-vis an individual physician by per capita distributions.

Caveats and Recommendations

Advisory Opinion Nos. 05-01 through 05-04 are expressly limited to their facts, and applicable only to the requesting parties. Moreover, the OIG makes it clear in each opinion that it is only approving *these arrangements*, each of which is subject to the strict safeguards described above. Programs that are more open-ended and indefinite regarding the savings to be shared or the term are not likely to be acceptable to the OIG, although the opinions did leave open the possibility of a program exceeding 1 year in length if appropriate safeguards were in place to prevent abuse.

Potential participants should also note that gainsharing payments from a hospital to a referring physician constitute a compensation arrangement subject to the federal Stark law patient referral prohibitions. Thus, such payments would have to be structured to satisfy one of the Stark statutory or regulatory exceptions to enable the participating physicians to continue to refer Medicare and Medicaid inpatients and outpatients patients to the hospital and to allow the hospital to bill for its covered services furnished to such patients.

In addition, physicians participating in a gainsharing arrangement with a tax-exempt hospital may already be (or may become by reason of the arrangement) "disqualified persons" in relation to the hospital for purposes of the IRS's excess benefit transaction regulations. Participating tax-exempt hospitals should consider taking the steps within their own organizations to qualify for the rebuttable presumption of reasonableness to protect against the possible imposition of excise taxes under those regulations.

Finally, on a positive note, even though the applicants were seeking opinions about cardiac service programs, there is no indication in the opinions that gainsharing programs with similar safeguards and applicable to other high-cost services (e.g., orthopedics) could not receive a favorable OIG opinion. Indeed, the gates may open wider to acceptance of gainsharing programs if Congress accepts MEDPAC's recommendations and permits CMS to authorize gainsharing programs, meaning removes legislatively the spectre of CMPs for such programs.

Until then, hospitals and physicians desiring to enter into gainsharing arrangements should proceed cautiously and under professional advice. Potential gainsharing program participants should seek their own advisory opinions from the OIG, may wish to seek Stark II advisory opinions from CMS as well, and should vet these transactions thoroughly with their governing boards to avoid unfavorable tax consequences.

THE STARK LAW

Under the Stark law, if a physician (or immediate family member of a physician) has a financial relationship with an entity, he or she may not make referrals to the entity for furnishing designated health services for which Medicare would make payment. Correspondingly, the entity may not present or cause to be presented a claim under Medicare, or a bill to any individual, third-party payer, or other entity for designated health services that were furnished pursuant to a prohibited referral.

In the case of physician services, the request by a physician for the item or service, including a consultation with another physician (and any tests or procedures ordered by or to be performed by or under the supervision of the other physician), constitutes a "referral" by a "referring physician." For other items, the request or establishment of a plan of care by a physician that includes a provision of the designated health services constitutes such referral. However, the following do not constitute a referral:

- A request by a pathologist for clinical diagnostic laboratory tests and pathological examination services,
  - By a radiologist for diagnostic radiology services
  - By a radiation oncologist for radiation therapy, if such services are furnished by or under the supervision of such pathologist, radiologist, or radiation oncologist pursuant to a consultation requested by another physician, if:
    - The request results from another physician's consultation, and
    - The tests or services are furnished by or under the supervision of the pathologist, radiologist, or radiation oncologist in his or her group practice.

For the purposes of the statute, a financial relationship that triggers the prohibition is a direct or indirect ownership or investment interest in the entity, or a direct or indirect compensation arrangement between the physician (or an immediate family member) and the entity. The ownership interest may be through equity, debt, or other means and includes an interest in an entity that holds an ownership or investment interest in any entity providing a designated health service.

The phrase *designated health service* is unique to the Stark law. The Stark law prohibits referrals for furnishing any designated health services that expressly include the following:

- Clinical laboratory services
- Physical therapy services
- Occupational therapy services
- Radiology or other diagnostic services
- Radiation therapy services
- Durable medical equipment
- Parenteral and enteral nutrients, equipment, and supplies
- Prosthetics, orthotics, or prosthetic devices
- Home health services
- Outpatient prescription drugs
- Inpatient and outpatient hospital services.

The Stark law however, does contain numerous exceptions. The first group of such exceptions applies to both ownership and compensation arrangement prohibitions. The ban on physician referrals does not apply in the case of physician services provided personally by (or under the personal supervision of) another physician in the same group practice as the referring physician.

Similarly, the ban is not applicable in the case of certain in-office ancillary services that are furnished personally by the referring physician, the physician who is a member of the same group practice as the referring physician, or individuals who are directly supervised by the physician or by another

physician in the group practice, and the services are furnished in a location specifically set forth in the statute. In addition, the ban does not reach in-office ancillary services that are billed by the physician performing or supervising the services, by a group practice of which the physician is a member under a billing number assigned to a group practice, or by an entity that is wholly owned by the physician or group practice.

The term *group practice* is narrowly and explicitly defined as a group of two or more physicians legally organized as a partnership, professional corporation, foundation, not-for-profit corporation, faculty practice plan, or similar association:

- In which each physician who is a member of the group substantially provides the full range of services that a physician routinely provides, including medical care, consultation, diagnosis, or treatment through the joint use of shared office space, facilities, equipment, and personnel
- For which substantial services of the physicians who are members of the group are provided through the group and are billed under a billing number assigned to the group, and amounts so received are treated as receipts of the group
- In which the overhead expenses and the income from the practice are distributed in accordance with methods previously determined
- In which no physician who is a member of the group directly or indirectly receives compensation based on the volume or value of referrals by the physician
- In which members of the group personally conduct no less than 75% of the physicianpatient encounters of the group practice
- In which the group's governance documents provide for centralized decision making by a centralized body

A physician in a group practice may be paid a share of overall profits of the group, or a productivity bonus, based on services performed or services incident to such personally performed services as long as the share or bonus is not determined in any manner that is directly related to the volume or value of referrals by the physician.

Another group of exceptions relates to compensation arrangements. The term *compensation arrangement* means any arrangement involving any remuneration between a physician (or an immediate family member) and an entity. *Remuneration* is broadly defined to include any remuneration paid directly or indirectly, overtly or covertly, in cash or in kind. Under this group of exceptions, the following are not considered to be illegal compensation arrangements:

- The rental of office space and equipment, within certain explicitly defined parameters
- Any amount paid by an employer to a physician who has a bona fide employment relationship with the employer for the provision of services if the employment is for identifiable services, the amount of the remuneration under the employment is consistent with the fair market value of services

and is not determined in a manner that takes into account the volume or value of any referrals by the referring physician, and the remuneration is provided pursuant to an agreement that would be commercially reasonable even if no referrals were made by the employer. The statute defines an *employee* as an individual who would be considered an employee under usual common law rules for determining an employer–employee relationship as applied pursuant to the Internal Revenue Code. (The statute expressly provides that the remuneration standard does not prohibit remuneration in the form of a productivity bonus based on services performed personally by the physician or an immediate family member of such physician.)

- Certain personal service arrangements for a period of at least 1 year. Under the exception for personal services arrangements, such relationships between DHS entities and physicians are permitted if the following occurs:
  - Each arrangement is in writing, signed by the parties, and specifies the services covered.
  - The arrangement covers all services to be furnished.[7]
  - The contract's aggregate services do not exceed that which is reasonably necessary for the legitimate business purposes of the arrangement.
  - The agreement is for at least 1 year, and in the event of termination prior to 1 year, the parties may not enter into a substantially similar agreement during the first year of the original agreement.
  - The compensation is set in advance, does not exceed fair market value, and except for a physician incentive plan,[8] does not take into account the volume or value of referrals or other business generated between the parties.
  - The services to do not involve the counseling or promotion of a business arrangement that violates either state or federal law.
- Remuneration that is provided by a hospital to a physician if such remuneration is not related to the provision of designated health services
- Physician recruitment in the case of remuneration that is provided by a hospital to a physician to induce the physician to relocate to the geographic area served by the hospital in order to be a member of the medical staff of the hospital if the following occurs:
  - The arrangement is in writing and signed by the parties.
  - The arrangement is not conditioned on the physician making referrals to the hospital.
  - The compensation is not based on referrals or business otherwise generated.
  - The physician is permitted to establish privileges at other hospitals as well as refer to other facilities.

The *geographic area* served by the hospital is defined as the area composed of the lowest number of contiguous zip codes from which the hospital draws at least 75% of its inpatients. A physician will be deemed to have "relocated" if the following occurs:

  - The physician moves his or her practice at least 25 miles.

or

- At least 75% of the revenue from physician's new practice location is generated from patients the physician did not see or treat at his or her old location. Residents and physicians in practice less than a year need not comply with the relocation requirement, and simply need to locate their new practices within the geographic area served by the hospital.

In addition, if the recruited physician is joining an existing practice, then the following must occur:

- The existing practice must sign the recruitment agreement if it is receiving payments from the hospital.
- All of the remuneration must remain with or pass through to the recruited physician except for "actual costs incurred" by the existing practice in recruiting the new physician.
- In the case of income guarantees, only the "actual additional incremental costs attributable to the recruited physician" may be allocated by the existing practice to the new physician.
- Records of the costs and passed-through amounts, must be kept for 5 years and made available to the DHHS upon request.
- The remuneration may not be determined based on referrals, or expected referrals, from the recruited physician (or the existing practice) or other business generated between the parties.
- The existing practice may not impose any additional practice restrictions on the recruited physician (e.g., a noncompete agreement), other than those relating to quality of care.
- The arrangement may not violate the anti-kickback statute.

Following enactment of the Stark law, the Health Care Financing Administration formulated a proposed rule, which was released in January 1998. The Final Rule was substantially modified and was released in two phases. Phase I was released on January 4, 2001.[9] Most of its provisions became effective January 4, 2002. Phase II was released on March 26, 2004.[10]

The Final Rule is lengthy and complex. The following sections discuss points that may apply to physician recruitment.

Medical Staff Incidental Benefits. The Final Rule provides clarification on certain incidental benefits given to medical staff members. In the past, there was some concern that free or discounted meals, free parking, drug samples, free coffee mugs, free note pads, free computer access to enhance medical records and educational information, or other similar physician benefits from a hospital might violate the Stark law. The Final Rule, however, allows these medical staff members incidental benefits, subject to the following:

- The benefits must be offered to all physicians on the staff of the hospital.
- The benefits must be offered regardless of volume or value of referrals from the physician or other business generated between the parties.
- The benefits must be offered only during periods when the medical staff members are making rounds or performing other duties that benefit the hospital.

- The benefits must be provided by the hospital and used by the medical staff only on the hospital's campus.
- The benefits must be reasonably related to the provision of, or designed to facilitate directly or indirectly the delivery of, medical services at the hospital.
- The value of the benefit should be less than $25 per occurrence.
- The arrangement must not violate the anti-kickback statute or any federal or state law or regulation governing billing or claims submission.

Under the Final Rule a hospital could give a physician either one noncash gift per year of up to $300 in value or two or more noncash gifts per year as long as the annual aggregate value of the gifts does not exceed $300. The Final Rule does not carve out an exception for free malpractice insurance coverage and free transcription services unless they are part of the usual employment benefit package and the physician is a hospital employee. Furthermore, the incidental benefits exception does not apply to cash payments. For example, paying a physician $20 per month to complete medical charts in a timely manner would appear to violate Stark II, whereas providing free food having a value of $20 to physicians during rounds would not violate Stark II. The Final Rule does not provide any exception or guidance for hospital waiver of deductibles or copayments if a staff physician is hospitalized. The Final Rule does confirm that free drugs, free training, or gifts provided to physicians by drug manufacturers are not prohibited under Stark II because drug manufacturers are not entities that furnish health services. Caution should be exercised, however, that the physician in receiving incidental benefits not violate other applicable laws and regulations, including, without limitation, the anti-kickback statute and the federal laws restricting the sale and distribution of drug samples.[11] The incidental benefits exception under the Final Rule applies only to individual physicians. For example, a gift by a hospital to a group practice would appear to violate Stark II, except for holiday parties and office equipment or supplies that are valued at not more than $300 per physician in the group, per year, but are, in effect, given or used as a group gift.

Compliance Training. In the past, there was some concern that giving physicians free or discounted training sessions concerning legal compliance might violate the Stark law. The final regulations, however, acknowledge that improving physician compliance is a worthwhile goal. Consequently, the Final Rule permits hospitals to provide free compliance training to physicians to help reduce potential fraud and overbilling within the Medicare system.

"Under Arrangements" Entities. In recent years, hospitals have outsourced an increasing number of services, and there has been concern that these arrangements might violate the Stark law when a physician is an owner or investor in the outsourcing entity. Typically, the outsourcing entity is subject to utilization review of a hospital, and customarily the hospital will do the billing for services rendered. Under the Stark law, these arrangements are not prohibited when the outsourcing entity is owned by physicians who also make referrals to the contracting hospital. CMS will treat "under arrangements" the same as a compensation rela-

tionship and will subject them to the same conditions (see "Fair Market Value" section below).

Academic Medical Centers. The Stark law now acknowledges the unique nature of academic medical centers, which often involve multiple-affiliated entities that jointly deliver health care services to patients. It cites an example of an academic setting where there are multiple components, such as a faculty practice plan, a medical school, a teaching hospital, and outpatient clinics. Referrals and monetary transfers among these various entities would appear to violate the Stark law. Under the Final Rule, however, these relationships and referrals would not violate the Stark law so long as certain conditions are met, including the following:

- The referring physician must be a bona fide employee of a component of an academic medical center on a full-time or substantial part-time basis.
- The referring physician must be licensed to practice medicine in the state.
- The physician must have a bona fide faculty appointment at the affiliated medical school and provide either substantial academic or substantial clinical teaching services or a combination of both for which the faulty member receives compensation as part of his or her employment relationship with the academic medical center. Note: The exception does not apply to payments to physicians who provide only occasional academic or clinical teaching services or who are principally community rather than academic medical center practitioners. This appears to present a problem for a physician who wishes to assist an academic medical center on a very limited basis (or less than "substantial part-time basis") if that physician refers patients to the academic medical center and if that physician receives compensation for his or her teaching duties.
- The total compensation paid for the previous 12-month period or fiscal year from all academic medical center components to the referring physician must be set in advance and, in the aggregate, cannot exceed fair market value for the services provided.
- The compensation paid to the physician must not be determined in a manner that takes into account the volume or value of any referrals or other business generated within the academic medical center.
- The compensation arrangement must not violate the anti-kickback statute, or any federal or state law or regulation governing billing or claim submission.

The academic medical center must also meet all of the following conditions:

- All transfers of money must (directly or indirectly) support the goal of teaching, indigent care, research, or community service.
- The relationship of the components must be set forth in writing and adopted by the governing body of each component. If the center is one legal entity, the financial reports of the components satisfy this requirement.

- All money paid to a referring physician for research must be used only to support bona fide research or teaching.

  Fair Market Value. Compensation arrangements between referring physicians (or their immediate family members) and hospitals are allowed under the Stark law if the following conditions are met:

- The agreement must be in writing and signed by the parties.
- The agreement must cover identifiable items or services and must be specified in the agreement.
- The agreement must cover all of the items or services to be provided by the physician (or immediate family member) to the entity.
- The agreement must specify the time frame for the arrangement and contain a termination clause, provided the parties may enter into only one arrangement covering the same items or services during the course of a year.
- An agreement may be made for less than 1 year and may be renewed any number of times if the terms of the arrangement and the compensation for the same items or services do not change.
- The compensation must be set in advance.
- The agreement must involve a transaction that is commercially reasonable and furthers a legitimate business purpose of the parties.
- The compensation must be consistent with fair market value and not be determined in a manner that takes into account the volume or value of any referrals.
- The services to be performed under the arrangement do not involve the counseling or promotion of a business arrangement or other activity that violates a state or federal law.
- It must not violate the anti-kickback statute or any federal or state law or regulation governing billing or claims submission.

Recent Enforcement of the Stark Law

The recent settlement between the United States and Tenet Healthcare is the largest recovery under the U.S. False Claims Act (FCA) from a single hospital arising out of alleged violations of the Stark law. There was no admission of liability by Tenet Healthcare under the settlement agreement, although the allegations in this whistleblower case included that North Ridge Medical Center in Fort Lauderdale, Florida (a Tenet Hospital), and its parent companies entered into a number of prohibited financial relationships with physicians in 1993 and 1994 and continued billing Medicare for referrals from these doctors through the late 1990s. The government also alleged that these violations of the Stark law give rise to violations of the FCA. The settlement agreement also resolved allegations that North Ridge Medical Center requested improper reimbursements on its annual cost reports, presumably costs associated with the prohibited payments to physicians.

The allegations in the case related to alleged Stark law violations included that North Ridge Medical Center paid physicians exorbitant rates to acquire their practices and as compensation for their continuing services in order to secure referrals from these physicians to the hospital. The hospital was previously owned by American Medical International, Inc. when the arrangements with these physicians were made during 1993 and 1994. After Tenet Healthcare purchased the hospital, it did not apparently unwind these physician arrangements when brought to its attention by the whistleblower in this case, who was the Chief Operating Officer of Physician Services in Florida for Tenet during 1996. There is apparently additional evidence that marked the referral patterns of the physicians before and after each acquisition and the relationship between physician compensation and the physician referral patterns to the hospital.

The settlement agreement also included a corporate integrity agreement (CIA) between the OIG, Tenet Healthcare Corporation, and North Ridge Medical Center. The CIA is for a minimum of 5 years, and requires the following:

- The establishment of a compliance officer and compliance committees throughout Tenet
- The development of written standards of conduct and policies and procedures for implementation of a compliance program
- The establishment of a training program with specified training in physician relationships, cost reporting, and specific compliance in contractual arrangements under the anti-kickback statute and the Stark law.

The CIA also obligates Tenet to undertake various reviews by independent review organizations as follows:

- Cost report preparation
- Cost report systems review
- Unallowable cost report review
- Physician relationships review

There is a specific requirement under the settlement agreement to engage a separate independent review organization to review hospital and physician relationships, which shall include, but shall not be limited to, the following:

- Physician recruitment and relocation payment
- Medical directorship arrangements
- Leases of office space and equipment to physicians
- Personal service agreements with physicians and physician groups
- Loans to physicians or physician groups
- Leases of space and equipment from physicians
- Physician practice acquisition
- Employment agreements with physicians or physician groups
- Joint ventures
- Services or supplies provided by Tenet or North Ridge to physicians or physicians groups (e.g., joint marketing, practice management, staffing,

malpractice insurance, continuing medical education, lab, pharmacy, transcription, sterilization, transportation)
• Gifts, travel, and entertainment provided to physicians and physician groups

United States v. McLaren Regional Medical Center is the seminal case regarding the court's application of the Stark law's fair market value exception. In this case, Family Orthopedic Realty, L.L.C. (FOR) and McLaren Regional Medical Center (McLaren) were charged with participating in a scheme that allegedly produced an improper financial and referral relationship between the owner of a building and a potential tenant. The government alleged that McLaren paid FOR remuneration disguised as a lease agreement in exchange for the referral of Medicare patients. The government charged both defendants with violating the False Claims Act proffering that the financial relationship violated Stark thereby making all Medicare claims tainted.

The defendants refuted the government's position by arguing that the lease agreement qualified within the fair market value safe harbor provision. Therefore, the issue before the court was whether the lease payments paid by McLaren to FOR represented the fair market value of the rental. An agreement will qualify within the safe harbor if the parties engaged in an arms length transaction, the value was consistent with the general market value of a similar item or location, and the value did increase or fluctuate based on a potential source of patient referrals to one party.[12]

First, the court examined the conduct of the parties during the formation of the lease to determine if McLaren and FOR engaged in an arms length transaction. The court examined the negotiation process by focusing on issues such as the length of the process, the amount of the rental fee, the length of the lease, the area calculation method, the timing of payments, compliance issues, and termination provisions to opine that the parties did engage in an arms length transaction.

Second, the court had to determine whether the agreed rental fee was consistent with the fair market value of similar lease space in similar areas. For this, the court relied on expert testimony. Each side presented experts that supported their side's position. The court concluded that it was not satisfied with the government's witnesses and that defendants experts' testimony was representative of the fair market value of the lease.

Lastly, the court examined if the value of the lease was influenced by possible patient referrals. Here, the government had the burden of establishing whether the lease rate was determined in a manner that took into account the value of patient referrals. To satisfy its burden the government pointed to the agreements exclusivity and noncompete provisions to establish that the value was influenced by referrals. Moreover, the government pointed to a contract provision that allowed McLaren to terminate the lease if FOR ever vacated the premises. This argument was premised on the notion that if FOR left the building it would no longer refer patients to McLaren.

However, the court did not find these arguments persuasive and stated:

> The government failed to present any evidence to establish that because of potential patient referrals, McLaren paid a higher rental rate than it otherwise would have paid, or that FOR . . . received a higher rate than it would have otherwise received because of any patient referrals that McLaren might have received.

Therefore, because the agreement was conducted at arms length, was not in excess of fair market value, and did not account for patient referrals, the lease agreement qualified for safe harbor protection and did not constitute a Stark violation. As a result the False Claims Act charge was dismissed.

REFERENCES

1. *Blue Cross and Blue Shield of Wisconsin v. The Marshfield Clinic*, No. 94-C-137-S, W.D. Wisconsin, 1994.
2. See Department of Justice and Federal Trade Commission, Antitrust Enforcement Policy Statements in the Health Care Area, September 15, 1993.
3. 60 Fed. Reg. 52014 and 60 Fed. Reg. 51808.
4. *Berlin v. Sarah Bush Lincoln Health Center*, 179 III.2d 1, 688 N.E. 2d 106 (1997).
5. For a good discussion of states where the corporate practice of medicine doctrine has been diluted or modified, *see* John Wiorek, "The Corporate Practice of Medicine: An Outmoded Theory in Need of Modification," *Journal of Legal Medicine*, 465, 475–84 (1987). *See also*, Dowell, "The Corporate Practice of Medicine Prohibition: A Dinosaur Awaiting Extinction," 27 *Journal of Health and Hospital Law*, 369 (1994).
6. 42 U.S.C 1395 nn (e)(5).
7. In order to meet this requirement, all separate agreements must incorporate each other by reference or cross-reference to a master list of contracts that is centrally maintained and updated and available for the Secretary's review upon request. In addition, a physician can furnish services through employees hired for that purpose, through a wholly owned entity, or through *locum tenens* physicians. 42 C.F.R. § 411.357(d)(ii).
8. An additional exception exists for physician incentive plans.
9. *Federal Register*, January 4, 2001, Volume 66.
10. *Federal Register*, March 26, 2004, Volume 69.
11. 21 U.S.C. Sec. 353(c) through (d).
12. 42 U.S.C. §1395nn(h)(3).

EXHIBIT 2-1   1991 FRAUD AND ABUSE SAFE HARBORS

U.S. Department of Justice
Antitrust Division
Office of the Assistant Attorney General

Washington, D.C. 20530
July 6, 1994

Eugene E. Olson, Esquire
Connolly, O'Malley, Lillis, Hansen & Olson
820 Liberty Building
418 Sixth Avenue
Des Moines, Iowa 50309

Dear Mr. Olson:

This letter responds to your request on behalf of the Collaborative Provider Organization, Inc., (CPO) for a statement pursuant to the Department of Justice's Business Review Procedure, 28 C.F.R. § 50.6, of the Department's current enforcement intentions concerning the CPO's proposal to establish a health care provider network in south-central Iowa. For the reasons set forth below, the department has no present intention of challenging the CPO's proposed activities under the antitrust laws.

From information provided by you, we understand that the CPO will be formed as a nonprofit Iowa corporation headquartered in Des Moines, which is located in Polk County, Iowa. The CPO, at least initially, intends to offer hospital and physician services to self-insured employers and other third-party payers in a 25-county area in south-central Iowa.[1]

The Des Moines General Hospital, an acute care facility licensed for 226 beds, is expected to be the initial hospital member of the CPO. There are three other entities operating general acute care hospitals in Des Moines: Broadlawns Medical Center (173 licensed beds); co-owned Iowa Lutheran Hospital and Iowa Methodist Medical Center (1053 licensed beds, combined); and co-owned Mercy Hospital Medical Center and Mercy Franklin Center (673 licensed beds, combined). Of the approximately 1400 physicians practicing in the 25-county area, 177 have expressed an interest in becoming members of the CPO, including 154 of the 957 physicians practicing in Polk County. The CPO anticipates that two or three rural hospitals located in the 25-county area may also join the CPO. The CPO will be nonexclusive: individual member providers are free to affiliate or contract with competing health care provider organizations and health insurance plans.

CPO members will not be directly involved in setting fees. The CPO will retain a third-party administrator who will survey CPO members and compile aggregate fee data to be used by the CPO in negotiating contracts for health care services. No CPO member will have access to another member's fees, pricing data, or other financial information.

The CPO will establish utilization standards and other measures to help contain health care costs. The physician members of the CPO will share risk through their provision of services at a capitated rate or on the basis of discounted fee-for-service rates with a 20% "withhold" of their fees, to be distributed to them only if cost containment and utilization goals are met. In this regard, a physician member who fails to meet the CPO's cost containment and utilization goals will initially receive counseling and be given a reasonable opportunity to conform to them. If the physician is unable or unwilling to take appropriate corrective action after this educational process, the physician will forfeit the withheld portion of compensation, which will be returned to the payor.

After careful consideration of the information you have provided, the department has concluded that it has no present intention of challenging the CPO's proposal, as set out in this letter, on antitrust grounds. The CPO appears to be a bona fide joint venture in which the participating physician members will share substantial financial risk by participating in capitated contracting arrangements, or

---

[1]The CPO will operate in a 25-county area surrounding Des Moines: Polk, Story, Boone, Jasper, Dallas, Warren, Adair, Appanoose, Clarke, Davis, Decatur, Greene, Guthrie, Lucas, Madison, Mahaska, Marion, Marshall, Monroe, Poweshiek, Ringgold, Tama, Union, Wapello, and Wayne ("25-county area").

offering discounted fee-for-service rates, with a substantial withhold that is payable to physicians only if cost containment goals are met. See September 15, 1993, Statement of Department of Justice and Federal Trade Commission Enforcement Policy on Physician Network Joint Ventures at 34-35, 40-43 ("Joint Enforcement Policy Statement"). The CPO, therefore, has the potential to be procompetitive by offering consumers of health care services in Des Moines and other areas of south-central Iowa an additional alternative health care delivery system. At the same time, however, the department would be concerned if the purpose or effect of the CPO's proposed activities were to facilitate collusion or otherwise reduce competition between or among market participants. Based on the information you have provided, however, the department has concluded that the CPO is unlikely to have such anticompetitive effects.

In conducting our competitive analysis of the CPO, we note that the CPO's potential operation in the 25-county area will likely involve its participation in several different relevant geographic markets. We will not discuss each one in this letter, however, but instead will focus our attention on the Des Moines, Polk County, area because that is where Des Moines General and most of the CPO's prospective physician members are located.

In the Des Moines, Polk County, area Des Moines General controls only 11% of the licensed general acute care hospital beds.[2] In addition, the information you provided notes that the CPO anticipates it will enroll less than 20% of all physicians licensed to practice in Polk County, including 20% or less of all the primary care physicians. The CPO also intends to enroll 20% or less of the physicians in 18 of 30 identified specialties, but would enroll a higher percentage of the physicians in 12 specialty areas.

The Joint Enforcement Policy Statement establishes a "safety zone" for physician networks that include 20% or less of the physicians in each physician specialty within the relevant market. The department does not believe, however, that the physician participation in excess of the 20% threshold in the 12 affected specialty areas presents significant anticompetitive concerns for several reasons. First, the CPO will include only 30% or less of the physician-specialists in six of these specialty areas. The representation above 30% in the other six specialty areas appears necessary to provide adequate coverage and choice for enrollees. Second, the CPO will be nonexclusive. Thus, its member providers, including its participating physicians, are free to affiliate with any current or future CPO competitor in the market. Finally, the CPO will not likely have a "spill-over" collusive effect in other areas of its physician members' practices because they will not have access to specific pricing data and will not be directly involved in negotiating fees.

For the foregoing reasons, the department has no present intention to challenge the CPO. In accord with our normal practice, however, the department remains free to bring whatever action or proceeding it subsequently concludes is required by the public interest if actual operation of the CPO proves anticompetitive in purpose or effect.

This statement of the department's enforcement intentions is made in accord with the Department's Business Review Procedure, 28 C.F.R. § 50.6, a copy of which is enclosed. Pursuant to its terms, your business review request and this letter will be made available to the public immediately. Your supporting documents will be publicly available within 30 days of the date of this letter, unless you request that any part of the material be withheld in accordance with Paragraph 10(c) of the Business Review Procedure.

Sincerely,

Anne K. Bingaman
Assistant Attorney General

---

[2]In its initial request, the CPO indicated that it might later subcontract with alternative health plans (AMPs) affiliated with Iowa Methodist Medical Center and Mercy Hospital Medical Center. The CPO, however, has to date undertaken no discussions with either AMP regarding the exact nature of its possible contractual arrangements and was not able to provide the department with information the department requested regarding such prospective contractual arrangements. Given that, the department is unable to state its current enforcement intentions with respect to these areas of the proposal.

AT
(202) 616-2771
TDD (202) 514-1888

- FOR IMMEDIATE RELEASE
- WEDNESDAY, JULY 6, 1994

DEPARTMENT OF JUSTICE WILL NOT CHALLENGE
DES MOINES AREA HEALTH CARE NETWORK

WASHINGTON, D.C.—The Justice Department today cleared the way for the Des Moines General Hospital and 177 physicians in south-central Iowa to offer a health care plan to business owners seeking new ways to cover their workers' medical needs.

The hospital and physician services network, to be called the Collaborative Provider Organization Inc. (CPO), would provide service over a 25-county area.

The proposal will provide an additional alternative health care delivery system and could increase competition and lower health care costs for consumers, said Anne K. Bingaman, Assistant Attorney General in charge of the Antitrust Division, in a business review letter.

Today's action is part of the administration's effort to encourage innovative arrangements between purchasers of medical services and health care providers to improve health care delivery at a reasonable cost, the department said.

The CPO will contract with payers at capitated, or per-subscriber rates, or on the basis of discounted fee-for-service rates. For those physicians compensated on a fee-for-service basis, the CPO will withhold 20% of their compensation, distributing it to them only if they meet certain cost containment and utilization goals.

Under the department's business review procedure, an organization may submit a proposed action to the Antitrust Division and receive a statement as to whether the division will challenge the action under the antitrust laws.

A file containing the business review request and the department's response may be examined in the Legal Procedure Unit of the Antitrust Division, Room 3235, Department of Justice, Washington, D.C., 20530. After a 30-day waiting period, the documents supporting the business review will be added to the file.

# # #

- 94-368
- 35952 Federal Register / Vol. 56, No. 145 / Monday, July 29, 1991/ Rules and Regulations

DEPARTMENT OF HEALTH AND HUMAN SERVICES
Office of Inspector General

42 CFR Part 1001

RIN 0991-AA49

Medicare and State Health Care Programs: Fraud and Abuse; OIG Anti-Kickback Provisions

AGENCY: Office of Inspector General (OIG), HHS.

ACTION: Final rule.

SUMMARY: This final rule implements section 14 of Public Law 100-93, the Medicare and Medicaid Patient and Program Protection Act of 1987, by specifying various payment practices which, although potentially capable of inducing referrals of business under Medicare or a State health care program, will be protected from criminal prosecution or civil sanctions under the anti-kickback provisions of the statute.

EFFECTIVE DATE: This regulation is effective on July 29, 1991.

FOR FURTHER INFORMATION CONTACT:
Thomas S. Crane or D. McCarty Thornton, Office of the General Counsel, (202) 619-0335.
Joel Schaer, Office of Inspector General, (202) 619-3270

SUPPLEMENTARY INFORMATION:

I. Background

A. The Medicare Anti-Kickback Statute

Section 1128B(b) of the Social Security Act (42 U.S.C. 1320a-7b(b)), previously codified sections 1877 and 1909 of the Act, provides criminal penalties for individuals or entities that knowingly and willfully offer, pay, solicit or receive remuneration in order to induce business reimbursed under the Medicare or State health care programs. The offense is classified as a felony, and is punishable by fines of up to $25,000 and imprisonment for up to 5 years.

This provision is extremely broad. The types of remuneration covered specifically include kickbacks, bribes, and rebates made directly or indirectly, overtly or covertly, or in cash or in kind. In addition, prohibited conduct includes not only remuneration intended to induce referrals of patients, but remuneration also intended to induce the purchasing, leasing, ordering, or arranging for any good, facility, service, or item paid for by Medicare or State health care programs.

Since the statute on its face is so broad, concern has arisen among a number of health care providers that many relatively innocuous, or even beneficial, commercial arrangements are technically covered by the statute and are, therefore, subject to criminal prosecution.

B. Public Law 100-93

Public Law 100-93, the Medicare and Medicaid Patient and Program Protection Act of 1987, added two new provisions addressing the Anti-Kickback Statute. Section 2 specifically provided new authority to the Office of Inspector General (OIG) to exclude an individual or entity from participation in the Medicare and State health care programs if it is determined that the party has engaged in a prohibited remuneration scheme. (Section 1128(b)(7) of the Act, 42 U.S.C. 1320a7(b)(7)). This new sanction authority is intended to provide an alternative civil remedy, short of criminal prosecution, that will be a more effective way of regulating abusive business practices than is the case under criminal law.

In addition, section 14 of Public Law 100-93 requires the promulgation of regulations specifying those payment practices that will not be subject to criminal prosecution under section 1128B of the Act and that will not provide a basis for exclusion from the Medicare program or from the State health care programs under section 1128(b)(7) of the Act.

C. Notice of Intent

The legislative history of section 14 of Public Law 100-93 indicates that Congress expected the Department of Health and Human Services to consult with affected provider, practitioner, supplier and beneficiary representatives before promulgating regulations. In order to most effectively address issues related to this provision, we published a notice of intent to develop regulations (52 FR 38794, October 19, 1987) soliciting comments from interested parties prior to developing a proposed regulation. As a result of that notice, the OIG received a number of public comments, recommendations and suggestions on generic criteria that can be applied to particular types of business arrangements in order to determine if such arrangements are inappropriate for civil or criminal sanctions.

D. Notice of Proposed Rulemaking

The proposed regulation designed to implement section 14 of Public Law 100-93 was developed by the OIG and published in the Federal Register on January 23, 1989 (54 FR 8033). The regulation sets forth various proposed business and payment practices, or "safe harbors," that would not be treated as criminal offenses under section 1128B(b) of the Act and would not serve as a basis for a program exclusion under section 1128(b)(7) of the Act. As a result of that proposed rulemaking, we received a total of 754 public comments for consideration.

II. Summary of the Proposed Rule

A. Business Arrangements Not Exempt

The proposed regulation indicated that in order for a business arrangement to comply with one of the 10 safe harbors, each standard of that safe harbor provision would have to be met. The proposed rule stated that if the business arrangement involves payments for different purposes (for example, a single payment for personal services and for equipment rental) then each payment purpose would be analyzed to determine if all the standards of each applicable safe harbor provision have been fulfilled. The proposed rule further specified that where individuals and entities have entered into arrangements that are covered by the statute and where they have chosen not to fully comply with one of the exemptions proposed in these regulations, they would risk scrutiny by the OIG and may be subject to civil or criminal enforcement action.

B. Need for Continuing Guidance

Since there may be a need for the department to respond to changes in health care delivery or business arrangements more quickly and informally than through the regulatory process to keep the industry abreast of our enforcement policy, the proposed rule invited public comment on how we can best achieve the dual goals of keeping the industry aware of our views of particular business practices, and assuring that our regulations remain current with new developments.

C. Notice to Beneficiaries

While we considered including in several of the proposed safe harbor provisions a requirement that a person notify each Medicare or Medicaid patient he or she refers to a related entity of the financial relationship that exists, we indicated that such notice requirements may be unduly burdensome compared with the potential benefits and, therefore, did not include the requirement in the safe harbors in the proposed regulation. Instead, we invited public comments on this issue.

D. Preferred Provider Organizations

We cited the increasing variety of arrangements among entities grouped under the generic headings *preferred provider organizations* (PPOs) or *managed care,* and that unlike HMOs, there is often no single entity that is recognized as the health care provider. The proposed regulations did not specifically delineate a safe harbor provision for these arrangements since we believed that one or more of the other proposed safe harbors would often cover relationships in preferred provider and managed care networks. We invited comments from the public, however, on the idea of adding additional safe harbors that would provide further protection to HMOs, PPOs, and other managed care plans.

E. Waiver of Coinsurance and Deductible Amounts for Inpatient Hospital Care

We noted that with the advent in 1983 of the prospective payment system for paying hospitals for inpatient care, some hospitals have advertised the routine waiver of Medicare coinsurance and deductible amounts as a means of attracting patients to their facilities. We solicited comments on defining a safe harbor for waiving coinsurance and deductible amounts that would be limited to inpatient hospital care, be available to all Medicare beneficiaries without regard to diagnosis or length of stay, and assure that any costs to the hospital of waiving the coinsurance and deductible amounts would not be passed on to any federal program as a bad debt or in any other way.

F. Proposed Safe Harbors

The regulation published on January 23, 1989, proposing to amend 42 CFR part 1001 by adding a new §1001.952, set forth "safe harbors" in 10 broad areas:

1. Investment Interests

To reflect the view that Congress did not intend to bar all investments by physicians in other health care entities to which they refer patients, a safe harbor provision was proposed for investment interests in large public corporations where such investments are available to the general public. This safe harbor described a minimum number of shareholders and a minimum number of assets the company must have in order to qualify under this provision.

Safe harbors for limited and managing partnerships were considered under the proposed regulation, but were not included. These areas were discussed in the preamble of the proposed rule, and we specifically requested public comments on adopting these practices as safe harbors.

2. Space Rental

While many rental arrangements are legitimate, many situations exist where rental payments are simply a device used to mask illegal payments intended to induce referrals. Accordingly, a safe harbor provision was proposed for rental arrangements if: (a) Access to the space is for periodic intervals and such intervals are set in advance in the lease, rather than based on the number of referred patients; (b) the lease is for at least one year so it cannot be readjusted on too frequent a basis to reflect prior referrals; and (c) the charges reflect fair market value.

3. Equipment Rental

With the understanding that the payment for the use of diagnostic and other medical equipment may simply be a vehicle to provide reimbursement for referrals, a safe harbor was proposed for certain situations involving equipment rentals similar to those applied to real estate rentals cited above.

4. Personal Services and Management Contracts

While health care providers often have arrangements to perform services for each other on a mutually beneficial basis, some of these arrangements may vary the payment with the volume of referrals. The proposed regulation sets forth a safe harbor provision for joint ventures and other arrangements involving payments for personal services or management contracts, but only if certain standards are met that limit the opportunity to provide financial incentives in exchange for referrals. This proposed provision required the services to be paid at fair market value, and was predicated on requirements similar to those set forth in the provisions for space and equipment rental.

5. Sale of Practice

Unlike the traditional sale of a practice by a retiring physician, a physician may sell, or appear to sell, a practice to a hospital while continuing to practice on its staff. A safe harbor provision was proposed for the sale of physician practices when occurring as the result of retirement or some other event that removes the physician from the practice of medicine or from the service area in which he or she was practicing, but not when the sale is for the purpose of obtaining an ongoing source of patient referrals.

6. Referral Services

Professional societies and other consumer-oriented groups often operate referral services for a fee. Because such a service fee could be construed as a payment in order to obtain a referral, we concluded that it was appropriate to establish a specific safe harbor for this type of practice. In order to safeguard against abuse, however, the provision is only available when several standards are met.

7. Warranties

It is in the public interest to have companies offer warranties as an inducement to the consumer to purchase a product. A safe harbor was proposed for such purposes.

8. Discounts

Safe harbors relating to discounts, employees, and group purchasing organizations are specifically required by statute. The discount exception was intended to encourage price competition that benefits the Medicare and Medicaid programs. The proposed discount provision was limited in application to reductions in the amount a seller charges for a good or service to the buyer. The discount could take the form of a specified price break or the inclusion of an extra quantity of the item purchased "at no extra charge." We did not propose to protect many kinds of marketing incentive programs such as cash rebates, free goods or services, redeemable coupons, or credits.

9. Employees

The proposed exception for employees permitted an employer to pay an employee in whatever manner he or she chose for having that employee assist in the solicitation of program business and applied only to bona fide employee–employer relationships.

10. Group Purchasing Organizations

The proposed group purchasing organization (GPO) exception was designed to apply to payments from vendors to entities authorized to act as a GPO for individuals or entities who are furnishing Medicare or Medicaid services. The proposed exception required a written agreement between the GPO and the individual or entity that specifies the amounts vendors will pay the GPO.

EXHIBIT 2-2 MANAGEMENT ADVISORY REPORT REGARDING HOSPITAL-BASED PHYSICIANS

DEPARTMENT OF HEALTH & HUMAN SERVICES   Office of Inspector General
                                                                         Memorandum

From   Richard P. Kusserow
            Inspector General

Subject   OIG Management Advisory Report: "Financial Arrangements
            Between Hospitals and Hospital-Based Physicians," OEI-09-89-00330

To   Gail R. Wilensky, PhD
            Administrator
            Health Care Financing Administration

This management advisory report alerts you to potential violations of the anti-kickback statute (statute), section 1128B of the Social Security Act (42 U.S.C. section 1320a-7b). We have identified potential violations in the financial arrangements between some hospitals and hospital-based physicians. These agreements: (1) require physicians to pay more than the fair market value for services provided by the hospitals, or (2) compensate physicians for less than the fair market value of goods and services that they provide to hospitals.

BACKGROUND

Hospital-based physicians include specialists such as anesthesiologists, emergency room physicians, pathologists, radiologists, and teaching physicians. Each of these specialties is dependent on the hospital environment to obtain referrals from other specialists practicing at their hospital. In turn, the hospitals are somewhat dependent on the hospital-based physicians because they provide essential services to the hospitals.

Hospitals recently began to view these physicians as potential new revenue sources. Some hospitals have reduced payments to hospital-based physicians, and some are requiring payments from those physicians.

Medicare pays for the services of hospital-based physicians in a variety of ways. Usually, Medicare pays physicians directly for the services delivered. However, when pathologists perform clinical laboratory services for hospital inpatients under part A, some portion of Medicare's payments to the hospital are for that pathology service. Different methods of payment may apply in each instance.

Medicare payments for anatomic pathology services are more complicated. Technical and professional components are paid separately. The former go directly to hospitals and the latter to the pathologist.

LEGAL CRITERIA

The statute makes it illegal to offer, pay, solicit, or receive remuneration for referring business payable under Medicare or Medicaid. Unlike most applications of the statute concerning Medicare compensation arrangements, the focus here is on the remuneration made to hospitals.

The statute is very broad, covering indirect or covert forms of remuneration, bribes, kickbacks, and rebates as well as direct or overt ones. Three significant cases have interpreted the statute.

In *United States v. Greber* 760 F.2d 68, 69 (3rd Cir.), cert. denied, 474 US. 968 (1985) the court held that, "if one purpose of the payment was to induce future referrals, the Medicare statute has been violated." The reasoning in *Greber* was adopted by the Ninth Circuit Court of Appeals in the *United States v. Kats* 871 F.2d 105 (9th Cir. 1989). In *Kats* the court found that the statute is violated unless the payments are "wholly and not incidentally attributable to the delivery of goods and services."

In *United States v. Lipkis* 770 E2d 1447 (1985), the Ninth Circuit Court of Appeals reviewed an arrangement between a medical management company that provided services to a physician's group and a clinical laboratory. The laboratory returned 20% of its revenues obtained from the physician group's referrals to the management company. The defendants alleged that these payments represented fair compensation for "specimen collection and handling services." *Ibid* at 1449. The court rejected this defense, noting "the fair market value of these services was substantially less than the [amount paid], and there is no question [the laboratory] was paying for referrals as well as the described services." *Ibid*. Thus, applying the reasoning of the Ninth Circuit Court of Appeals in *Lipkis*, an inference can be drawn that illegal remuneration occurs when a contract between a hospital and hospital-based physicians calls for the rental of space or equipment or provision of professional services on terms other than fair market value.

If a provider's conduct falls within the purview of the statute, it can be prosecuted unless the conduct meets a statutory exception or "safe harbor" (when finalized). It should be observed that there is no statutory exception or contemplated "safe harbor" provision that applies to the conduct described herein.

ANALYSIS

Contracts that require physicians to split portions of their income with hospitals are highly suspect, although not per se violations of the statute. Usually there is little basis to require hospital-based physicians to turn over a percentage of their earnings to the hospital. In addition, in many arrangements the fees hospitals receive are vastly in excess of the value of the services (such as billing services) they provide to the hospital-based physicians.

EXAMPLES OF AGREEMENTS

We have reviewed many agreements that provide payments or remuneration to hospitals in excess of the fair market value of the services provided by them. Because many of these arrangements may violate the statute, disclosure of the terms of these agreements are rare, and therefore it is very difficult to establish the prevalence of these agreements. Several medical societies and anonymous parties have shown the following contract provisions without identifying names and locations:

- A group of emergency room physicians pays a hospital half of its cash receipts exceeding $600,000 annually.
- A hospital provides no, or token, payback to pathologists for part A services in return for the opportunity to perform part B services at that hospital.
- Radiologists must pay 50% of their gross receipts to a facility's endowment fund.
- Thirty-three percent of all profits above a set amount must be paid by a radiology group to a hospital for its capital improvements, equipment, and other departmental expenditures.
- A radiologist group was required to purchase radiology equipment and agreed to donate the equipment to the hospital at the termination of the contract. The hospital has an unrestricted right to terminate the contract at any time.
- When net collections for a radiology group exceed $230,000, 50% is paid to the hospital, and the hospital reserves the right to unilaterally adjust the distributions if it determines that the physician group has not fulfilled the terms of the contract.
- A radiologist group pays 25% of the profits exceeding $120,000 to the hospital for capital improvements. Fifty percent of the profits exceeding $180,000 go to this purpose.
- A radiology group pays for facilities, services, supplies, personnel, utilities, maintenance, and billing services furnished by the hospital on a fee schedule that begins at $25,000 for 1989, and rises to $100,000 by 1993. Payments are due only if the radiologist's gross revenue exceeds $1,000,000 in the previous year.

CONCLUSION

All of these examples appear to violate the statute because they provide compensation to the hospitals that exceeds the fair market value of the services the hospitals provide under the contracts. It also appears the payment of the remuneration is intended to provide the hospital-based physician with referrals from the other physicians on the hospital's medical staff.

These illegal financial arrangements may have several unfortunate results. The remuneration gives the hospitals a financial incentive to develop policies and practices that encourage greater utilization of the services of hospital-based physicians. Additionally, hospital-based physicians faced with lowered incomes may be encouraged to do more procedures in order to offset the payments to the hospitals. These problems are among the recognized purposes of having the anti-kickback statute on the books in the first place.

Illegal arrangements may also complicate the development of physician fee schedules if physician practice costs are artificially inflated by arrangements not based on fair market values.

RECOMMENDATION

The HCFA should instruct its contractors to: (1) notify physicians and hospitals about potential legal liability when they enter into agreements not based on the fair market value of necessary goods and services exchanged; and (2) refer identified cases to the Office of Inspector General for possible prosecution or sanctions.

To reduce potential legal liability, all contracts between hospitals and hospital-based physicians should do the following:

- Be based on the fair market value of services (The nature and value of all services performed should be stated separately, and the fair market value should be documented.)
- Be unrelated to physician income or billings (These agreements are not *per se* illegal but are suspect.), and
- Be limited to goods and services necessary for the provision of medical services by the hospital-based physicians and typical of what hospitals provide hospital-based physicians.

It should be noted explicitly that these criteria do not establish a "safe harbor." Compliance with these criteria will not immunize parties from liability under the statue.

We would appreciate your comments on this report within 30 days. If you have any questions please contact me or have your staff contact Barry Steeley at FTS 646-3138.

Reprinted from Jan. 31, 1991, memorandum

EXHIBIT 2-3   MAY 1992 SPECIAL FRAUD ALERT REGARDING PHYSICIAN INCENTIVES

OFFICE OF INSPECTOR GENERAL

Hospital Incentives to Physicians—Special Fraud Alert

The Office of Inspector General was established at the Department of Health and Human Services by Congress in 1976 to identify and eliminate fraud, abuse, and waste in Health and Human Services programs and to promote efficiency and economy in departmental operations. It carries out this mission through a nationwide program of audits, investigations, and inspections. To help reduce fraud in the Medicare and Medicaid programs, the Office of Inspector General is actively investigating violations of the Medicare and Medicaid Anti-Kickback Statute, 42 U.S.C. Section 1 320a-7b(b). Among other things, the statute penalizes anyone who knowingly and willfully solicits, receives, offers, or pays remuneration in cash or kind to induce or in return for the following:

A. Referring an individual to a person for the furnishing or arranging for the furnishing of any item or service payable under the Medicare or Medicaid program, or
B. Purchasing, leasing, or ordering or arranging for or recommending purchasing, leasing, or ordering any good, facility, service, or item payable under the Medicare or Medicaid program.

Violators are subject to criminal penalties, or exclusion from participation in the Medicare and Medicaid programs, or both. In 1987, Section 14 of the Medicare and Medicaid Patient and Program Protection Act, P.L. 100-93, directed this department to promulgate "safe harbor" regulations in order to provide health care providers with a mechanism to assure them that they will not be prosecuted under the anti-kickback statute for engaging "safe harbor" regulations on July 29, 1991 (42 C.F.R. sec. 1001.952, 56 Fed. Reg. 35, 952). The scope of the anti-kickback statute is not expanded by the "safe harbor" regulations; these regulations give those in good faith compliance with a "safe harbor" the assurance that they will not be prosecuted under this statute.

Why Do Hospitals Provide Economic Incentives to Physicians?

As many hospitals have become more aggressive in their attempts to recruit and retain physicians and increase patient referrals, physician incentives (sometimes referred to as *practice enhancements*) are becoming increasingly common. Some physicians actively solicit such incentives. These incentives may result in reductions in the physician's professional expenses or an increase in his or her revenues. In exchange, the physician is aware that he or she is often expected to refer the majority, if not all, of his or her patients to the hospital providing the incentives.

Why Is It Illegal for Hospitals to Provide Financial Incentives to Physicians for Their Referrals?

The Office of Inspector General has become aware of a variety of hospital incentive programs used to compensate physicians (directly or indirectly) for referring patients to the hospital. These arrangements are implicated by the anti-kickback statute because they can constitute remuneration offered to induce, or in return for, the referral of business paid for by Medicare or Medicaid. In addition, they are not protected under the existing "safe harbor" regulations.[1]

---

[1]The department is considering seeking public comment on the advisability of granting protection under the "safe harbor" regulations for certain hospital incentives for physicians starting a new practice. However, such a concept would have no legal effect whatsoever until promulgated as a final regulation.

These incentive programs can interfere with the physician's judgment of what is the most appropriate care for a patient. They can inflate costs to the Medicare program by causing physicians to inappropriately overuse the service of a particular hospital. The incentives may result in the delivery of inappropriate care to Medicare beneficiaries and Medicaid recipients by inducing the physician to refer patients to the hospital providing financial incentives rather than to another hospital (or nonacute care facility) offering the best or most appropriate care for that patient.

Suspect Hospital Incentive Arrangements—What to Look For

To help identify suspect incentive arrangements, examples of practices that are often questionable are listed below. Please note that this list is not intended to be exhaustive but, rather, to suggest some indicators of potentially unlawful activity:

- Payment of any sort of incentive by the hospital each time a physician refers a patient to the hospital
- The use of free or significantly discounted office space or equipment (in facilities usually located close to the hospital)
- Provision of free or significantly discounted billing, nursing, or other staff services
- Free training for a physician's office staff in areas such as management techniques, CPT coding, and laboratory techniques
- Guarantees that provide that, if the physician's income fails to reach a predetermined level, the hospital will supplement the remainder up to a certain amount
- Low-interest or interest-free loans, or loans which may be "forgiven" if a physician refers patients (or some number of patients) to the hospital
- Payment of the cost of physician's travel and expenses for conferences
- Payment for a physician's continuing education courses
- Coverage on hospitals' group health insurance plans at an inappropriately low cost to the physician
- Payment for services (which may include consultations at the hospital) that require few, if any, substantive duties by the physician, or payment for services in excess of the fair market value of services rendered

Financial incentive packages that incorporate these or similar features may be subject to prosecution under the Medicare and Medicaid Anti-Kickback Statute, if one of the purposes of the incentive is to influence the physician's medical decision as to where to refer his or her patients for treatment.

What to Do If You Have Information About Hospitals That Offer These Types of Incentives to Physicians

If you have information about hospitals that offer the types of incentives described above to physicians, contact any of the regional offices of the Office of Investigations of the Office of Inspector General, U.S. Department of Health and Human Services, at the following locations:

Regions	States Served	Telephone
Boston	MA, VT, NH, ME, RI, CT	(617) 565-2660
New York	NY, NJ, PR, VI	(212) 264-1691
Philadelphia	PA, MD, DE, WV, VA	(215) 596-6796
Atlanta	KY, GA, NC, SC, FL, TN, AL, MS	(404) 331-2131
Chicago	IL, MN, WI, MI, IN, OH	(312) 353-2740
Dallas	TX, NM, OK, AR, LA	(214) 767-8406
Kansas City	MO, KS	(816) 426-3811
Denver	CO, UT, WY, MT, ND, SD, IA, NE	(303) 844-5621
San Francisco	CA, NV, AZ, HI	(415) 556-8880
Seattle	WA, OR, ID, AK	(206) 533-0229
Washington, DC	DC & Metropolitan areas of VA & MD	(202) 619-1900

EXHIBIT 2-4 DECEMBER 1992 THORNTON LETTER TO IRS

DEPARTMENT OF HEALTH & HUMAN SERVICES

Office of the Secretary
Office of the General Counsel
Washington, D.C. 20201

DEC 22 1992

Mr. T. J. Sullivan
Technical Assistant (Health Care Industries)
Office of the Associate Chief Counsel
(Employee Benefits and Exempt Organizations)
Internal Revenue Service
Washington, D.C. 20224

Dear Mr. Sullivan:

You have informally inquired about our views concerning the application of the Medicare and Medicaid Anti-Kickback Statute, 42 U.S.C. 1320a-7b(b), to certain types of situations involving the acquisition of physician practices. In the situations in question, the physician practices would be acquired either by a hospital or by another entity that would also acquire one or more hospitals (and potentially other health care providers as well). The physicians from these practices would continue to treat patients and be affiliated (through an employment relationship or otherwise) with the hospital or other entity that acquired their practices. The acquisition of the physician practices could arise through a number of different methods or arrangements and the resulting or ensuing relationships or affiliations could vary. However, the end result in each case would be the common ownership or control of both hospitals and physician practices by a single entity. We are responding to your inquiry in general terms and not in reference to any specific fact pattern(s).

Typically, in the case of the acquisition of a physician practice by a hospital or other entity, there is a large, up-front payment to the physician, often of many hundreds of thousands of dollars or more. This sum is asserted to be payment for the purchase of the assets of the practice. There are also payments made to the physician subsequent to the sale of the practice in which the physician becomes employed by the hospital or entity or otherwise enters into a contract to provide services to patients. These payments are asserted to be compensation for services rendered to patients by the physician.

As you know, the anti-kickback statute provides for penalties against anyone who knowingly and willfully solicits, receives, offers, or pays remuneration, in cash or in kind, to induce or in return for:

A. Referring an individual to a person for the furnishing or arranging for the furnishing of any item or service payable under the Medicare or Medicaid programs, or
B. Purchasing, leasing, or ordering or arranging for or recommending purchasing, leasing, or ordering any good, facility, service, or item payable under the Medicare or Medicaid programs.

Persons who violate the anti-kickback statute are subject to criminal penalties and/or exclusion from participation in the Medicare and Medicaid programs. The anti-kickback statute sets forth certain specific exceptions to the general prohibition against remuneration, and specifically authorizes this department to promulgate, by regulation, additional payment practices (known as "safe harbors") that will be immune from prosecution. The department published final "safe harbor" regulations on July 29, 1991 (42 C.F.R. 1001.952, 56 Fed. Reg. 35,952) setting forth 11 regulatory exceptions to the anti-kickback statute. Among the safe harbors included in the regulations were provisions relating to employees and sale of practitioner practices. Additional safe harbor provisions relating to managed care entities were published as final regulations (with comment period) on November 5, 1992 (57 Fed. Reg. 52,723).

We have significant concerns under the anti-kickback statute about the type of physician practice acquisitions described in your inquiry to us. Frequently, hospitals seek to purchase physician practices as a means to retain existing referrals or to attract new referrals of patients to the hospital. Such purchases implicate the anti-kickback statute because the remuneration paid for the practice can constitute illegal remuneration to induce the referral of business reimbursed by the Medicare or Medicaid programs.[1] We believe the same concerns raised by hospital purchases of physician practices could also arise where another entity (such as a foundation) purchases a physician practice, when such foundation also owns or operates a hospital that benefits from referrals from those physicians.

In particular, we are concerned that the remuneration paid in connection with or as a result of the acquisition of a physician's practice could serve to interfere with the physician's subsequent judgment of what is the most appropriate care for a patient. The remuneration could result in the delivery of inappropriate care to Medicare or Medicaid beneficiaries by inducing the physician to utilize the affiliated hospital rather than another hospital or less costly facility that may provide better or more appropriate care. It could also have the effect of inflating costs to the Medicare or Medicaid programs by causing physicians to inappropriately overuse the services of a particular hospital (or other affiliated provider). This higher cost could occur directly because of the higher rates of that hospital or the ordering of unnecessary services, or the higher cost could occur indirectly as a result of lessened competition in the marketplace. Finally, these arrangements could significantly interfere with a beneficiary's freedom of choice of providers. All these considerations are the very abuses that the anti-kickback statute was designed to prevent. We recently addressed these same types of possible abuses in an Office of Inspector General Special Fraud Alert entitled "Hospital Incentives to Physicians." A copy of that fraud alert is enclosed for your information.

The following are specific aspects of physician practice acquisition or subsequent activities that may implicate or result in violations of the anti-kickback status. Our comments focus primarily on two broad issue categories: (1) the total amount paid for the physician practice and the nature and type of items for which the physician receives payment; and (2) the amount and manner in which the physician is subsequently compensated for providing services to patients.[2]

Under the anti-kickback statute, either of the above categories of payment could constitute illegal remuneration. This is because under the anti-kickback statute, the statute is violated if one purpose of the payment is to induce the referral of future Medicare or Medicaid program business. *United States v. Greber*, 760 F.2d 68, 69 (3rd Cir. 1985) cert. denied, 474 U.S. 988 (1985); *United States v. Kats*, 871 F. 2d 105, 108 (9th Cir. 1989). Thus, it is necessary to scrutinize the payments (including the surrounding facts and circumstances) to determine the purpose for which they have been made. As part of this undertaking, it is necessary to consider the amounts paid for the practice or as compensation to determine whether they reasonably reflect the fair market value of the practice or the services rendered, in order to determine whether such items in reality constitute remuneration for referrals. Moreover, to the extent that a payment exceeds the fair market value of the practice or the value of the services rendered, it can be inferred that the excess amount paid over fair market value is intended as payment for the referral of program-related business. *United States v. Liykis*, 770 F. 2d 1447 (9th Cir. 1985).

When considering the question of fair market value, we would note that the traditional or common methods of economic valuation do not comport with the prescriptions of the anti-kickback statute. Items ordinarily considered in determining the fair market value may be expressly barred by the anti-kickback statute's prohibition against payments for referrals. Merely because another buyer may be

---

[1] Since tax-exempt hospitals are generally required to participate in the Medicare and Medicaid programs as a condition of obtaining or maintaining their tax-exempt status, the anti-kickback statute is necessarily a significant issue to be addressed by them.

[2] We would also note that while the anti-kickback statute contains a statutory exemption for payments made to employees by an employer, the exemption does not cover any and all such payments. Specifically, the statute exempts only payments to employees that are for the purpose of compensating such employees for the referral of patients who would likely not be covered by the employee exemption.

willing to pay a particular price is not sufficient to render the price paid to be fair market value. The fact that a buyer in a position to benefit from referrals is willing to pay a particular price may only be a reflection of the value of the referral stream that is likely to result from the purchase.[3]

Accordingly, when attempting to assess the fair market value (as that term is used in an anti-kickback analysis) attributable to a physician's practice, it may be necessary to exclude from consideration any amounts that reflect, facilitate, or otherwise relate to the continuing treatment of the former practice's patients. This would be because any such items only have value with respect to the ongoing flow of business to the practice. It is doubtful whether this value may be paid by a party who could expect to benefit from referrals from that ongoing practice.[4] Such amounts could be considered as payments for referrals. Thus, any amount paid in excess of the fair market value of the hard assets of a physician practice would be open to question. Similarly, in determining the fair market value of services rendered by employee or contract physicians, it may be necessary to exclude from consideration any amounts that reflect or relate to past or future referrals or any amounts that reflect or are affected by the expectation or guarantee of a certain volume of business (by either the physician or the hospital). Specific items that we believe would raise a question as to whether payment was being made for the value of a referral stream would include, among other things, the following:

- Payment for goodwill
- Payment for the value of the ongoing business unit
- Payment for covenants not to compete
- Payment for exclusive dealing agreements
- Payment for patient lists
- Payment for patient records

Payments for the above types of assets or items are questionable where, as is the case here, there is a continuing relationship between the buyer and the seller, and the buyer relies (at least in part) on referrals from the seller.

We believe a very revealing inquiry would be to compare the financial welfare of the physicians involved before and after the acquisition. (One can expect to find projections on this subject among materials given to prospective physician participants in these arrangements.) If the economic position of these physicians is expected to significantly improve as a result of the acquisition, it is likely that a purpose of the acquisition is to offer remuneration for the referrals that these physicians can make to the buyer. Another revealing inquiry would be to compare referral patterns before and after the acquisition, specifically, whether the sellers become increasingly "loyal" to the buyer. (Obviously, this inquiry would only occur if the acquisition took place, but it is a potential topic to study in the future to the extent acquisitions occur and are subject to audit or investigation by the Internal Revenue Service.)

---

[3]This deviation from the normal "economic" model was made expressly clear in the safe harbor provisions. For purposes of determining the value of space or equipment rentals, "fair market value" is specifically defined to exclude the "additional value one party . . . would attribute to the property [equipment] as a result of its proximity or convenience to sources of referrals or business otherwise generated." 42 C.F.R. 1001.952(b) and (c), 56 Fed. Reg. 35971-35973, 35985.

[4]We note that these physician practice acquisitions do not fall within the parameters of the existing safe harbor provisions on the sale of practitioner practices. In the final safe harbor regulations, we expressly declined to expand the scope of the safe harbor to cover purchases of physician practices by hospitals or other types of entities or to situations in which the seller remains in a continuing position to make referrals or influence referrals to the buyer because of our concerns that many of such purchases were in fact merely attempts to provide remuneration in return for a future stream of referrals. See Preamble to the final safe harbor regulations, 56 Fed. Reg. at 35975. We also attempted to deal with arrangements that have the potential to lock in a referral stream in the safe harbor provisions dealing with joint ventures. See 42 C.F.R. 1001.952(a), 56 Fed. Reg. 35, 984-85.

In sum, these arrangements raise grave questions of compliance with the anti-kickback statute. We believe that many of these arrangements are merely sophisticated disguises to share the profits of business at a hospital with referring physicians, in order to induce the physicians to steer referrals to the hospital.

We hope this letter has provided helpful information in response to your informal inquiry.

Sincerely,

McCarty Thornton, Associate General Counsel
Inspector General Division

Enclosure

Retyped with permission of the Department of Health & Human Services

EXHIBIT 2-5 ANALYSIS SECTION OF POLK COUNTY *v.* PETERS DECISION

LUFKIN DIVISION

FILED
U.S. DISTRICT COURT
EASTERN DISTRICT OF
TEXAS

AUG 28 1992
MURRAY L. HARRIS, Clerk
BY DEPUTY Patricia Durden

POLK COUNTY, TEXAS d/b/a
POLK COUNTY MEMORIAL HOSPITAL
V. § CIVIL ACTION NO. 9:92CV45
KENNETH W. PETERS, M.D.

V. ANALYSIS

Although this is a case of first impression in that it involves physician recruitment by a hospital and the physician's referral of surgical patients to that hospital rather than a kickback, the Court is persuaded that the Agreement is well within the purview of 42 U.S.C. 1395(b) (1983). *See Harvey L. Timkin, Medicare Fraud and Abuse,* 62 Wis.L.J. 13 (1989); (Incentive programs directly or indirectly aimed at inducing doctors to refer patients to a hospital violate the anti-kickback statute since the hospital provides a benefit to the doctor, therefore satisfying the remuneration requirement, in return for inducing referrals); *Francis J. Hearn, Caring for the Health Care Industry: Government Response to Medicare Fraud and Abuse,* S. J. Contemp. Health L. & Policy 175 (1989). ("If any form or remuneration is given to the recruited physician, then technically the recruitment program has violated the Medicare anti-kickback provision.")

It is undisputed that the hospital agreed to and did provide remuneration to Defendant in the form of an interest free loan. It is also undisputed that the hospital agreed to provide free office space, rent and utility subsidies, and reimbursement for malpractice insurance. It is clear that these remunerations were subject to Defendant's referral of patients to the hospital absent exceptional circumstances. Furthermore, no effort beyond the Tom Gilbert letter was made to collect the money due under the Agreement until years after the due date, when Defendant had become embroiled in other litigation with the hospital. Finally, the Court takes judicial notice of its own records in *Peters v. Lake Livingston, et al.,* cause no. L-88-179-CA. REX. 181, D. Ex 81. The hospital's original stated reason for termination of Defendant's medical staff privileges was his failure to utilize it as his "primary hospital."

While the hospital may well have been motivated to a greater or lesser degree by a legitimate desire to make better medical services available in the community, there can be no doubt that the benefits extended to Defendant were, in part, an inducement for him to refer patients to the hospital. The Court must, therefore, find that the Agreement made on the basis of this action violates 42 D.S.C. S1395nn(b).

In conclusion, it follows under the applicable Texas law that the Agreement, being illegal, is void and unenforceable. *See E. G. Segal v. McCall, 184 S. W. 188 (Tex. 1916); David Gavin Co. v. Gibson (Tex. Civ. App. Houston 14 1989); Savin Corp. v. Copy Distributing Co., 715 S.W.2d 590 (Tex. Civ. App - Corpus*

Christi, 1986). Indeed, the policy against aiding in the enforcement of an illegal contract is such that a party that has inserted an illegal provision for its own benefit may nevertheless defend against a suit for breach of contract on the basis of the illegality. *Biray, Inc. v. Cathodic Protection Service, 307 S.W. 2d 570,* (Tex. Civ. App. *14 1974).* Accordingly it is

ORDERED, ADJUDGED, and DECREED that Plaintiff take nothing by this suit.

Retyped Analysis section of public document: Memorandum Opinion of U.S. Magistrate Judge Judith K. Guthrie in Polk County v. Peters *(1992).*

EXHIBIT 2-6   PHYSICIAN RECRUITMENT GUIDELINES

(Exhibit 1 to Closing Agreement with the Hermann Hospital Estate)
Hermann Hospital Estate hereby adopts the following guidelines effective immediately:

HOSPITAL PHYSICIAN RECRUITMENT GUIDELINES

I. Definitions

- Existing physician—Nonemployee physician having medical staff privileges at Hospital
- Newly recruited physician—Nonemployee physician not yet having medical staff privileges at Hospital
- Permissible recruit—Physician who either (a) is a recent graduate of a residency or fellowship program, whether or not in the Hospital's community, or (b) has not previously practiced in Hospital's community or been affiliated with another hospital service in all or part of the Hospital's community
- Permissible incentive—A provision of cash, credit, goods, services, or other valuable rights to a physician in exchange for the physician's agreement to relocate into or remain within Hospital's community, if provided in an amount and manner that does not confer prohibited inurement or more than incidental private benefit upon the physician. Incentives shall not be permissible and shall be presumed to confer prohibited inurement or more than incidental private benefit upon physicians unless such incentives are provided in accordance with the specific rules set forth in section II, below.
- Community—Designated geographical area comprising or existing within confines of Hospital's primary and secondary service area as defined by Hospital.
- Recruiting fees or costs—Fees or costs paid to recruiting companies, expenses of travel, moving, and relocation, and the dollar cost of any other incentives, provided to or on behalf of, or in connection with, a permissible recruit

II. Hospital Will Provide No Incentives to Physicians That Are Not Permissible Incentives

A. Retention incentives of any kind provided to existing physicians are not permissible incentives.
B. Permissible incentives do not include recruitment or retention incentives provided to other than permissible recruits.
C. Recruitment incentives offered to a permissible recruit will not be considered permissible incentives unless there is a demonstrable community need for the physician as evidenced by one or more of the following:
   1. A population-to-physician ratio in the community that is deficient in the particular specialty (with reference to the ideal ratio set forth in GMENAC reports) of the physician being recruited
   2. Demand for a particular medical service in the community coupled with a documented lack of availability of the service or long waiting periods for the service, if the physician is being recruited to increase availability of that service
   3. Designation of the community (or that portion of the community that the physician is serving) at the time the recruitment agreement is executed as a health professional shortage area (HPSA) as defined in 42 CFR 5.1–5.4
   4. A demonstrated reluctance of physicians to relocate at the Hospital due to the Hospital's physical location (this criterion is intended to refer to a hospital located in a rural or economically disadvantaged inner city area)
   5. A reasonable expected reduction in the number of physicians of that specialty serving in Hospital's service area due to the anticipated retirement within the next 3-year period of physicians presently in the community

      6. A documented lack of physicians serving indigent or Medicaid patients within Hospital's service area, provided that newly recruited physicians commit to serving a substantial number of Medicaid and charity care patients.

D. In connection with providing permissible incentives to a physician, Hospital may obligate the physician to fulfill any or all of the following stipulations or duties, among others:
      1. Relocation to service area of Hospital
      2. Establishment of a full-time private practice
      3. Continued presence in the community for a specified period
      4. Maintenance of license to practice
      5. Acceptance of Medicaid and charity patients
      6. Emergency room duty or other rotations
      7. Performance of community or medical teaching
      8. Performance of necessary administrative duties
      9. Maintenance of staff privileges
     10. Maintenance of a practice in the specialty for which recruited

E. Incentives may not be conditioned on a requirement or understating that the physician admit or refer patients to Hospital, or on any prohibition or restriction upon the ability of the physician to obtain or maintain staff privileges at other hospitals or to treat patients at or admit patients to other hospitals.

F. A physician to whom incentives, other than those described in paragraphs G, J, and K, are provided must agree to a periodic accounting to Hospital and to allow Hospital to inspect the physician's financial books and records as a condition to receipt of any such incentive. For incentives described in paragraphs J and K, Hospital shall obtain documentation of expenses from physician prior to providing the allowed reimbursements.

G. Permissible incentives include loans, lines of credit, or loan guarantees offered to physicians, but only if such loans, lines of credit, or loan guarantees, are (a) documented and evidenced by an executed promissory note; (b) adequately secured (such as by accounts receivable and/or office equipment); and (c) bear interest at a reasonable rate reflecting market conditions (e.g., prime plus 1% or 2%, or the applicable federal rate). Any loan forgiveness component will be conditioned upon the continued presence of the physician in practice in the community and will be ratable for a period of not less than 4 years, with the time period specified by contract at the time the loan or loan guarantee is made. A demonstrable need for the particular physician and the amount of the particular incentive shall be evidenced when provision is made for forgiveness of a loan.

H. Permissible incentives include reasonable income guarantees offered to permissible recruits, subject to all the following conditions:
      1. Such income guarantee is for a period of 2 years or less.
      2. No off-agreement benefits are offered or provided.
      3. All terms are agreed to in advance in writing and are not modified over the life of the agreement.
      4. In the event periodic income guarantee advances are made to the physician, they will be structured as a loan or loans bearing a reasonable rate of interest, with any loan terms or loan forgiveness complying with paragraph G above.
      5. Where the income guarantee is for a net income amount, a reasonable fixed ceiling amount must be placed on allowable expenses and amounts for which advances may be made.
      6. The guarantee represents all or part of a compensation package that is reasonable in its entirety.

I. The following shall be permissible incentives only if no comparable and related value through an alternative incentive mechanism, such as an income guarantee or a forgiven loan, as described in paragraphs G and H, respectively, is otherwise provided to the permissible recruit receiving such assistance:
      1. Reasonable subsidies paid or provided, or other similar financing arrangement for medical office space rent, overhead expenses (such as utilities), or rental of equipment for a permissible recruit; however, no such subsidy may be provided unless the rental amount is (but for the subsidy) at fair rental value, and in no event may such subsidy be provided for more than 2 years.

    2. Reasonable subsidized equipment purchases or other assistance in acquiring equipment on behalf of a permissible recruit, but only if free or reduced cost use by the physician does not exceed 2 years. If title is transferred to the physician at the end of the period of free or reduced cost use, Hospital will receive payment for such equipment's fair market value from the physician.

    3. No assistance in acquiring equipment or space may be provided if it entails a conveyance or lease of such equipment or office space with a leaseback to Hospital.

J. Permissible incentives include payment of actual moving expenses and relocation costs, subject to reasonable limits and, in any case, a reasonable fixed ceiling amount. Hospital may require return of any such moving expenses or relocation costs in the event the newly recruited physician does not remain in Hospital's service area for a specified period of time.

K. Reasonable interview travel expenses may be reimbursed to permissible recruits.

L. Permissible incentives shall not include travel and continuing education expenses for any nonemployee physician where such expenses are primarily related to the physician's private practice of medicine.* Educational and related expense reimbursements, however, are permissible in the case of nurses and nurse anesthetists in exchange for future employment commitments, especially if Hospital's service area is experiencing a documented nursing shortage.

M. *Permissible* shall not include the payment or subsidized provision of private practice start-up or maintenance assistance, such as consulting services to assist in practice management, or other practice management design plans, if an income guarantee has been or will be provided to the same physician.*

N. Permissible incentives shall not include Hospital subsidization of salary and benefit costs for the support personnel of a nonemployee physician in his or her private practice.*

O. Permissible incentives shall not include the payment or provision, directly or indirectly, of malpractice insurance for the current private practice of a nonemployee physician. Coverage with respect to a physician's bona fide duties as medical director for Hospital, or any other activity undertaken for or on behalf of the Hospital that is distinct from his or her private practice, is permissible. Reasonable payment for tail coverage in the case of a permissible recruit who is relocating is permissible. For purposes of this paragraph and the following paragraph, Hospital shall not appoint a medical director, full- or part-time, unless there is a legitimate and demonstrable business purpose for doing so.*

P. Except with respect to a physician's bona fide duties as medical director for Hospital, or any other activity undertaken for or on behalf of the Hospital that is distinct from his or her private practice, permissible incentives shall not include subsidized parking, telephone allowances, including cellular car phones, car allowance, health insurance, or payment of medical society dues or licensing fees.*

Q. Signing bonuses or other bonus payments are not permissible incentives and will not be offered or made.

R. Where a permissible recruit is recruited to enter an existing physician's established medical practice, Hospital shall pay no more than 50% of the recruiting fees or costs associated with that physician.

S. Permissible incentives shall not include the conveyance or promise of a future conveyance of a Hospital outpatient department (such as Hospital clinics or centers) to a physician. Hospital shall maintain proper records of fees due for patient utilization of outpatient departments, as well as other overview safeguards, to ensure that such outpatient departments are operated for the benefit of Hospital and its community and are not effectively operated as the private practices of physicians.

T. Recruiting fees or costs shall in no event be paid to existing physicians, but such fees or costs may be paid to outside search consultants.

---

*This paragraph is not intended to prevent payment for or inclusion of these items as allowable expenses subject to the reasonable fixed ceiling amount referred to in paragraph II.H.5 above.

U. Although management may negotiate recruitment agreements within these guidelines, Hospital board approval and review by Hospital's legal counsel or tax advisor shall be obtained prior to execution for each specific financial package provided to each individual recruited physician.

V. All incentives provided to physicians will be reported on Form W-2 or Form 1099.

W. These physician recruitment guidelines apply to and are binding on each and every current and after-created subsidiary or controlled affiliate of Hospital, or common parent, that recruits physicians.

X. Each incentive arrangement with each physician shall be memorialized in writing, and no off-agreement incentives or benefits shall be offered or provided. Each such agreement with each physician shall contain a clause allowing Hospital to terminate the agreement and recover from the physician any payment that is determined by a court or government agency to be illegal or inconsistent with Hospital's tax-exempt status.

Y. In addition to such other records as may be required, Hospital will maintain complete and accurate records documenting amounts paid and other incentives provided to permissible recruits, and community need, to ensure compliance with these guidelines.

Z. Failure to comply with any provision in the above Physician Recruitment Guidelines may be found to constitute prohibited inurement and excessive private benefit that is inconsistent with Hospital's continued status as an organization described in section 501(c)(3) of the Internal Revenue Code; however, it is not intended that any such failure would constitute prohibited inurement or excessive private benefit other than as determined under the federal tax laws in effect at the time of such failure.

AA. The above-described Physician Recruitment Guidelines shall be modified to the extent Congress or the IRS legislatively or administratively, as the case may be, establishes different physician recruitment standards for tax-exempt hospitals.

ADOPTED this 16th day of September 1994.

Reprinted with permission from Daily Tax Report, No. 200, pp. L-3–L-5 (Oct. 19, 1994). Copyright 1994 by The Bureau of National Affairs, Inc. (800 372-1033). http://www.bna.com.

Source: 1990 Update: Report of the Graduate Medical Education National Advisory Committee. US Department of Health and Human Services.

EXHIBIT 2-7   ANNOUNCEMENT 95-25 (NOW KNOWN AS REV. RUL. 97-21)

_____

_____

_____

_____

Section 501.—Exemption From Tax on Corporations, Certain Trusts, Etc.

26 CFR 1.501(c)(3)–1: Organizations organized and operated for religious, charitable, scientific, testing for public safety, literary, or educational purposes, or for the prevention of cruelty to children or animals.

Tax consequences of physician recruitment incentives provided by hospitals described in section 501(c)(3) of the Code. This ruling provides examples illustrating whether nonprofit hospitals that provide incentives to physicians to join their medical staffs or to provide medical services in the community violate the requirements for exemption as organizations described in section 501(c)(3) of the Code.

Rev. Rule. 97–21

ISSUE

Whether, under the facts described below, a hospital violates the requirements for exemption from federal income tax as an organization described in § 501(c)(3) of the Internal Revenue Code when it provides incentives to recruit private practice physicians to join its medical staff or to provide medical services in the community.

FACTS

All of the hospitals in the situations described below have been recognized as exempt from federal income tax under § 501(a) as organizations described in § 501(c)(3) and operate in accordance with the standards for exemption set forth in Revenue Ruling 69–545, 1969–2 C.B. 117. The physicians described in the following recruiting transactions do not have substantial influence over the affairs of the hospitals that are recruiting them. Therefore, they are not disqualified persons as defined in § 4958, nor do they have any personal or private interest in the activities of the organizations that would subject them to the inurement proscription of § 501(c)(3). Furthermore, in Situations 1, 2, and 4, the physicians have no preexisting relationship with the hospital or the members of its board. For purposes of this revenue ruling, the physician recruiting activities described in Situations 1, 2, 3, and 4 are assumed to be lawful. However, because the Internal Revenue Service does not have jurisdiction regarding whether the activities described in Situations 1, 2, 3, and 4 are lawful under the Medicare and Medicaid Anti-Kickback Statute, 42 U.S.C. § 1320a–7b(b), taxpayers may not rely upon the facts or assumptions described in this ruling for purposes relating to that statute.

Situation 1

Hospital A is located in County V, a rural area, and is the only hospital within a 100 mile radius. County V has been designated by the U.S. Public Health Service as a health professional shortage area for primary medical care professionals (a category that includes obstetricians and gynecologists). Physician M recently completed an OB/GYN residency and is not on Hospital A's medical staff. Hospital A recruits Physician M to establish and maintain a full-time private OB/GYN practice in its service area and become a member of its medical staff. Hospital A provides Physician M a recruitment incentive package pursuant to a written agreement negotiated at arm's length. The agreement is in accordance with guidelines for physician recruitment that Hospital A's board of directors establishes, monitors, and reviews regularly to ensure that recruiting practices are consistent with Hospital A's exempt purposes. The agreement was approved by the committee appointed by Hospital A's board of directors to approve contracts with hospital medical staff. Hospital A does not provide any recruiting incentives to Physician M other than those set forth in the written agreement.

In accordance with the agreement, Hospital A pays Physician M a signing bonus, Physician M's professional liability insurance premium for a limited period, provides office space in a building owned by Hospital A for a limited number of years at a below market rent (after which the rental will be at fair market value), and guarantees Physician M's mortgage on a residence in County.

Hospital A also lends Physician M practice start-up financial assistance pursuant to an agreement that is properly documented and bears reasonable terms.

Situation 2

Hospital B is located in an economically depressed inner-city area of City W. Hospital B has conducted a community needs assessment that indicates both a shortage of pediatricians in Hospital B's service area and difficulties Medicaid patients are having obtaining pediatric services. Physician N is a pediatrician currently practicing outside of Hospital B's service area and is not on Hospital B's medical staff. Hospital B recruits Physician N to relocate to City W, establish and maintain a full-time pediatric practice in Hospital B's service area, become a member of Hospital B's medical staff, and treat a reasonable number of Medicaid patients. Hospital B offers Physician N a recruitment incentive package pursuant to a written agreement negotiated at arm's length and approved by Hospital B's Board of Directors. Hospital B does not provide any recruiting incentives to Physician N other than those set forth in the written agreement.

Under the agreement, Hospital B reimburses Physician N for moving expenses as defined in § 217(b), reimburses Physician N for professional liability tail coverage for Physician N's former practice, and guarantees Physician N's private practice income for a limited number of years. The private practice income guarantee, which is properly documented, provides that Hospital B will make up the difference to the extent Physician N practices full-time in its service area, and the private practice does not generate a certain level of net income (after reasonable expenses of the practice). The amount guaranteed falls within the range reflected in regional or national surveys regarding income earned by physicians in the same specialty.

Situation 3

Hospital C is located in an economically depressed inner-city area of City X. Hospital C has conducted a community needs assessment that indicates indigent patients are having difficulty getting access to care because of a shortage of obstetricians in Hospital C's service area willing to treat Medicaid and charity care patients. Hospital C recruits Physician O, an obstetrician who is currently a member of Hospital C's medical staff, to provide these services and enters into a written agreement with Physician O. The agreement is in accordance with guidelines for physician recruitment that Hospital C's board of directors establishes, monitors, and reviews regularly to ensure that recruiting practices are consistent with Hospital C's exempt purpose. The agreement was approved by the officer designated by Hospital C's board of directors to enter into contracts with hospital medical staff. Hospital C does not provide any recruiting incentives to Physician O other than those set forth in the written agreement. Pursuant to the agreement, Hospital C agrees to reimburse Physician O for the cost of 1 year's professional liability insurance in return for an agreement by Physician O to treat a reasonable number of Medicaid and charity care patients for that year.

Situation 4

Hospital D is located in City Y, a medium- to large-size metropolitan area. Hospital D requires a minimum of four diagnostic radiologists to ensure adequate coverage and a high quality of care for its radiology department. Two of the four diagnostic radiologists currently providing coverage for Hospital D are relocating to other areas. Hospital D initiates a search for diagnostic radiologists and determines that one of the two most qualified candidates is Physician P.

Physician P currently is practicing in City Y as a member of the medical staff of Hospital E (which is also located in City Y). As a diagnostic radiologist, Physician P provides services for patients receiving care at Hospital E, but does not refer patients to Hospital E or any other hospital in City Y. Physician P is not on Hospital D's medical staff. Hospital D recruits Physician P to join its medical staff and to provide coverage for its radiology department. Hospital D offers Physician P a recruitment incentive package pursuant to a written agreement, negotiated at arm's length and approved by Hospital D's board of directors. Hospital D does not provide any recruiting incentives to Physician P other than those set forth in the written agreement.

Pursuant to the agreement, Hospital D guarantees Physician P's private practice income for the first few years that Physician P is a member of its medical staff and provides coverage for its radiology department. The private practice income guarantee, which is properly documented, provides that Hospital D will make up the difference to Physician P to the extent the private practice does not generate a certain level of net income (after reasonable expenses of the practice). The net income amount guaranteed falls within the range reflected in regional or national surveys regarding income earned by physicians in the same specialty.

Situation 5

Hospital F is located in City Z, a medium- to large-size metropolitan area. Because of its physician recruitment practices, Hospital F has been found guilty in a court of law of knowingly and willfully violating the Medicare and Medicaid Anti-Kickback Statute, 42 U.S.C. § 1320a–7b(b), for providing recruitment incentives that constituted payments for referrals. The activities resulting in the violations were substantial.

LAW

Section 501(c)(3) provides, in part, for the exemption from federal income tax of corporations organized and operated exclusively for charitable, scientific, or educational purposes, provided no part of the organization's net earnings inures to the benefit of any private shareholder or individual.

Section 1.501(c)(3)–1(d)(2) of the Income Tax Regulations provides that the term *charitable* is used in § 501(c)(3) in its generally accepted legal sense. The promotion of health has long been recognized as a charitable purpose. *See Restatement (Second) of Trusts*, §§ 368, 372 (1959); 4A Austin W. Scott and William F. Fratcher, *The Law of Trusts* §§ 368, 372 (4th ed. 1989); and Rev. Rule. 69–545, 1969–2 C.B. 117. Under the common law of charitable trusts, all such organizations are subject to the requirement that their purposes may not be illegal. *See Restatement (Second) of Trusts* § 377 (1959); 4A Austin W. Scott and William F. Fratcher, *The Law of Trusts* § 377 (4th ed. 1989); *Bob Jones University v. U.S.*, 461 U.S. 574, 591 (1983); Rev. Rule. 80–278, 1980–2 C.B. 175; Rev. Rule. 80–279, 1980–2 C.B. 176.

Section 1.501(c)(3)–1(c)(2) states that an organization is not operated exclusively for charitable purposes if its net earnings inure in whole or in part to the benefit of private shareholders or individuals.

Section 1.501(a)–1(c) defines "private shareholder or individual" as referring to persons having a personal and private interest in the activities of the organization.

Section 1.501(c)(3)–1(d)(1)(ii) states that an organization is not organized exclusively for any of the purposes specified in § 501(c)(3) unless it serves public, rather than private interests. Thus, an organization applying for tax exemption under § 501(c)(3) must establish that it is not organized or operated for the benefit of private interests.

Rev. Rule. 69–545, 1969–2 C.B. 117, holds that a nonprofit hospital that benefits a broad cross section of its community by having an open medical staff and a board of trustees broadly representative of the community, operating a full-time emergency room open to all regardless of ability to pay, and otherwise admitting all patients able to pay (either themselves, or through third-party payers such as private health insurance or government programs such as Medicare) may qualify as an organization described in § 501(c)(3). The same standard has been used by the courts as the basis for evaluating whether health maintenance organizations qualify for exemption as organizations described in § 501(c)(3). *Sound Health Association v. Commissioner*, 71 T.C. 158 (1978), acq. 1981–2 C.B. 2; *Geisinger Health Plan v. Commissioner*, 985 F.2d 1210 (3rd Cir. 1993), *rev'g* 62 T.C.M. (CCH) 1656 (1991).

Rev. Rule. 72–559, 1972–2 C.B. 247, holds that an organization that provides subsidies to recent law school graduates during the first 3 years of their practice to enable them to establish legal practices in economically depressed communities that have a shortage of available legal services and to provide free legal service to needy members of the community may qualify as an organization described in § 501(c)(3).

Rev. Rule. 73–313, 1973–2 C.B. 174, holds that attracting a physician to a community that had no available medical services furthered the charitable purpose of promoting the health of the community. In Rev. Rule. 73–313, residents of an isolated rural community had to travel a considerable distance to obtain care. Faced with the total lack of local services, the community formed an organization to raise funds and build a medical office building to attract a doctor to the locality. (No hospitals or existing medical practices were involved.) The ruling states that certain facts are particularly relevant: (1) the demonstrated need for a physician to avert a real and substantial threat to the community; (2) evidence that the lack of a suitable office had impeded efforts to attract a physician; (3) the arrangements were completely at arm's length; and (4) there was no relationship between any person connected with the organization and the recruited physician. The ruling states that, under all the circumstances, the arrangement used to induce the doctor to locate a practice in the area "bear[s] a reasonable relationship to promotion and protection of the health of the community" and any private benefit to the physician is incidental to the public purpose achieved. It concludes that the activity furthers a charitable purpose and the organization qualifies for exemption as an organization described in § 501(c)(3).

Rev. Rule. 75–384, 1975–2 C.B. 204, holds that an organization whose primary activity is sponsoring antiwar protest demonstrations in which demonstrators are urged to commit violations of local ordinances and breaches of the public order does not qualify as an organization described in § 501(c)(3) because its activities demonstrate an illegal purpose that is inconsistent with charitable purposes.

Rev. Rule. 80–278, 1980–2 C.B. 175, and Rev. Rule. 80–279, 1980–2 C.B. 176, discuss the qualification as organizations described in § 501(c)(3) of organizations that conduct environmental litigation and environmental dispute mediation. In holding that these organizations may qualify, the rulings state

that, in determining whether an organization meets the operational test, the issue is whether the particular activity undertaken by the organization appropriately furthers the organization's exempt purpose. The rulings state that an organization's activities will be considered permissible under § 501(c)(3) if the following conditions are met: (1) the purpose of the organization is charitable; (2) the activities are not illegal, contrary to a clearly defined and established public policy, or in conflict with express statutory restrictions; and (3) the activities are in furtherance of the organization's exempt purpose and are reasonably related to the accomplishment of that purpose.

ANALYSIS

To meet the requirements of § 501(c)(3), a hospital that provides recruitment incentives to physicians must provide those incentives in a manner that does not cause the organization to violate the operational test of § 1.501(c)(3)–1. Whether the recruitment incentives cause the organization to violate the operational test is determined based on all relevant facts and circumstances. When a § 501(c)(3) hospital recruits a physician for its medical staff who is to perform services for or on behalf of the organization, the organization meets the operational test by showing that, taking into account all of the benefits provided the physician by the organization, the organization is paying reasonable compensation for the services the physician is providing in return. A somewhat different analysis must be applied when a § 501(c)(3) hospital recruits a physician for its medical staff to provide services to members of the surrounding community but not necessarily for or on behalf of the organization. In these cases, a violation will result from a failure to comply with any of the following four requirements:

First, the organization may not engage in substantial activities that do not further the hospital's exempt purposes or that do not bear a reasonable relationship to the accomplishment of those purposes. As discussed in Rev. Rule. 80–278 and Rev. Rule. 80–279, in determining whether an organization meets the operational test, the issue is whether the particular activity undertaken by the organization is appropriately in fur-

therance of the organization's exempt purpose.

Second, the organization must not engage in activities that result in inurement of the hospital's net earnings to a private shareholder or individual. An activity may result in inurement if it is structured as a device to distribute the net earnings of the hospital. *See Lorain Avenue Clinic v. Commissioner*, 31 T.C. 141 (1958); *Birmingham Business College, Inc. v. Commissioner*, 276 F.2d 476 (5th Cir. 1960).

Third, the organization may not engage in substantial activities that cause the hospital to be operated for the benefit of a private interest rather than public interest so that it has a substantial nonexempt purpose. Section 1.501(c)(3)–1(d)(1)(ii).

Finally, the organization may not engage in substantial unlawful activities. As discussed in Rev. Rule. 75–384, Rev. Rule. 80–278, and Rev. Rule. 80–279, the conduct of an unlawful activity is inconsistent with charitable purposes. An organization conducts an activity that is unlawful and therefore not in furtherance of a charitable purpose, if the organization's property is to be used for an objective that is in violation of the criminal law. Activities can accomplish an unlawful purpose through either direct or indirect means.

Situation 1

Like the organization described in Rev. Rule. 73–313, Hospital A has objective evidence demonstrating a need for obstetricians and gynecologists in its service area and has engaged in physician recruitment activity bearing a reasonable relationship to promoting and protecting the health of the community in accordance with Rev. Rule. 69–545. As with the subsidies provided to the recent law school graduates in Rev. Rule. 72–559, the payment of a bonus, the guarantee of a mortgage, the reimbursement of professional liability insurance, the provision of subsidized office space for a limited time, and the lending of start-up as recruitment incentives are reasonably related to causing Physician M to become a member of Hospital A's medical staff and to establish and maintain a full-time private OB/GYN practice in Hospital A's service area. The provision of the incentives under the circumstances described furthers the charitable purposes served by the hospital and is consistent with the requirements for exemption as an organization described in § 501(c)(3).

Situation 2

Like Hospital A in Situation 1, Hospital B has objective evidence demonstrating a need for pediatricians in its service area and has engaged in physician recruitment activity bearing a reasonable relationship to promoting and protecting the health of the community in much the same manner as the organization described in Rev Rul. 73-313. As with the recruitment incentive package provided by Hospital A, the payment of moving expenses, the reimbursement of professional liability tail coverage, and the provision of a reasonable private practice income guarantee as recruitment incentives are reasonably related to causing Physician N to become a member of Hospital B's medical staff and to establish and maintain a full-time private pediatric practice in Hospital B's service area. Thus, the recruitment activity described furthers the charitable purposes served by the hospital and is consistent with the requirements for exemption as an organization described in § 501(c)(3).

Situation 3

In accordance with the standards for exemption set forth in Rev. Rul. 69-545, Hospital C admits and treats Medicaid patients on a nondiscriminatory basis. Hospital C has identified a shortage of obstetricians willing to treat Medicaid patients. The payment of Physician O's professional liability insurance premiums in return for Physician O's agreement to treat a reasonable number of Medicaid and charity care patients is reasonably related to the accomplishment of Hospital C's exempt purposes. Because the amount paid by Hospital C is reasonable and any private benefit to Physician O is outweighed by the public purpose served by the agreement, the recruitment activity described is consistent with the requirements for exemption as an organization described in § 501(c)(3).

Situation 4

Hospital D has objective evidence demonstrating a need for diagnostic radiologists to provide coverage for its radiology department so that it can promote the health of the community.

The provision of a reasonable private practice income guarantee as a recruitment incentive that is conditioned upon Physician P obtaining medical staff privileges and providing coverage for the radiology department is reasonably related to the accomplishment of the charitable purposes served by the hospital. A significant fact in determining that the community benefit provided by the activity outweighs the private benefit provided to Physician P is the determination by the board of directors of Hospital D that it needs additional diagnostic radiologists to provide adequate coverage and to ensure a high quality of medical care. The recruitment activity described is consistent with the requirements for exemption as an organization described in § 501(c)(3).

Situation 5

Hospital F has engaged in physician recruiting practices resulting in a criminal conviction. As in Rev. Rul. 75-384, the recruiting activities were intentional and criminal, not isolated or inadvertent violations of a regulatory statute. An organization that engages in substantial unlawful activities, including activities involving the use of the organization's property for an objective that is in violation of criminal law, does not qualify as an organization described in § 501(c)(3). Because Hospital F has knowingly and willfully conducted substantial activities that are inconsistent with charitable purposes, it does not comply with the requirements of § 501(c)(3) and § 1.501(c)(3)-1.

HOLDING

The hospitals in Situations 1, 2, 3, and 4 have not violated the requirements for exemption from federal income tax as organizations described in § 501(c)(3) as a result of the physician recruitment incentive agreements they have made because the transactions further charitable purposes, do not result in inurement, do not result in the hospitals serving a private rather than a public purpose, and are assumed to be lawful for purposes of this revenue ruling.

Hospital F in Situation 5 does not qualify as an organization described in § 501(c)(3) because its unlawful physician recruitment activities are inconsistent with charitable purposes.

SCOPE

This ruling addresses only issues under § 501(c)(3) in the described situation. No inference is intended as to any other issue under any other provision of law, including any issue involving worker classification, income tax consequences to the physicians, and application of the Medicare and Medicaid Anti-Kickback statute, 42 U.S.C. §1320a-7b(b).

DRAFTING INFORMATION

The principal author of this revenue ruling is Judith E. Kindell of the Exempt Organizations Division. For further information regarding this revenue ruling contact Judith E. Kindell on (202) 622-6494 (not a toll-free call).

EXHIBIT 2-8   EXPEDITED BUSINESS REVIEW APPROVAL REQUEST—
COLLABORATIVE PROVIDER ORGANIZATION, INC.

CONNOLLY, O'MALLEY, LILLIS, HANSEN & OLSON
ATTORNEYS AT LAW
820 LIBERTY BUILDING
418 SIXTH AVENUE
DES MOINES, IOWA 50309

February 9, 1994

Assistant Attorney General
Antitrust Division
United States Department of Justice
10th and Constitution Avenue N.W.
Washington, D.C. 20530

In re: Expedited Business Review Approval Request—
          Collaborative Provider Organization, Ind.

Ladies and Gentlemen:

Pursuant to the Department of Justice's Expedited Business Review Procedure announced on December 1, 1992 [58 Red. Reg. 6132 (1993)], our law firm is requesting the department's review of an Iowa nonprofit corporation's anticipated activities in the area of health care. This request is made pursuant to the Expedited Review Procedure and 28 CFR §50.6. Our request is made upon the basis of the best information known to date and upon reasonable estimates of future activity. Where possible, the proposed entity will implement any suggested modifications that address any antitrust concerns of the department.

We verify that this Expedited Business Review procedure has been invoked in good faith and we have made a diligent search for documents and information required to be submitted pursuant to 28 CFR §50.6 and, where possible, have provided complete disclosure of all responsive material.

1. Name and Address

The name of the proposed entity is Collaborative Provider Organization, Inc. The principal place of business would be Des Moines, Iowa. Collaborative Provider Organization, Inc. (hereafter referred to as CPO) would be an Iowa nonprofit organization under the Iowa Non-Profit Corporation Act (Chapter 504A of the Iowa Code, 1993). There would be no shareholders of the corporation; however, as permitted by the Iowa Non-Profit Corporation Act, there would be corporation members. No dividends or profits would be distributed to members. Member classifications would be as follows:

A. Class A members. Class A members would be limited to allopathic (MD) and osteopathic (DO) physicians meeting all of the following qualifications: (1) the physician shall hold an unrestricted Iowa medical license; (2) the physician shall be a member in good standing on the medical staff of an acute care hospital in the State of Iowa; (3) the physician shall have current and unrestricted Federal (DEA) and State of Iowa Narcotic Registrations; and (4) the physician shall be in the active medical practice in the State of Iowa, either full-time or part-time.
B. Class B members. Class B members would be limited to acute care hospitals in the State of Iowa which are duly licensed by the state and are accredited by either the Committee of the Joint Commission on the Accreditation of Hospitals Organization (JCAHO) or the American Osteopathic Association (AOA) or which are state certified for Medicare.

2. Persons Expected to Participate

The Class A members of the CPO who are expected to participate in the venture would be approximately one hundred seventy (170) physicians in specialties as set forth on Exhibit A attached hereto. The Class B members who are expected to participate are Des Moines General Hospital, a duly licensed 226 bed hospital located at 603 East 12th Street, Des Moines, Iowa (the founding Class B member), as well as possibly two or three small rural hospitals.

Class A members would be required initially to file an application fee of one hundred fifty dollars ($150). Annual membership fees would be established by resolution of the governing board. Class B members would pay an initial application fee of one thousand dollars ($1000) and thereafter an annual fee which in the aggregate for all Class B members would equal the total fees paid by Class A Members. The Class B annual fees would be prorated among members based on gross revenue attributable to all Class B hospital inpatient and outpatient care regardless of source.

The Class A members would provide health care to the public in the form of professional services. The Class B members would provide health care services to the public, primarily in the area of inpatient and outpatient hospitalization care.

3. Objective of the Venture

The objectives of the proposed venture would be as follows:

A. To create a health care provider organization with a substantial emphasis on primary care physicians. The term *primary care physician* shall mean physicians specializing in and holding themselves out to the public as practicing predominantly in the areas of family practice, general practice, general internal medicine, as well as general pediatrics.
B. To contract or subcontract with other entities such as insurance companies, employers, accountable health plans (AHPs), and other groups for the furnishing of health care services. The CPO, with the assistance of a third-party administrator, would negotiate with these organizations for the furnishing of these health care services.
C. Although the CPO would initially be limited to contracting on behalf of CPO members for health care services, the CPO may in the future establish a management service organization or other integrated delivery system such as an accountable health plan (AHP).
D. The CPO would also actively seek to protect the rights of patients to choose their own physicians and hospitals.
E. The CPO would help physicians and hospitals from being unfairly eliminated or locked out of health care markets by other competitors.
F. The CPO would assist health care providers in furnishing high-quality, cost-effective, and competitive health services within the State of Iowa. This would be accomplished, in part, through the services of a third-party administrator, a utilization management committee, a quality management committee, and a credentials committee.
G. The CPO would offer a mechanism for physicians and hospitals to act as partners in creating structures of managed care and providing for risk sharing.
H. The CPO would offer the opportunity for physicians and hospitals to interact directly with local businesses and employers to offer "bundled" sets of medical and surgical services under a simplified and unified bill.
I. The CPO would offer the ability for physicians and hospitals to deal directly, constructively, and efficiently with other managed care entities.

As discussed above, the CPO would have a definite primary care gatekeeper emphasis consistent with trends throughout the United States. The CPO, however, would not exclude nonprimary care providers.

The geographical market for the CPO is anticipated to be the following counties within the State of Iowa: Polk, Story, Boone, Jasper, Dallas, Warren, Adair, Appanoose, Clarke, Davis, Decatur, Greene, Guthrie, Lucas, Madison, Mahaska, Marion, Marshall, Monroe, Powesheik, Ringgold, Tama,

Union, Wapello, and Wayne counties. A map showing the market area is attached hereto as Exhibit B.

Although interest has been expressed by additional health care providers such as psychologists, chiropractors, podiatrists, and physical therapists, the CPO will narrow its focus and concentrate its efforts at the present time in the areas of allopathic and osteopathic physicians as well as hospitals.

Membership in any particular class would generally be denied to a prospective member if the CPO at the time of the member's application determines, upon consultation with legal counsel, that granting membership would create antitrust or anticompetitive risk.

4. Products or Services

The CPO would not manufacture products but would assist health care providers in furnishing high-quality, cost-effective, and competitive health services in the State of Iowa. The services rendered by the CPO would consist of contracting on behalf of members for either discounted fee for services or for a capitated fee structure that the CPO hopes will be more competitive and more cost-effective than other competing health care providers. As discussed above, the CPO could possibly in the future establish a more integrated delivery system, such as an accountable health plan (AHP) or even a health maintenance organization (HMO).

5. Extent to Which Members in the CPO Currently Market Services

Each prospective member in the CPO presently negotiates his or her own individual contracts with insurance companies, employers, and other organizations. Upon implementation of the CPO, the contracting would be done by the CPO with the assistance of a third-party administrator, thus allowing for greater efficiency and reducing repetitive contract discussions with multiple parties. Members of the CPO will not have to spend considerable time in negotiating contracts individually which will, in turn, allow the health care provider to devote more time to delivery of health care. This should also simplify matters for the consumer (employers, insurance companies, etc.).

6. The Identity and Competitive Significance of Persons Who Participate in the Relevant Product and Geographical Market

In the relevant market area defined above in paragraph 3, there are a total of approximately 1428 osteopathic and allopathic physicians and 28 hospitals. Of the physicians in the relevant market, approximately 677 are primary care physicians (as defined under the CPO proposed structure). The CPO reasonably anticipates that no more than thirty percent (30%) of the primary care physicians in the relevant market would join the proposed CPO. At the present time thirteen percent (13%) of the primary care physicians in the relevant market have formally expressed an interest in CPO membership. A breakdown of each specialty is shown in the attached Exhibit A.

The relevant market area is highly competitive regarding health care, especially in the greater Des Moines, Polk County area. Within Polk County there are the following hospitals:

	Name	*Licensed Beds*
A.	Broadlawns Medical Center	173
B.	Des Moines General Hospital	226
C.	Iowa Lutheran Hospital	343
D.	Iowa Methodist Medical Center	710
E.	Mercy Hospital Medical Center	555
F.	Veterans Administration Hospital	155
G.	Mercy Franklin Hospital	118

Two of the above hospitals (Methodist and Lutheran) have merged effective November 22, 1993, under a new corporate structure known as Iowa Health System. Mercy Hospital has recently announced the acquisition of Mercy Franklin Hospital.

Descriptions of existing or proposed organized delivery systems, accountable health plans, or other similar ventures in the relevant market area are set forth in the attached Exhibit C, which is an excerpt from the October 1993 edition of *Focus on Health Care* published by the Iowa Hospital Education and Research Foundation.

7. Restrictions on Ability of Participants to Compete with the Venture

As can be seen by the attached articles of incorporation as well as the proposed by-laws of the CPO (Exhibits D and E attached hereto), the CPO is nonexclusive, and there is no limitation on the ability of any member to join other organizations or other competing entities. Paragraph F of Article IV of the proposed by-laws provides:

> Application or approval for membership in the corporation shall not prevent any person or entity within any class of membership from participating in any preferred provider organizations, physician hospital organizations, organized delivery systems, independent practice associations, or other health care provider organizations or any other contractual relationship in addition to the corporation.

Paragraph B of Article IV provides that:

> A member may elect not to participate in any contract if, within ten (10) business days of the member's receipt of a copy of such contract, the member sends a written notice to the corporation by certified mail, return receipt requested, of the member's election not to participate in the contract.

8. Restrictions on the Flow of Information from the Venture to Its Members

Section 3 of Article VIII of the proposed CPO by-laws provided as follows:

> The board shall have the authority to retain a third-party administrator (TPA) to create a database, prepare statistical analyses, and furnish recommendations to enable the corporation to negotiate contracts for health care and to help carry out the purposes for which the corporation was formed, all consistent with antitrust laws and other applicable federal and state laws. All information obtained by the TPA shall be proprietary and confidential. As a condition of membership, each member covenants and agrees that, except for the final statistical analysis and recommendations of the TPA, no member shall have access to any disaggregated information held by the TPA or any accounting firm, actuary, or research firms providing services to the TPA

Paragraph G of Article IV provides as follows:

> No member shall have access to another member's patient fee or pricing information or other financial information, including, but not limited to, salary and fringe benefits for associates or employees. Furthermore, no member shall have access to any data or information gathered by a third-party administrator (TPA) as described below in Article VIII, Section 3.

9. Ten Largest Customers (Projected) for Services to Be Offered by the Venture

The CPO will either (1) coordinate the offering of health care services to small and medium-sized employers and companies having 25–50 employees or subcontractors with the two presently identified accountable health care plans (AHPs) established separately by Iowa Methodist Medical Center and Mercy Hospital Medical Center; or (2) the CPO may in the future create a third AHP in the market and coordinate the offering of services to small and medium-sized employers and companies having 25–50 employees. If a third AHP is established by the CPO, marketing would be done primarily through independent insurance agents as well as offering the health care services directly to employers in conjunction with one or more tertiary care hospitals. The annual purchases of the CPO's services is unknown at this time.

The proposed CPO has not yet retained the services of a third-party administrator, actuary, consultant, or management company. Therefore, it is very difficult to project financial costs in connection with the venture. The founding Class B member, Des Moines General Hospital, has recently implemented a preferred provider organization for its employees that offers some insight into the financial aspects of health care organization in general terms.

The Des Moines General Hospital preferred provider organization (PPO) has 535 persons who are covered, including dependents of employees. The PPO is administered by Benefits Administration of America, Inc., which charges administrative fee of approximately $14,000 per month. Claims paid by the Hospital for participants average approximately $86,000 per month. These costs, however, are not entirely typical of all employee groups in the market area. Employees of hospitals, and their dependents, tend to be high health care utilizers. It has been projected that health care employees and their dependents will utilize health care services 25–30% more than other comparable nonhealth care employee groups.

10. Requirements for Entry into Any Relevant Product or Geographic Market and the Identity of Persons Believed to Be Positioned to Enter into the Market

The key to the operation of the proposed CPO will be a sound base of primary care physicians serving in a gatekeeper role supported by nonprimary care specialists. In addition, primary care hospitals will be an important factor as well as a contractual relationship for services with tertiary hospitals in the greater Des Moines area. It is also anticipated that there will be several rural community hospitals seeking membership, which will also help the CPO serve rural areas of Iowa. Knoxville Community Hospital in Marion County and Lucas County Hospital have both expressed an interest in joining the CPO.

11. Business Efficiencies That Are Likely to Flow from the Venture

Business efficiencies of the CPO would include the following:

A. Each physician member will be relieved of the burden of dealing with provider contracts individually. The CPO will perform this service with the assistance of a third-party administrator.
B. Through the assistance of a third-party administrator, the CPO can perform services more efficiently and in a more businesslike manner. Many of the prospective CPO members do not have the level of expertise or time necessary to cope with the myriad of provider contracts being negotiated or offered in the relevant market area. Many prospective members are sole practitioners or are in small practice groups isolated in rural areas.
C. The CPO, through the assistance of the third-party administrator and other consultants, will track clinical outcomes and be able to more efficiently and economically provide appropriate health care services.
D. The CPO, through the committee structures, third-party administrator, and other consultants, will manage resource utilization, help reduce unnecessary services, and help enhance quality care.
E. The CPO would review the credentials of all members. A committee of CPO members would be established for this purpose.
F. The CPO would help ensure that a patient would have a choice of his or her own physician and should be able to stay with that physician during the course of treatment where possible. By reducing referrals to other physicians or other groups, where medically appropriate, the CPO hopes to eliminate unnecessary services and thus reduce costs.

12. All Documents Reflecting the Formation of the Venture

Attached to this letter as Exhibits D and E are the following:

A. Articles of incorporation of Collaborative Provider Organization, Inc. These articles were filed with the Iowa Secretary of State on November 30, 1993. Although the articles have been filed, the organization has not formally been organized, no officers have been selected, and no persons have been accepted for membership in the organization. The initial board of directors established in the articles of incorporation has met and has authorized the Request for Expedited Business Review as contained in this letter.
B. Proposed by-laws of the organization. The by-laws are in preliminary draft form and have not been adopted. The organization does not anticipate adopting by-laws until completion of the Expedited Business Review.

13. Documents Concerning the Business Plans or Strategy for the Venture

The CPO at this time does not have a marketing or business plan other than what has been described in this letter.

14. Documents Prepared Within Two Years Reflecting the Business Plans of Any Venture Participant

The CPO at this time does not have a marketing or business plan other than what has been described in this letter.

15. Documents Discussing or Relating to Legality or Illegality Under the Antitrust Laws of the Venture or Competition or the Price of Any Product or Service

No such documents exist; however, the issue of antitrust has been discussed in the organizational meetings with prospective members, and, as a result, a decision was made to request an expedited review procedure.

16. Documents Showing the Person or Firms Expected to Exchange Information

As previously discussed, paragraph G of Article IV provides that:

> No member shall have access to another member's patient fee or pricing information or other financial information, including, but not limited to, salary and fringe benefits for associates or employees. Furthermore, no member shall have access to any data or information gathered by a third-party administrator (TPA) as described below in Article VIII, Section 3.

Section 3 of Article VIII provides that:

> The board shall have the authority to retain a third-party administrator (TPA) to create a database, prepare statistical analyses, and furnish recommendations to enable the corporation to negotiate contracts for health care and to help carry out the purposes for which the corporation was formed, all consistent with antitrust laws and other applicable federal and state laws. All information obtained by the TPA shall be proprietary and confidential. As a condition of membership, each member covenants and agrees that, except for the final statistical analysis and recommendations of the TPA, no member shall have access to any disaggregated information held by the TPA or any accounting firm, actuary, or research firms providing services to the TPA.

17. The Purpose and Objectives of the Information Exchange

The purpose and objectives of the information exchange involving the third-party administrator or other related consultant is to create a database, prepare statistical analyses, and furnish recommendations to enable the CPO to negotiate contracts for health care and to help carry out the purposes for which the corporation was formed. By gathering this information, the third-party administrator will be in a position to provide a final statistical analysis and recommendations as to how the CPO and the members can compete more aggressively in the market (e.g., provide health care services at a cost lower than competitors).

18. The Nature, Type, Timeliness, and Specificity of the Information to Be Obtained

The third-party administrator will assimilate information concerning utilization, quality standards, cost to purchase services, both corporate and individual, fees, charges, and clinical outcomes. The third-party administrator will compile this data and compare it with standards for individual persons and potential purchasers of services. Although several potential third-party administrators have been identified, no final decision has been made pending the Expedited Business Review.

19. The Method by Which Information Will Be Exchanged

See answers to paragraphs 16, 17, and 18 above.

20. The Characteristics of the Market

As described above, the market is extremely competitive. In Polk County, Iowa, Iowa Lutheran Hospital and Iowa Methodist Medical Center have merged effective November 22, 1993, to form an organization having the most licensed beds in the central Iowa area. Mercy Hospital recently announced the acquisition of the former Westside Hospital (now known as Mercy Franklin Hospital). Both Iowa Methodist Medical Center and Mercy Hospital Medical Center have announced the formation of accountable health plans, and they are actively recruiting physicians to those plans.

Furthermore, there is cross-staffing at hospitals within the great Des Moines area, and it is very common for a physician to have staff privileges at several, if not all, of the area hospitals. Some of these characteristics are described in Exhibit C, which has previously been mentioned in this letter. Furthermore, managed care organizations (such as HMOs) are increasing their share of the relevant market.

21. The Identity and Competitive Significance of Persons That Participate in the Relevant Market but Will Not Participate in the Information Exchange

The total number of physicians in the relevant market area is 1428. Of this number, approximately 677 are primary care physicians. At the present time, approximately fifty-two percent (52%) of the Class A physician members of the proposed CPO will be primary care physicians. The balance will be nonprimary specialists. The vast majority of physicians in the relevant market area will not be participating in the CPO. The assumption is that they already are or will be participating in comparable organizations (whether it be an AHP, HMO, physician–hospital organization, or other similar entity). These nonmember persons would not be participating in the information exchange.

22. The Ten Largest Customers in Any Market That Will Be Involved in the Exchange of Information

No specific companies or customers have been identified by the proposed CPO; however, it is anticipated that small to medium-sized employers and companies having 25–50 employees will be the primary emphasis of the CPO.

23. Describe All Safeguards That Are Planned to Prevent Disclosure of Specific Information to Competitors

As stated above, the third-party administrator will create a database, prepare statistical analyses, and furnish recommendations in a confidential fashion. Except for the final statistical analysis and recommendations, no member shall have access to any disaggregated information held by the third-party administrator or any accounting firm, actuary, or research firms providing services. It is anticipated that the CPO would establish rules and regulations prohibiting the disclosure of information to competitors. By the terms of the proposed by-laws, all members must abide by the rules and regulations. Furthermore, no member shall have access to another member's patient fee or pricing information.

Please contact the undersigned if you have any questions concerning this matter. Thank you for your consideration.

Very truly yours,

Eugene E. Olson
For the Firm

EXHIBIT 2-9 TWENTY KEY IRS CLASSIFICATION FACTORS FOR DETERMINING INDEPENDENT CONTRACTOR STATUS

Sixteen factors demonstrating an employer-employee relationship (versus an independent contractor relationship), with sufficient "control" exerted by the hospital:

- **Instructions**—The hospital can require physicians to comply with instructions about when, where, and how the work is to be done.
- **Training**—The hospital provides training for the physicians.
- **Integration**—The hospital integrates the physician's services into its regular business operations.
- **Services rendered personally**—The hospital requires the physician to perform the services personally, versus the physician utilizing help of others without hospital's knowledge or approval.
- **Hiring of assistants**—The hospital, not the physician, hires, supervises, and pays for assistants to the physician.
- **Continuing relationship**—The hospital uses the physician's services in an ongoing or frequently occurring basis.
- **Set hours**—The hospital sets the hours the physician is to work.
- **Full-time basis**—The hospital requires the physician to work on substantially a full-time basis for the hospital.
- **On-premises services**—The hospital requires the physician to perform his or her services on hospital premises.
- **Order/sequence**—The hospital dictates the order or sequence in which the physician will complete duties.
- **Reports**—The hospital requires the physician to submit specific reports on services performed (i.e., account for work done).
- **Payments**—The hospital makes regular, periodic payments to the physician for performance of services, in contrast to lump sum payments for specific services or projects completed.
- **Expenses**—The hospital pays for or reimburses the physician for expenses related to his or her duties.
- **Equipment/supplies**—The hospital, in contrast to the physician, supplies the equipment and supplies necessary for the physician to perform his or her duties.
- **Right to discharge**—The hospital retains the right to discharge the physician from his or her duties prior to the completion of the project or term of the contract, independent of performance standards.
- **Right to quit**—The physician retains the right to quit at any time prior to the completion of the project or term of the contract.

The following four factors demonstrate an independent contractor relationship (versus an employer-employee relationship), with sufficient "independence" maintained by the physician:

- **Investment**—The physician invests in the equipment and/or premises required to perform his or her services.
- **Profit or loss**—The physician can suffer a loss or realize a profit as a result of the services performed (rather than merely suffer nonpayment if he or she does not perform the services as expected).
- **Multiple employers**—The physician performs similar services for more than one unrelated hospital or entity at the same time.
- **Availability to general public**—The physician's services remain available to the general public, rather than just through the hospital.

Adapted from the Internal Revenue Service, Revenue Ruling 87-41.

Part III

Recruitment Policy Development

The vast majority of healthcare centers are trying their best to comply with the government's ambiguous rules and regulations for recruiting physicians, but the task requires some forethought and planning. The purpose of this section is to assist organizations in developing written policies that will be consistent with the guidelines.

The following topics will be presented:

- Reasons for creating a physician recruitment policies document
- Development sequence
- Contents of the policies document

REASONS FOR CREATING A PHYSICIAN RECRUITMENT POLICIES DOCUMENT

Creating a physician recruitment policies document offers many advantages to a hospital. Among these are:

- **Documentation**—Having a written set of recruitment policies that emphasize adherence to current IRS and OIG regulations can provide some protection in the event of an audit of a hospital's recruitment activities. This protection originates both from having a set of approved guidelines for hospital personnel to follow and having written documentation contained in the physician recruitment policies document itself.

- **Internal hospital issues**—A physician recruitment policies document can be of great assistance to the chief executive officer and other hospital personnel in responding to requests from physicians and other parties. If anyone makes an unusual or unreasonable request for assistance, it is very valuable to be able to reference an existing set of policies as the reason for denying the request. Doing so can defuse politically dangerous issues. These policies can alter the disappointed physician's opinion that this was an arbitrary personal rejection by the CEO and substantiate that it was a non-personal administrative decision based on approved policy.
- **Clarification of board's role**—One universal tenet contained in every recruitment policies document is affirmation of the governing board's role as the ultimate governing authority for all recruitment activities. Language contained in a physician recruitment policies document can reaffirm and clarify this concept of "overriding board governance."
- **Consensus building**—Having the medical staff, governing board, and hospital management involved in the design and drafting of a physician recruitment policies document can be an important initial step in building consensus regarding the purpose, scope, and direction of a hospital's recruitment program. When recruitment policies are set down in writing, all individuals concerned with recruitment are able to remain focused on an agreed-upon course of action.
- **Expedite decision making**—A hospital that has an established set of physician recruitment policies and approved contract language in place is in a much better position to draft recruitment contracts that can be approved expeditiously. The physician recruiter who is forced to operate without such policies frequently cannot tell the physician candidate what incentives the hospital is willing to offer and may have to withdraw a portion of the offer when senior management or the governing board subsequently rejects it. Even if this does not occur, the contract drafting and contract approval process is often much more protracted without an established physician recruitment policies document in place.
- **Education**—One of the sections recommended for inclusion in a physician recruitment policies document is a statement that members of the hospital's governing board and hospital management have "awareness" concerning the general rules and regulations governing physician recruitment. A spin-off benefit of creating a recruitment policies document is that both hospital management and members of the governing board are compelled to become more familiar with the legal environment in which these activities occur.
- **Community need study**—In the course of developing physician recruitment policies, a hospital quickly becomes aware of the critical importance of the "community need" doctrine and the necessity of having a current quantitative physician manpower ("community need") study available. For those hospitals that do not have a current physician manpower study, drafting a physician recruitment policies document often provides the impetus to complete or update such a study.
- **Recruitment committee structure**—Many hospitals do not have a formal vehicle (i.e., recruitment committee) in place that sets policies and

supervises ongoing recruitment activities. Creating a physician recruitment policies document often highlights the need for a permanent oversight body and leads to the formation of a recruitment committee.

- **Legal counsel**—The IRS has stated clearly that independent legal counsel should review physician recruitment contracts in advance on behalf of the hospital. Thus, it is important to involve legal counsel early in the recruitment process.

DEVELOPMENT SEQUENCE

Although there is no blueprint for developing written physician recruitment policies, a logical sequence of events for hospitals to replicate might involve the following steps:

1. Create a physician recruitment policies document commissioned by the board of trustees.
2. Form a temporary recruitment policies task force.
3. Select a recruitment policies task force, ideally with representation from medical staff, the community, senior hospital management, and the board of trustees.
4. Establish via the task force the scope and general content of the physician recruitment policies.
5. Complete the initial draft version of the physician recruitment policies, either internally or with outside assistance.
6. Review the initial draft version of the physician recruitment policies by legal counsel.
7. The recruitment policies task force approves the final draft of the physician recruitment policies.
8. The board of trustees approves the final draft of the physician recruitment policies.
9. Dissolve the recruitment policies task force.
10. Form permanent physician recruitment committees.

CONTENTS OF A PHYSICIAN RECRUITMENT
POLICIES DOCUMENT

Similar to the development sequence, no standard outline exists for the contents of a physician recruitment policies document. The content, length, degree of detail, and other aspects of each recruitment policy document should be customized to fit the needs and objectives of each individual hospital.

For example, a large institution with extensive recruitment activities located in a state or city with a history of above-average legal scrutiny (e.g., Pennsylvania or Orange County, California) may require a lengthy, detailed document. Conversely, a small rural hospital, located in a state having a historically low legal profile (e.g., North Dakota or Montana) may need only a very short, concise document.

Based on these considerations, the following is a reasonable list of the major sections of a physician recruitment policies document:

I.   Preliminary Statements
     A. Preamble
     B. Statement of Awareness
II. Supervision of Recruitment Activities
     A. Board of Trustees
     B. Role of the Governing Board
III. Overview of Standard Contractual Elements
IV. Policies Applying to Specific Recruitment Incentives
V.   Supporting Exhibits

The following sections track this format, discussing physician recruitment policies and contracting in detail. Sample language is provided that may be suitable for writing these policies. In all legal matters, however, obtain the advice and counsel of an experienced attorney who specializes in healthcare law.

PRELIMINARY STATEMENTS

Preamble

Any physician recruitment policies document should ideally begin with a preamble statement. The preamble links each hospital's charitable mission (described in its mission statement) and its role as an important community healthcare resource to the recruitment process.

The following text provides an example of a preamble statement from a physician recruitment policies document.

Sample Language

An important goal of the Hospital's overall mission is to provide high-quality care to residents in the Hospital's service area consistent with community standards. One way to achieve this mission and fulfill statutory and legal obligations is to assist in the coordinated development of a highly qualified medical staff that can meet the healthcare needs of the patients located in the Hospital's service area.

The purpose of the Hospital's physician recruitment program is the continuation of its charitable, not-for-profit role in providing quality health care to the Hospital's service area. In fulfilling this role, the Hospital recognizes the necessity to recruit new physicians to the community where there is a demonstrated need for such physicians.

In recognition of the fact that these needs cannot always be met through random seeking of privileges by physicians in the community, the Hospital has recognized that it will periodically need to assist in the recruitment of qualified physicians to the medical staff. This can be accomplished through employing physicians, recruiting physicians who are relocating from outside the area into existing local practices, establishing entirely new practices in the community, and a variety of other methods.

To identify acceptable and permissible physician recruitment transactions, the Hospital Board has directed that a policy document be drafted. The overriding purposes of this document are to set forth policies that coincide as closely as possible with existing federal and state regulations and provide coordinated direction to the Hospital personnel in their recruitment efforts so that both the goals and mission of this Hospital and the needs of the community are met.

From time to time, the Hospital, in consultation with legal counsel, will revise these guidelines to comply with any changes in applicable laws and regulations or governmental interpretations of the same. In the implementation of these guidelines, it will be the policy of the Hospital to consult regularly with legal counsel.

Statement of Awareness

A second preliminary statement that should be included in any physician recruitment policies document is a statement of awareness. This statement reaffirms that hospital management and members of the governing board have taken the time and effort to become familiar with current laws and regulations pertaining to physician recruitment activities.

It is sometimes useful to document that the hospital has made available some literature pertaining to this topic or had legal counsel make an educational presentation on recruitment laws and regulations to both hospital personnel and hospital board members.

An example of a statement of awareness from a physician recruitment policies document is provided below.

Sample Language

The Hospital will use its best efforts to abide by all local, state, and federal laws and regulations and will seek to minimize the risk of legal and/or regulatory exposure. The Hospital will use its best efforts to ensure that no activity is undertaken that would directly compromise the Hospital's tax-exempt status as a 501(c)(3) organization or certification as a Medicare/Medicaid provider or knowingly expose the Hospital to unreasonable regulatory action or investigation.

The policies adopted in this document have been drafted and implemented to comply reasonably with known laws and regulations. Should changes in applicable laws and regulations affect the policies contained in this document, they will be modified as required to conform to these changes.

As one best-effort measure to comply with existing laws and regulations that pertain to physician recruitment, all appropriate Hospital Personnel involved with physician recruitment and all Board members have been given a copy of [name of document or review article distributed to hospital personnel].

These individuals have been specifically directed by the Hospital's Chief Executive Officer to read the above-mentioned document thoroughly, become familiar with the current laws and regulations, and consult with the Hospital's legal counsel with any questions that they may have on this subject.

SUPERVISION OF RECRUITMENT ACTIVITIES

Board of Trustees

The continuing corporate scandals during recent years have created significant ongoing pressure to strengthen honesty and integrity and promote compliant and ethical behavior in corporate America, including in the health-care industry. The advent of corporate liability disasters such as Enron, World-Com, Arthur Andersen, and Health South has precipitated legislation and enforcement action aimed at curbing corporate malfeasance. The passage of the Sarbanes-Oxley Act of 2002 in conjunction with the U.S. Sentencing Guideline Amendments and the Department of Justice (DOJ) *Principles of Federal Prosecution of Business Organizations* ("Thompson memo"), are intended to combat conflict of interest and promote independent decision making for business organizations and highlight the need for these organizations to implement effective compliance and ethics programs. Self-governance, self-reporting, and the acceptance of responsibility are the new building blocks of the organizational culture expected to result from these reordered enforcement priorities. The fact of the matter is that the federal government expects modern business organizations to become partners in combating misconduct and promoting corporate compliance and ethical behavior, and this has elevated the need for hospital organizational governing authorities to ensure compliant recruitment practices.

The New Era of Corporate Responsibility

The federal government established the themes of corporate compliance and independent decision making and minimization of conflicts of interests as the hallmark of corporate responsibility in the healthcare industry with the passage of such legislation as the Health Care Quality Improvement Act of 1986 and Health Insurance Portability and Accountability Act of 1996 (HIPAA). These statutory enactments provide substantial resources for investigating and prosecuting healthcare fraud; such activities commenced in a widespread fashion during the mid 1990s. The legacy of enforcement of the healthcare fraud and abuse laws has encouraged, and even mandated, the themes of compliance and independent decision making, and it has minimized conflicts of interest and promoted best practices for governance of health-care organizations, which all occurred prior to the passage of the

Sarbanes-Oxley Act. The enforcement actions that have set the federal and state government's agenda over the past decade in the healthcare industry have raised the stakes for not only public companies but also for private and not-for-profit organizations providing healthcare goods and services (i.e., hospitals). This corporate experience in health care has been a preview of the expectations that exist for the rest of corporate America as reflected in the passage of the Sarbanes-Oxley Act, the enforcement policies reflected in the DOJ's Thompson memo and the U.S. Sentencing Guideline Amendments effective in November 2004.

Sarbanes-Oxley Overview and Sentencing Guideline Amendments Raise the Stakes for All Business Organizations

In the summer of 2002, President Bush signed the Sarbanes-Oxley Act in an effort to foster greater financial accuracy and curb corporate malfeasance. This was the first attempt to govern corporate conduct by imposing criminal liability directly on executives for investor fraud outside the healthcare industry. The purpose of the reform was to change the way business organizations conduct their business, while simultaneously assigning a greater level of accountability to corporate boards and executives.

Among other things, the act ensures that corporations make a commitment to ethical conduct and improve self-governance practices. Self-governance mandates that corporations strive to not only be in compliance with the letter of the law, but with the spirit of the law as well. If the goal of the organization is to only comply with the law, there is a good chance it will miss its mark set by the act, the sentencing guideline amendments, and federal government enforcement policy.

In 1991, few could have predicted the profound impact that the U.S. Organizational Sentencing Guidelines would have in the area of corporate governance and compliance. The ability of an organization to detect and ferret out illegal activities has become paramount in the effort to keep corporate America honest. The guidelines introduced the concept of the compliance program as a means for an organization to reduce its criminal culpability through preventative behavior. Under the guidelines, organizations with an existing compliance program are eligible for a culpability score reduction at sentencing. However, at its inception, organizations were unclear as to who within the organization was ultimately responsible for the implementation and oversight of a compliance program, and what constituted an effective program.

The duty of oversight for such a program did not effectively enter the realm of the corporate boardroom until the decision in *re: Caremark International, Inc.* In *Caremark*, the Delaware Chancery Court noted that a failure by the board of directors to assure the existence of an adequate information reporting system implemented to provide senior management and the board with timely and accurate information relating to legal compliance might in some situations be treated as a violation of an individual director's duty of care. This decision was responsible for bringing compliance into the boardroom in a direct way by elevating it to the level of a fiduciary obligation for individual board members. After this decision, the implementation and oversight of a compliance program in no uncertain terms became the obligation of the board and high-level management. After *Caremark*, the remaining issue was what constituted an effective program.

In early 2004, at the direction of the Sarbanes-Oxley Act, the U.S. Sentencing Commission met to review and amend the existing guidelines. The commission's objective was to strengthen the guidelines by enhancing the need for effective compliance, while ensuring that it was sufficient to deter and punish organizational misconduct. An advisory group recommended overall revisions to the sentencing guidelines to highlight the importance of structural safeguards designed to prevent and detect criminal conduct and specifically recommended a regime of internal crime prevention and self-policing. The recent amendments significantly encourage business organizations to partner with the federal government in a program of crime control and provide strong incentives for such organizations to self-police, self-report, and to cooperate in investigations of its own wrongdoing.

Although the U.S. Sentencing Guideline Amendments are not necessarily new concepts to the area of corporate compliance and certainly not in the healthcare industry, it strengthens and specifically clarifies the original seven elements of a compliance program for organizations contained in the original guidelines. Rather than redraft the elements of a successful compliance program, the advisory group focused its efforts on what makes a program "effective." The amendments outline that an effective compliance and ethics program means the "prevention and detection of criminal conduct" coupled with the "promotion of an organizational culture that encourages ethical conduct and a commitment to compliance with the law." The amendments place a great deal of importance on ethical behavior, organizational responsibility, and risk assessment. No longer is compliance with the law the yardstick to measure the effectiveness of a program. Strict legal compliance must be accompanied by a strong commitment to ethical behavior and a proactive management style that addresses areas of key concern and known risk.

The Sentencing Guidelines Amendments adopt a "carrot and stick" approach in the criminal penalty structure for business organizations. The ability of a business organization to implement and sustain an effective corporate compliance program can literally mean the difference between its survival or its demise under the new amendments. The fulfillment of the expectations of the amendments for compliance can not only influence the government's decision on bringing charges against a business organization, but also has the potential to reduce an organization's culpability score, in terms of dollars, from astronomical amounts to virtually zero. Furthermore, compliance with the Sentencing Guideline Amendments will also be attractive for courts as a requirement for probationary sentences for a business organization. Accordingly, it is the standard by which business organizations should measure the effectiveness of its compliance programs.

The Content of the Sentencing Guideline Amendments

The U.S. Sentencing Guideline Amendments codifies the *Caremark* principles by assigning oversight and responsibility to high-level personnel of the organization and by providing that the "organizational leadership shall be knowledgeable about the content and operation of the program to prevent and detect violations of the law." Additionally, the organization's governing authority shall be knowledgeable and shall exercise reasonable oversight with respect to the implementation and effectiveness of the compliance program with responsibility to "ensure the implementation and effectiveness of the program." This amendment also requires that the individual responsible for compliance (i.e., compliance officers) be given adequate resources and authority to carry out such responsibility and provides that such individuals shall report directly to the governing authority.

The amendments mandate that compliance responsibility should not be delegated to individuals who have committed crimes or engaged in activities inconsistent with the goals of the program. Organizations should implement a hiring and promotion screening process to determine if the individual has engaged in prior misconduct and determine if that conduct was inconsistent with the goals of compliance.

The Sentencing Guideline Amendments also add to the compliance training requirement and specifically extend this requirement to upper-level management of an organization, as well as the organization's employees and agents.

The Sarbanes-Oxley Act along with the Sentencing Guideline Amendments and the DOJ prosecution guidelines has placed enormous pressure on directors of business organizations to devise internal controls for effective compliance programs. The complexities associated with compliance mean that sophisticated business organizations maintain a code of conduct and ethics as part of their corporate compliance program and furthermore requires that such programs be effective in detecting and preventing activities that can give rise to liability for the organization.

In today's climate, a corporation simply cannot run the risk of not implementing an effective governance and compliance program. It is clear from what has been learned in the healthcare industry that all business organizations should be taking steps to implement internal controls to prevent and detect noncompliant activity and promote positive business practices. Corporate boards need to be more diligent about oversight of high-ranking company executives and ensure that they have compliance programs that can detect corporate fraud. The benefits of these compliance programs are simply too great to ignore. The lesson that should be learned from legislation such as Sarbanes-Oxley and its sentinel effect is that companies, large or small, both public and private, must take efforts to ferret out wrongful conduct or likely suffer the consequences of failing to do so.

Role of the Governing Board

A hospital's governing board is ultimately responsible for all recruitment activities conducted by the hospital and to ensure it is consistent with the law and best compliance practices. As a consequence, any and all recruitment activities conducted by hospital personnel or by agents of a hospital may be delegated to others only through board-approved policies or through committees commissioned by the hospital's governing board. The governing board is ultimately responsible for any and all hospital recruitment activities; therefore, it is prudent that oversight structures be in place to provide a framework within which all activities occur. Many hospital boards find committees to be the most effective and efficient manner in which to manage the recruitment oversight process, although they should report to high-level management personnel in the organization, who in turn, report directly to the board of directors.

There are two aspects to delegated recruitment oversight by a hospital's governing board:

- Monitoring overriding policies for the hospital's recruitment program
- Monitoring day-to-day activities of the hospital's recruitment program (i.e., the recruitment process itself)

A single recruitment committee may accomplish both of these functions, or a hospital may wish to create two committees with separate functions:

- Recruitment policy committee
- Recruitment activities committee

The following are some basic issues that hospitals have to consider when forming recruitment committees:

- Number of committees
- Names of the committees
- Functions of the committees (e.g., setting overriding policies, approving individual physician contracts, monitoring day-to-day activities)
- Relationship of the committees to the hospital's governing board (e.g., the committee exists as a subcommittee of the governing board or as an independent hospital committee)
- Degree of independent authority and autonomy the recruitment committee has from the governing board
- Committee structure (e.g., number of members, composition by membership category, length of term, chairmanship)
- Financial authorization limits (e.g., maximum amount of support per physician, annual financial approval caps)

No matter how the recruitment committee structure is established, it must be continually emphasized to all involved with the recruitment process that any substantial deviation from established recruitment policy may occur only after approval by the board of directors.

The following sections provide examples of language from a physician recruitment policies document where the hospital's board designated two separate committees to supervise recruitment policies and ongoing recruitment activities.

Governing Board's Authority Affirmed

Sample Language_____

- Overall responsibility and authority for all recruitment activities conducted by the Hospital resides with the Board of Trustees.
- Any and all recruitment activities conducted by Hospital personnel or by agents of the Hospital may be delegated only by the Hospital Board to others through Board-approved policies or Board-designated committees.
- Any deviation from established recruitment policies may be permitted only after approval by the Board of Trustees.
- Although the Hospital Board retains ultimate responsibility and authority for establishing and monitoring physician recruitment policy, it has been determined that both the Hospital's and the community's needs regarding physician recruitment can best be served by establishing Board-commissioned recruitment committees.

Committee #1: The Recruitment Policy Committee

Sample Language_____

The Hospital's Board has directed that a Recruitment Policy Committee (RPC) be established to carry out various duties relating to overall Hospital recruitment policy. The RPC will exist as a permanent Board-commissioned body and will report recommended actions to the overall Hospital Board for approval.

Composition. The RPC will consist of five (5) voting and two (2) non-voting members:

- The Hospital's Chief Executive Officer
- A member-at-large from the community, appointed to a one- (1) year term by the Chairman of the Hospital Board
- The Director of Physician Support Services
- A member-at-large from the Hospital's Senior Management team, appointed by the Hospital's Chief Executive Officer
- A member-at-large from the Hospital's Board, appointed by the Chairman of the Hospital Board. This member-at-large will serve on the RPC for a one- (1) year term and will serve as the Chairman of the RPC during that time.
- In addition, the Hospital's Legal Counsel and the current Chief of the Medical Staff shall serve as nonvoting, ex officio members of this committee.

Responsibilities. This Committee shall have the following responsibilities:

- The RPC will commission, review, and edit a physician recruitment policies document for the Hospital. The final recommended version of this document will be sent to the overall Hospital Board for final approval.
- From time to time, the RPC will review any needed deletions, alterations, or additions to established Hospital recruitment policies and send its recommendations regarding same to the overall Hospital Board for final

approval. The most current version of the physician recruitment policies document will then be amended to reflect these changes once they are approved.

- On an annual basis, or more often if needed, the RPC will review, with the assistance of the Hospital's Legal Counsel, the entire physician recruitment policies document for compliance with changing regulations and legal precedent in the area of physician recruitment and support arrangements. Following this review, recommended additions, deletions, or other alterations will be sent to the overall Hospital Board for approval.
- On an annual basis the RPC will commission, review, and approve an update of the Hospital's quantitative Community Need Analysis.
- If the Hospital does not have a baseline Community Need Analysis, the RPC will commission senior Hospital management to complete such an analysis. Upon completion, the Community Need Analysis will be reviewed and approved by the RPC.

Committee #2: The Recruitment Activities Committee

Sample Language_____

- To carry out effectively the day-to-day activities necessary for the Hospital to fulfill its role in the medical staff, the Hospital Board has commissioned a second recruitment committee, the Recruitment Activities Committee (RAC). The RAC will exist as a permanent Board-commissioned body and will report specified actions to the Finance Subcommittee of the Hospital's Board. The RAC will be free to make independent decisions and take actions on specific recruitment initiatives within the policies and guidelines set out in this document, as well as to request that the Board approve any deviations from currently approved recruitment policy.
- The Recruitment Activities Committee will consist of five (5) voting members:
  - The Director of Physician Support Services, who will also serve as permanent Chair of this Committee
  - The Hospital's Chief Financial Officer
  - Two members-at-large from the active medical staff, appointed for one- (1) year terms by the Chief of the Hospital's Medical Staff
  - A member-at-large from the community the Hospital serves. This community member-at-large may not be a Hospital employee, a member of the Hospital's Medical Staff, or a current Hospital Board Member, and must reside within the Hospital's service area. This community member-at-large will be appointed for a two- (2) year term by the Chairman of the Board of Trustees.

Responsibilities. This Committee shall have the following responsibilities:

- Approving or rejecting specific recruitment contracts. The RAC may approve contracts only as long as all of the terms of each contract adhere to the Board-approved physician recruitment policies currently in force. All approved contracts must be reported to the full Hospital Board at its next scheduled meeting.

- Transactions approved by the RAC that conform to Hospital recruitment policies shall not require full Board approval unless the dollar amount of the commitment to a particular physician or medical practice exceeds $250,000, or unless Board authorization is otherwise necessary for legal implementation and documentation of the transaction.

- Transactions and physician support services that conform to established Hospital recruitment policies and guidelines shall not require full Board approval unless the dollar amount of the commitment to a particular physician or medical practice exceeds $250,000 or unless Board authorization is otherwise necessary for legal implementation and documentation of the transaction.

- If, after review, the RAC feels that contractual terms have merit but deviate from approved physician recruitment policies, the RAC may request an approval of the deviation. This request from the RAC will be communicated to the Chairman of the Recruitment Policy Committee, who will be required to convey the request to the overall Hospital Board for approval or rejection.

- The Hospital's Chief Financial Officer, as a member of the RAC, will report the financial terms of all executed recruitment contracts to the Finance Subcommittee of the Hospital's Board. These reports will be for informational purposes only.

- The RAC will present a quarterly written report to the Finance Subcommittee of the Hospital's Board. This report will be prepared by the Chairman of the RAC. The quarterly report will summarize the financial status of all ongoing (active) recruitment contracts, including funds advanced, adherence to financial reporting requirements, and status of repayments.

- The Chairman of the RAC will have ongoing monitoring responsibilities and will report all nonfinancial compliance matters to the RAC, as needed.

- The RAC will not have the authority or responsibility to control day-to-day recruitment activities carried out by Hospital personnel (e.g., site visits, contract negotiations, and acquisition of search firm contracts). Responsibility and authority for conducting these activities will reside with the Director of Physician Support Services, who will report to the Hospital's Chief Executive Officer.

OVERVIEW OF STANDARD CONTRACTUAL ELEMENTS

In view of the rapidly evolving and certainly more complex regulatory environment facing hospitals, constructing a recruitment contract that is both legal and competitive is becoming more difficult. One way to accomplish both of these goals is to adhere to a well-planned contractual format.

Although there can be no rigid standard format for all hospital recruitment contracts, most comprehensive recruitment contracts contain at least eight contractual elements, as described below.

Element I—Recitals

Most contracts contain a series of factual statements, or "recitals," that explain the overriding reasons for striking the agreement. Recitals should be placed near the beginning of the agreement, after the date and identification of the parties involved in the transaction. Each recital statement customarily begins with the word "whereas."

This part of the contract should at least include statements alluding to the physician's desire to relocate and need for assistance to relocate his or her practice to a hospital's service area.

*Sample Contract Language*_____

WHEREAS, Physician presently maintains a private medical practice in [City and State], which is outside of Hospital's service area; and

WHEREAS, Physician has expressed an interest and desire to establish a private practice and provide medical services to persons residing in Hospital's service area, and has requested assistance from Hospital in relocating to this service area.

- Language establishing a hospital's not-for-profit status

*Sample Contract Language*_____

WHEREAS, the Hospital is a [Name of State] not-for-profit corporation recognized as exempt from income tax pursuant to Section 501(c)(3) of the Internal Revenue Code. The Hospital is organized and operated for the purpose of promoting and providing health care services to the public.

- Language linking the charitable, scientific, and educational mission of a hospital to recruitment activities

*Sample Contract Language*_____

WHEREAS, the Hospital has determined that it is in the public interest and consistent with the Hospital's charitable, scientific, and educational purposes for it to encourage and assist qualified physicians to practice in the [Name of Service Area] area.

- The community's need for additional physicians in the recruit's specialty. *Note that including language referencing community need or community benefits in the Recitals section further documents that a hospital has an appropriate "paper trail" to justify recruitment of each physician.*

*Sample Contract Language*_____

WHEREAS, the Hospital has documented that the [Name of Service Area] area is medically underserved with respect to the presence and availability of physicians specializing in [Name of Recruited Physician's Specialty]. In addition, the Hospital's Medical Staff Development Plan calls for the recruitment of physicians to serve the public within the [Name of Service Area] area.

Element II—Obligations of the Hospital

Every contract should include a detailed enumeration of both the incentives to be provided and the conditions under which the benefits are to be granted. Specifically, the following should be included:

- Specification of the benefits to be provided by a hospital and the terms under which the benefits are to be provided
- Specification of any other obligations of a hospital

Sample Contract Language

Hospital shall lend sums of money to Physician to guarantee that for the first year of practice, commencing on or about [Practice Starting Date], Physician shall receive actual net compensation, before payment of withholding taxes, equal to [Amount of Guarantee] per year. Hospital shall also reimburse Physician for the actual cost of a professional mover to relocate Physician's furniture and personal belongings from [Present Location] to [Area Where Hospital is Located]. These moving expenses shall be subject to prior review and written approval of Hospital's Chief Financial Officer, but in no event shall they exceed $_____.

Element III—Obligations of the Physician

The obligations of a physician must be defined with the same degree of detail as a hospital's obligations.

Specification of the physician's obligations should include, at a minimum, the following:

- Establishment of a private practice of medicine in a hospital's service area for rendering of medical services on a full-time basis

Sample Contract Language

Physician shall practice medicine on a full-time basis and shall maintain regular office hours for the public as are usual and customary in the greater [Name of Service Area or City] area for physicians in the specialty of [Name of Physician's Specialty].

- Maintenance of a license to practice medicine with no restrictions or limitations

Physician shall maintain his license in the State of [Name of State] in good standing throughout the term of this Agreement with such licensure not containing any restrictions or conditions that affect Physician's ability to practice medicine.

- Maintenance of current drug registrations

Sample Contract Language

Physician shall maintain current and unrestricted federal (DEA) and state narcotic registrations.

- Maintenance of active membership on a hospital's medical staff

Sample Contract Language

Physician shall maintain Active Status on the Medical Staff of Hospital in good standing throughout the term of this Agreement.

- Compliance with a hospital's bylaws and all other rules, regulations, and procedures of a hospital and its medical staff

Sample Contract Language

Physician agrees to comply at all times during the term of this Agreement with the following, which may be amended or adopted from time to time by the Hospital: (a) Hospital Bylaws; (b) the Medical Staff Bylaws of Hospital; (c) all other rules, regulations, procedures, and policies of Hospital and the Medical Staff; (d) all applicable federal, state, and local laws and regulations; and (e) all policies, rules, and procedures of any and all authorities relating to licensure and regulation of the medical services provided by Physician.

- Compliance with all ethical and legal standards relating to the practice of medicine

Sample Contract Language

Physician shall at all times engage in his or her profession in accordance with the generally accepted standards of Physician's profession and shall faithfully adhere to the standards and principles of medical ethics of the American Medical Association and all other associations or boards concerned with Physician's area of medical expertise.

- Maintenance of malpractice insurance coverage with such minimum amounts and limits as required by a hospital

Sample Contract Language

Physician shall obtain and maintain malpractice insurance with the minimum limits of _____ Dollars ($_____) per occurrence and _____ Dollars ($_____) in aggregate, or in such other amounts as required by Hospital throughout the term of this Agreement. Upon request of Hospital from time to time, Physician shall furnish adequate proof of such insurance coverage to Hospital.

- Compliance with certain Medicare and Medicaid requirements. *Note that Section 1395(X)(V), subparagraph (I) of the Social Security Act concerns access by the Comptroller General to physician records. See Exhibit 3-1, Access to Records, for a copy of this requirement.*

Sample Contract Language

Physician recognizes that Hospital is a participant in various third-party payment programs including, without limitation, Medicare and Medicaid, as well as various managed care programs, in which participation is essential to the ability to deliver health care. Physician agrees to cooperate fully with Hospital and provide assistance for participation in payment associated with such programs. Such cooperation shall include, but is not be limited to, the following:

1. Physician agrees that, if this Agreement is subject to Social Security Act 1395 (x)(V)(I), as it may be amended from time to time, Physician shall perform the obligations as may be from time to time specified for sub-contractors in the Social Security Act and the regulations promulgated pursuant thereto.
2. Physician agrees to make available at the Hospital such information and records as Hospital may reasonably request to facilitate Hospital's compliance with the requirements of the Medicare Conditions of Participation and the Medicaid Provider Agreement and, if applicable, to facilitate Hospital's substantiation of its reasonable costs in accordance with the requirements applicable to Hospital pursuant to the Medicare and Medicaid programs.
3. Physician must agree to treat federal health care program patients in a nondiscriminatory manner.

- If the recruited physician is to be a hospital employee, compliance with additional regulations and standards.

Sample Contract Language

Furthermore, Physician shall comply with all applicable statutes, rules, regulations, and standards of any governmental authorities and accreditation bodies that relate to Physician and Hospital.

Element IV—Prohibitions against Requiring Certain Obligations

It is equally important to include the following statements that specifically prohibit requiring certain obligations from a physician:

- There must not be any requirement that a recruited physician make referrals to, be in a position to make or influence referrals to, or otherwise generate business for a hospital as a condition for receiving the recruitment incentives.
- The amount or value of the recruitment incentives provided by a hospital must not vary based on the volume, or value of any referrals to, or business otherwise generated for a hospital by a recruited physician.

Sample Contract Language

Hospital and Physician understand and agree that nothing contained in this Agreement shall in any way require or suggest that Physician refer patients or admit patients to the Hospital at any time whatsoever. Physician shall be absolutely free to refer or admit patients to any hospital or other healthcare facility that Physician, in consultation with Physician's patients, deems appropriate without loss of any benefits whatsoever under this Agreement.

- A recruited physician must not be restricted from establishing medical staff privileges at, referring any patients or services to, or otherwise generating any business for any other hospital or health care organization of his or her choosing.

Sample Contract Language

Although Physician shall be required to maintain active professional staff privileges in his or her specialty at the Hospital and fulfill the obligations of a staff member as defined by the Professional Staff Bylaws, Physician shall be completely free to maintain professional staff privileges at any other area hospital and healthcare facility of his or her choosing.

Element V—Terms of Financial Benefits

The majority of financial benefits provided to a recruited physician are usually conveyed through a "start-up" or "income guarantee" loan. A hospital should specify the exact terms of the loan, including the following:

- A statement that this is, in fact, a loan that must eventually be paid back
- Specification of any required collateral, promissory notes, or credit reports
- The method in which money is to be advanced (lent)
- A statement that the benefits are not to exceed a term of three years

Sample Contract Language

Hospital shall lend Physician sums of money to guarantee that for the first year of practice, Physician shall receive actual net compensation, before payment or withholding of taxes, equal to [Amount of Monthly Net Income Guarantee] per year after payment of the Overhead Expenses, computed on a monthly basis.

For example, if Physician has an annual Income Guarantee in the amount of $80,000, and monthly Overhead Expenses are $3,400, the income guarantee would be computed as follows:

$5000 Monthly Gross Receipts
–3400 <u>Monthly Overhead Expenses</u>
$1600 Actual Net Compensation from Practice

$6666 Monthly Income Guaranty
–1600 <u>Actual Net Compensation from Practice</u>
$5066 Amount of Loan Funds Advanced by Hospital

Payment of any loan monies to be advanced by Hospital to Physician shall occur on or before the fifteenth (15th) day of each month provided Physician's monthly "Verification of Receipts and Overhead Expenses" report has been received by Hospital.

- The maximum term of the payout and payback (repayment) periods must be defined. *Note that for a more detailed specification and sample contract language on Repayment, see the "Practice Start-up Loans and Income Guarantee Loans" on page 98.*
- Each contract should specify a cap on the total funds that can be advanced.
- The monthly administrative verification of gross receipts and overhead expenses must be described.

Sample Contract Language

Beginning on [First Day of Loan] and each month thereafter for one (1) year, Physician shall verify in writing to Hospital, Physician's reasonable Overhead Expenses in a "Verification of Receipts and Overhead Expenses" report of the Hospital's design. This report shall be received on or before the fifteenth (15th) day of each month.

Overhead Expenses shall mean those reasonable costs and expenses directly related to operation of the practice. These costs and expenses include the following:

1. Office rent and utilities
2. Property insurance
3. Professional liability insurance premiums or other insurance required by this contract
4. Health and accidental disability insurance
5. Employee salaries, payroll taxes, and reasonable fringe benefits
6. Office and clinical supplies
7. Telephone costs

Reasonable Overhead Expenses shall not include any personal expenses such as personal automobile, personal debt or loans, and payments to Physician's deferred compensation plan.

- The interest rate to be charged and terms of its accrual must be specified.
- The interest rate must be consistent with current commercial market rates (e.g., 1–2% above national prime lending rate, commercial market rates charged by local banks).
- The administrative oversight requirements by a hospital must be specified (e.g., periodic review of the physician's books and records to verify the continued advancement of funds).

Sample Contract Language

Hospital shall have reasonable access to Physician's financial records and reports during normal business hours to verify the Overhead Expenses and the amount of the loan guarantee income as well as to audit Physician for compliance under Section [Number of Pertinent Section], above.

If a hospital offers an alternative to cash as the means of repayment, usually by "forgiving" a portion of the loan through continued hospital and community service, the following should apply:

- Where there is an alternate method of repayment through service, there must be a true community need or additional community benefits conveyed by a physician during each year of the loan forgiveness.
- The specific services driving forgiveness must be delineated. *Note that it will be important to notify each physician that all forgiven amounts will generate an IRS Form 1099 by the hospital and will likely be treated as income to the physician by the IRS.*
- The services should be of a manner that is above and beyond the services that a physician would engage in as a normal part of conducting a medical practice. (An example of a forgiveness service might be requiring a physician to participate in supervision of a hospital's family practice residents.)

For a more detailed description of alternate repayment methods, see "Start-Up and Income Guarantee Loans" on p. XX.

Element VI—Conditions of Termination or Default

- Each agreement should contain language describing those events that would immediately terminate the contractual relationship. Any of these events would typically trigger a cessation of further support by a hospital and also cause immediate or accelerated repayment of funds advanced to a recruited physician.
- The hospital's policy regarding default under a physician's recruitment contract should provide that reasonable collection efforts will be taken in the event of nonpayment by a physician, including, if necessary, legal action to collect all sums owing.
- Hospitals should be aware that if defaults are ignored, especially monetary defaults, the federal government could view such action as payment for patient referrals to the hospital or as a violation of the prohibition against

private inurement or private benefit concerning a tax-exempt Section 501(c)(3) hospital corporation.

- Events triggering termination or default should include, at a minimum, the following:
  - ○ Physician leaving a hospital's service area
  - ○ Physician ceasing to operate a full-time practice in a hospital's service area for any reason (e.g., disability, voluntary cessation)
  - ○ Physician ceasing to retain an unrestricted license to practice medicine in the state (i.e., license revocation, surrender, or suspension)
  - ○ Physician ceasing to retain staff privileges at a hospital through revocation, nonrenewal, resignation, or suspension of staff privileges for more than 60 days
  - ○ Physician failing to personally staff a specified weekly average of hours in his or her private office
  - ○ Physician failing to secure and maintain appropriate and adequate insurance (i.e., minimum amounts and limits as required by a hospital) to cover medical malpractice, personal property loss, and other insurable professional risk for which the physician is responsible
  - ○ Physician failing to participate actively on medical staff committees to which he or she is assigned. "Active participation" is defined by attendance minimums contained in the Medical staff bylaws of a hospital.
  - ○ Physician failing to perform any other obligations, duties, or conditions to be observed or performed by a physician
  - ○ On occurrence of physician's death

All of these events are subject to specific time limits before going into effect, such as "disabled for more than 30 days."

Sample Contract Language

If Physician shall fail or refuse to perform all of his or her obligations or meet his or her duties under this Agreement, Hospital shall give Physician written notice specifying the nature of such failure or refusal. If Physician does not substantially cure such failure or refusal within thirty (30) days after receipt of the notice, Hospital shall have the right, upon further written notice to Physician, to declare Physician in default and to terminate this Agreement immediately.

However, if Physician's license to practice medicine in the State of [Name of State] is restricted, revoked, canceled, surrendered, or suspended so that Physician does not maintain the ability to practice medicine in a full and unrestricted manner and such condition continues for more than a thirty-(30) day continuous period, this Agreement may, at the option of the Hospital, be summarily terminated by giving notice of the termination to Physician.

If Physician ceases the practice of medicine in the Hospital's service area, this Agreement may be summarily terminated by giving notice to Physician. Upon such termination, no further forgiveness of the loans shall accrue, and thereafter the then-remaining unpaid and unforgiven portions thereof shall be paid in full in accordance with their terms, and the payment of any other sums by Hospital hereunder shall also terminate.

- There should also be a separate "termination/acceleration clause" in the event that any future state or federal legislation, regulation, statute, or governmental interpretation makes any part of the agreement invalid or jeopardizes a hospital's tax-exempt status.

Sample Contract Language

In the event of future legislation, government rule or regulation, policy, or governmental interpretation thereof that applies to this Agreement and prohibits or invalidates any of its provisions, or causes either the Hospital or Physician not to qualify under or otherwise be in violation of any Medicare or Medicaid reimbursement regulations, or if the Hospital's continuing ability to qualify as a tax-exempt 501(c)(3) corporation is in jeopardy at any time as determined by the Hospital, then the parties hereto shall either forthwith cause to be made to this Agreement such amendments as may be reasonably required to bring its terms back into compliance or, in the alternative, terminate this Agreement. In the event of termination, Physician shall immediately pay back all sums of money owed to the Hospital, including interest, unless other means of repayment are approved by the Hospital.

Element VII—Miscellaneous Concluding Statements

Each contract should contain a variety of standard legal statements. The specific clauses to be included depend on current laws and regulations, as well as on the opinion of legal counsel. At a minimum, however, each contract should include statements relating to the following:

- The fact that the contract constitutes the "entire agreement" between the parties (i.e., there are no additional verbal agreements or understandings not included in the contract). *The language terminating prior agreements is especially important in cases in which the recruited physician has received a letter of intent or similar document, and the final contractual terms differ from those contained in the letter of intent.*

Sample Contract Language

This Agreement constitutes the entire understanding between the parties, and all prior negotiations and understandings between the parties have been merged into this Agreement. There are no understandings, representations, or agreements—either oral, written, or implied—other than those set forth herein; and all prior agreements are expressly terminated as of the effective date of this Agreement. Waiver of any provision of this Agreement shall not be deemed a waiver of future compliance therewith, and such provisions shall remain in full force and effect.

- Language specifying that no part of the agreement can be modified without the written consent of both parties

*Sample Contract Language*_____

No amendment, waiver, change, modification, or termination of any of the terms, provisions, or conditions of this Agreement shall be effective unless made in writing and signed or initialed by all parties.

- The person or place where any required notice is to be delivered

*Sample Contract Language*_____

Until changed by a similar notice in writing, written notices given or required to be given under this Agreement shall be deemed duly served when personally received by one of the parties set forth below; or in lieu of such personal service, when deposited in the U.S. mail, by certified mail, postage prepaid, return receipt requested, or with a recognized overnight courier such as Federal Express, Airborne, or UPS, and addressed as follows:
If sent to Hospital:

[Name, Title, and Business Address of Hospital's Representative]

If sent to Physician:

[Name, Degree, and Business Address of Physician]

- Language addressing assignment of rights and duties

*Sample Contract Language*_____

Physician shall not assign any rights nor delegate any duty under this Agreement. Physician, however, at any time may form a professional corporation of which Physician retains controlling interest and to which Physician may assign rights and delegate all duties under this Agreement. If a professional corporation is formed, Physician shall remain personally responsible and obligated as a guarantor of the obligations of the corporation to the Hospital. In the event of any such assignment, Hospital shall be notified in advance in writing, and this Agreement shall be amended to the extent necessary to reflect the formulation of the professional corporation as a party to this Agreement.

Element VIII—Exhibits

Frequently, the body of a recruitment agreement will reference specific documents or require completion of additional legal instruments. Hospitals should attach copies of pertinent documents as exhibits to recruitment agreements when appropriate. Examples of such exhibits include the following:

- Excerpts from a hospital's medical staff development plan substantiating the quantitative community need for the recruited physician
- A copy of the promissory note
- A copy of Form UCC-1 (financing statement) if used to secure a loan
- A copy of a mortgage if used to secure a loan

Exhibit 3-2, found at the end of this section, provides a sample of a complete physician recruitment contract containing all eight standard contractual elements. This is only a sample of a recruitment contract and should not be considered a "model" or "recommended" contract for individual hospitals. Always consult legal counsel about drafting physician recruitment contracts.

POLICIES APPLYING TO SPECIFIC RECRUITMENT INCENTIVES

The following sections address specific recruitment incentives in detail. It is important to remember that in addition to the specific requirements and legal documentation discussed in each section, each of these incentives also must adhere to the "General Guiding Principles" described in Part I of this book.

Practice Start-Up Loans and Income Guarantee Loans

Any hospital should be able to offer a start-up or income guarantee loan to qualified recruits, provided that this benefit is clearly structured as a loan that must be paid back in cash or through an alternative form of repayment (e.g., a specific work-off arrangement). Automatic forgiveness and other arrangements that eliminate specific payback requirements are not truly loan agreements and should not be offered as benefit options.

Provision of start-up or income guarantee loans to recruited physicians is an area that is receiving increased scrutiny from federal agencies. The May 1992 Special Fraud Alert (see Exhibit 2-3) listed "income . . . guarantees" and "low-interest or interest-free loans, or loans which may be 'forgiven' if a physician refers patients to the hospital," as 2 of 10 "suspect" arrangements between physicians and hospitals.

Requirements

All start-up loans and income guarantee loans should be extended to physicians pursuant to the following requirements and conditions:

- The loan rates, terms, and conditions must be reasonable and consistent with commercial market rates, terms, and conditions. These should include an interest rate of at least the prevailing prime rate plus 1–2%, or a commercially reasonable local market ("fair market") rate. The loan documents should also provide for adequate security to ensure the loan's repayment (e.g., financing statement regarding accounts receivable, equipment).

- Any variance in loan rates, terms, and conditions from commercially reasonable loan arrangements must be treated as income to the physician and reported in a timely fashion on the appropriate federal income tax reporting form (e.g., IRS Form 1099). *It is especially important that every hospital also inform physicians of any amounts that the IRS is likely to consider personal income, which will trigger income tax liability for these physicians. This notification should be made in writing to the physician, preferably before any funds are advanced.*
- The loan must have a payback requirement.
- The payout ("income support" or "draw") portion of the loan must be no more than 24 months in duration.
- The total term of the loan (payout and payback portions) must be 60 months or less. If the loan is forgivable, it must be worked down over at least 4 years.
- There must be a cap on the total amount of the loan.
- Interest should be computed from the first day any funds are advanced and must accrue throughout all sections of the loan (i.e., from the date the loan is funded).
- Generally, there will be no payments of principal or interest during the first year, although interest should continue to accrue. In the second year, monthly payments of interest only may be made. Beginning in the third year, monthly payments of principal and interest should be made over 3 years or less, depending on the size of the loan and a physician's ability to repay the loan.
- There must be no "related referral requirement" contained in the loan documents or implied outside their context. Any physician should be free to refer patients to any hospital and to join the staffs of any other hospitals he or she desires without any loss of benefits under the recruitment agreement.
- There must be no influence exerted whatsoever as to where a physician refers his or her patients for treatment. The hospital should inform every physician about the Fraud and Abuse Statute contained in the Social Security Act and also warn that any solicitation or receipt of incentives in exchange for referrals would be a violation of the act and subject to criminal charges, civil monetary penalties, and exclusion from the Medicare program. This last sanction potentially applies to both physicians and hospitals.
- A hospital should attempt to obtain a physician's personal guarantee and a security interest in collateral sufficient in value to secure the full repayment of the loan.
- In determining whether to extend a loan, a hospital should perform due diligence as to a physician's creditworthiness, including considering each physician's history of payment on any prior loans.

- Specifically, it is best if each physician agrees to a preapproval credit search and periodic review of records according to the following guidelines:
  - Each physician should agree to a credit search and demonstrate a satisfactory credit risk profile to be eligible for a loan.
  - Each physician should be required to submit a net worth statement at the initiation of a loan.

Sample Contract Language

Prior to the advancement of any loan funds under this Agreement, Physician shall agree to allow Hospital to demonstrate a satisfactory credit risk profile of Physician through a credit search by a professional credit agency.

Physician also agrees to submit a Net Worth Statement to Hospital prior to advancement of any loan funds.

- Each physician should agree to a review of books and records (personal, professional corporation, etc.) by the hospital at specified times before and during the loan payout. This inspection should be conducted no less than every 6 months during the payout section of the loan. Usually, the hospital's chief financial officer is responsible for implementing this provision.

Sample Contract Language

Hospital shall have reasonable access to Physician's financial records and reports during normal business hours to verify the overhead expenses and the amount of loan funds advanced to guarantee income, as well as to audit Physician for compliance with obligations listed in Section [Location of Pertinent Section of the Contract], above.

- There should be documentation that financial arrangements are prudent from an investment standpoint and that any income guarantees are reasonable.
- There should be documentation of the need to recruit physicians in that particular specialty to a hospital and its service area community.
- There should be documentation that, in its determination of the loan amount, a hospital considered the reluctance of a physician to initiate or relocate his or her practice in an unfamiliar area, as well as documentation of the competitive recruitment efforts of other hospitals in the area, the state, and the nation.

Legal Documentation

Legal documentation of loan arrangements should include a loan agreement setting forth, at a minimum, the following:

- Loan amount and interest rate
- Repayment requirements
- Event triggering immediate repayment (termination events)

- Security for the loan, preferably including at least a life insurance policy securing the unpaid loan balance

Sample Contract Language

The policy shall name the Hospital as the beneficiary. Physician shall furnish Hospital with a Certificate of Insurance or other satisfactory evidence to show that the policy is in effect and that the beneficiary cannot be changed, nor can the policy be terminated or canceled without prior notice to and approval of Hospital.

Until all loans described in this Agreement are either repaid or forgiven in whole, Physician shall obtain and keep in force a decreasing term life insurance policy on his life in an amount at least equal to the unpaid principal and accrued interest on the loan from the Hospital.

If Physician should die before full payment of the loan or before it becomes fully forgiven by the Hospital pursuant to the above conditions, the insurance proceeds shall be considered as liquidated damages and shall also be paid to the Hospital to fully discharge Physician's indebtedness to the Hospital.

Physician shall furnish Hospital with the Certificate of Insurance or other evidence that the policy is in effect within thirty (30) days of the effective date of this Agreement. If Physician fails to provide satisfactory evidence of insurance by that time, no additional funds will be advanced until such time as evidence of insurance is provided:

- Conditions of loan and borrower's affirmative covenants, including physician obligations under basic contract requirements, as applicable
- That there are no related referral requirements or restrictions on where the physician refers patients
- Events of default
- A promissory note. (See Exhibit 3-3, Example of a Practice Support Promissory Note.)

Sample Contract Language

Contemporaneously with the effective date of this Agreement, Physician shall execute a promissory note in an amount equal to the maximum amount that may be disbursed pursuant to the terms described in Section [Location of Pertinent Section] of this Agreement. The promissory note shall be in the form attached hereto as Exhibit [Location of Pertinent Exhibit].

- A security agreement against personal property or fixtures, or mortgage or second mortgage against any real estate owned by the physician, setting forth, at a minimum, the following:
  - Grant of security interest and description of collateral in which security interest is granted
  - Specification of the obligations secured
  - The borrower's representations and warranties
  - Events of default and rights of parties.

State laws vary concerning required documents. Please consult hospital or other legal counsel for specific requirements for each transaction.

- In case of loan guarantee, documents listed above should exist between the bank extending the loan and the physician. The bank and the hospital enter into a guarantee agreement. To the extent the guarantee agreement is secured, there would be a separate security agreement between the hospital and the physician, subordinated to the security interest granted the bank and Form UCC-1.
- Form UCC-1 (see Exhibit 3-4 for Example Form UCC-1)

*Sample Contract Language*_____

Physician shall grant a Form UCC-1 (UCC Financing Statement) to help secure the loan.

Physician shall also grant a mortgage on any real estate owned by Physician to help secure the loan.

- Each start-up loan proposal should be accompanied by specific documentation regarding the nonmonetary value of each applicant to each hospital and community; that is, documentation on how the recruit's presence in the hospital's service area will "increase efficiency and enhance productivity for the hospital" (per GCM 39498).

Traditional Repayment

Start-up and income guarantee loans traditionally are repaid in cash, with interest. Repayment language should reflect the following:

- The accrual rate of the interest on loan funds advanced

*Sample Contract Language*_____

All loan amounts owing to Hospital by Physician shall accrue interest from the date the funds are advanced, at the rate of two (2) points above the prime rate as published in the *Wall Street Journal*, on January 1, 20___, and adjusted annually.

- The terms of repayment

*Sample Contract Language*_____

From [Starting Date of Loan] until [12th Month of Loan], there shall be no payments of principal or interest due.

From [13th Month of Loan] until [24th Month of Loan], payment shall be made for interest only on the first day of each month.

From [25th Month of Loan] until [Last Month of the Loan], repayment of principal and interest shall be made in equal monthly installments amortized over [Number of Years] years.

- Any penalties for failure to make full and timely payments
- The terms for early repayment based on excess earnings during the guaranty period

Sample Contract Language

If, in any month during the first twelve (12) months following Physician's commencement of his or her Practice in accordance with Section [Number of Pertinent Section] of this Agreement, Net Income of Physician exceeds [Amount of Monthly Income Guarantee], Physician shall repay outstanding amounts previously paid by Hospital pursuant to Section [Number of Pertinent Section] above to the extent of such excess. Physician shall make such payment to Hospital upon Hospital's receipt of the monthly "Verification of Receipts and Overhead Expenses" report.

Alternative Repayment ("Loan Forgiveness")

As noted in the introduction to this section, the concept of automatic forgiveness of loans should not be permitted with respect to transactions entered into by a hospital. However, a hospital can make arrangements with physicians for the physician to repay the loan by service in kind, more commonly known as "work-off."

Loan forgiveness should adhere to the following principles:

- The work-off must be a service above and beyond the service that the physician would normally conduct as part of a routine medical practice.
- The amount of the loan offset by the work-off should be reasonably correlated with actual services provided and time spent.
- The work-off activities themselves should be designed to enhance the health care and health status of the community or a segment thereof.
- At the time any portion of the loan is forgiven, make sure that there continues to exist a quantitative community need for the physician or that significant community benefits continue to be conveyed. These should be reevaluated annually to ensure the continuing community need or benefits at the time the loan amount is being forgiven.
- Also, if the physician ceases to have active privileges at a hospital but continues to practice in the service area and continues to meet the forgiveness criteria, forgiveness must continue as community benefits (versus specific benefits to the hospital) continue to be conveyed.

Sample Contract Language

As an alternative means of repayment of loans, the Hospital shall acknowledge that one fifth (1/5) of the principal balance and accrued interest on the Promissory Note from Physician to Hospital has been paid beginning on [Date] and one fifth (1/5) of the principal balance and accrued interest on [Anniversary of Date] of each year thereafter if Physician has met all of the following requirements:

- Physician shall be in full-time practice of medicine in [City and State], and Physician's services are available to the public as described in this agreement.
- Physician shall work a normal workweek as may be required of other physicians in the area who practice in Physician's specialty.
- Physician shall in no way restrict the number of Medicare and Medicaid patients who are seen or treated by Physician.
- Physician shall accept patients referred by the Hospital's referral service regardless of the patient's ability to pay.
- Physician shall not limit the number of indigent or charitable patients seen or treated. Physician shall keep a record of all such patients and make those records available to the Hospital upon request.
- Physician shall assist the Hospital in its educational program regarding residents so as to enhance the Hospital's position as a teaching institution. The educational duties of Physician shall be mutually agreed upon by Physician and the Hospital's Director of Medical Education.
- Physician shall be placed on the on-call list of the Hospital's emergency room and, when called and when available, shall see and treat patients in the emergency room regardless of the patients' ability or inability to pay for service.
- Physician, if requested, shall assist in fundraising efforts for the Foundation in order to promote the charitable and educational purposes of the Foundation and the Hospital.
- Physician shall provide reasonable assistance to the Hospital in its physician recruitment programs.
- Physician shall maintain active professional staff privileges in Physician's specialty at Hospital and fulfill the obligations of a staff member as defined by the Professional Staff Bylaws; however, there shall be no requirements whatsoever concerning where Physician shall admit patients.

The following items also should be addressed in view of current tax and safe harbor considerations:

- The recruited physician should be carefully advised that the hospital cannot give him or her tax advice or legal advice, including any advice concerning forgivable loans.

To help avoid future ill will, the physician should be told in advance that an IRS Form 1099 will be issued for each year that a loan is forgiven. The physician should be alerted that the loan forgiveness probably will constitute taxable income in the years it is forgiven. It should be documented in the agreement that the physician was instructed to consult with his or her own tax and legal advisors for advice.

Sample Contract Language

Physician acknowledges and agrees that Physician has not relied on any representation or advice from Hospital or Hospital representatives concerning any legal or tax matters. Physician shall be solely responsible to obtain

Physician's own independent tax and legal advice concerning all aspects of this Agreement.

- In the last several years, the IRS has audited recruited physicians' income tax returns to see if they are reporting the income from recruitment incentives. IRS agents may request that hospitals furnish copies of recruitment contracts that, in turn, will be compared with the physician's tax returns.
- It is important to reemphasize that activity outside a safe harbor does not necessarily make that activity illegal. In view of the fact that the safe harbor regulations are narrow in scope, however, hospitals should be extremely careful if they wish to consider forgivable loans in the future. If a forgivable loan is necessary to recruit a physician seriously needed by the community, the loan should be implemented only after consultation with legal counsel specializing in health law.

SUPPORTING EXHIBITS

General Principles

In general, smaller, one-time payments may be preferable to loans, loan guarantees, and other types of recruitment and support arrangements that involve an ongoing, long-term financial commitment by a hospital.

Some one-time payments (e.g., signing bonuses) are apt to be more suspect to the OIG and IRS than payments for incentives such as relocation expenses. Signing bonuses are more suspicious because they cannot be traced to money that actually has been expended, as opposed to incentives, such as relocation expenses, on which the physician has actually expended money. As a general rule, signing bonuses should be carefully avoided. (See earlier discussion regarding the Hermann Hospital IRS Closing Agreement on p. XX.)

Requirements

One-time payments should be consistent with the following terms and conditions:

- The reasonableness of the payment or payments must be considered in combination with any other recruitment incentives being extended to a physician (i.e., overall reasonableness doctrine).
- The terms and conditions of any one-time payment to a physician should be documented in an agreement with the physician.
- If a separate loan for other reasons is being extended to a physician, one-time payment can be made a part of the loan, subject to all the requirements discussed herein for loans, and should be incorporated in the legal documentation needed for loans.
- No payment should be made until after the physician has executed the recruitment incentive agreement.

Reimbursement of Relocation Expenses

A hospital may wish to consider a reimbursement package for reasonable expenses incurred by physicians relocating to a hospital's service area. If a physician is moving his or her residence and a practice from outside the geographic area served by a hospital, then the payments should be characterized as relocation expenses. A limit or cap should be placed on the amount to be reimbursed. A hospital should retain the right to approve all expenses, either prospectively or after being given receipts.

It is important that documentation relative to the commercial reasonableness of relocation expenses is obtained and periodically updated. It is important that this documentation verify that the relocation expenses are structured parallel to recognized commercially reasonable relocation programs in a hospital's service area. Examples of such documentation could include relocation packages offered to key executives at large local corporations or comprehensive relocation services offered by national home equity companies.

Requirements

Any relocation expense reimbursement package should adhere to the following:

- There should be a cap on the amount of reimbursement provided.
- A hospital should, at a minimum, require repayment on a pro rata basis of relocation monies advanced by the hospital if a recruit leaves its service area before a certain period of time has elapsed (e.g., within the first 12 months).
- Relocation expense reimbursement should consider the following:
  - Reimbursement for the actual and reasonable charges of a professional mover to relocate the physician's property to a hospital's service area
  - Reimbursement of personal automobile expenses at a reasonable specified rate per mile, as well as the cost of hotel accommodations during trips to locate suitable housing, survey professional office space, or attend to other business related to relocation
  - Reimbursement of the cost of temporary lodging for up to a specified number of weeks for a physician and his or her family, in the event that a physician does not immediately secure a permanent residence in the hospital's service area
- It is important that there be no implication of "related referral requirements."
- The community need or benefit standards must be met.

Legal Documentation

- The specific types of relocation expenses eligible for reimbursement should be described.
- Expenses should ideally be subject to prospective review and approval to be eligible for reimbursement.
- There should be a payment cap on total expenses.

*Sample Contract Language*_____

In consideration for Physician locating a practice in Hospital's service area, Hospital agrees to reimburse Physician for the actual and reasonable costs of a professional mover to transfer Physician's furniture and personal belongings from [Present Location] to [Hospital's Service Area]. These moving expenses shall be subject to the prior review and written approval of Hospital's Chief Financial Officer before the Hospital shall be obligated to make actual payment.

In addition, Hospital shall pay Physician for reasonable expenses incurred in connection with house-hunting trips between [Present Location] and [Hospital's Service Area]. These expenses, however, shall be subject to the prior review and written approval of Hospital's Chief Financial Officer before Hospital is obligated to make payment. In no event shall the total expenses reimbursed and paid by Hospital under this paragraph exceed the sum of [Amount of Payment Cap].

If temporary housing is needed to complete relocation of Physician and Physician's immediate family to [Name of Service Area], then Hospital shall pay up to [Financial Cap in Dollars] per month for temporary housing, but not to exceed [Time Cap in Months] months.

- A hospital may wish to include a clause stipulating minimum time that must be spent in the service area to qualify for full reimbursement.

*Sample Contract Language*_____

Relocation expenses need not be repaid to Hospital, provided that Physician remains available to Hospital's service area in the full-time practice of Physician's specialty for a period of at least two (2) years following the effective date of this Agreement.

- Each hospital should include language stipulating pro rata recapture of reimbursed relocation expenses should a physician leave the service area or cease practice prematurely.

*Sample Contract Language*_____

If physician leaves the Hospital's service area or ceases the full-time practice of medicine in Physician's specialty prior to the passage of two (2) years after the effective date of this Agreement, Physician shall repay the Hospital on a pro rata basis for all sums of money advanced to Physician for relocation and moving. If, for example, Physician ceases the full-time practice of Physician's specialty after one (1) year, Physician shall repay the Hospital one half of the moving and house-hunting expenses.

Signing or Recruitment Bonus

A signing or recruitment bonus payment is a controversial type of incentive. The Hermann Hospital Closing Agreement with the IRS prohibited signing bonuses or other bonus payments. Consequently, hospitals should avoid such bonuses and should consider them a high-risk activity.

If a hospital nevertheless feels that paying a bonus is necessary to recruit a physician, it should consider the following suggestions:

- The reasonableness of the bonus payment must be considered in combination with any other recruitment incentives being offered (i.e., overall reasonableness doctrine).
- The terms and conditions of the signing bonus should be documented in a written agreement with the physician.
- No monies should be advanced to the physician until after the physician has executed the agreement.
- A specific dollar limit should be placed on how much the hospital will pay as a signing bonus.
- A hospital should require repayment of signing bonus monies, at least on a pro rata basis, if a recruited physician prematurely leaves the local service area before a certain amount of time has elapsed (e.g., within the first year of practice).
- There must be no implication of "related referral requirements."
- Any recruit receiving a signing bonus should meet community need or benefit standards.

Legal Documentation

- The agreement should include a description of the community need for a physician, and anticipated community benefits should be included in the agreement.

Sample Contract Language_____

Hospital has established through its Physician Manpower Study that there exists a shortage of practitioners in Physician's specialty in the [Geographic Location] area, and that the access to care in Physician's specialty will be increased through the recruitment of Physician to the [Geographic Location].

- The agreement should detail specific terms of the payment.

Sample Contract Language_____

The hospital shall pay a one-time Recruitment Incentive Bonus payment to Physician in the amount of [Amount of the Signing Bonus]. These funds shall be advanced to Physician no later than thirty (30) days from the effective date of this Agreement.

- A hospital may wish to include language stipulating the minimum time that must be spent in the service area to qualify for "forgiveness" of the signing bonus.

Sample Contract Language_____

The recruitment Incentive Bonus payment need not be repaid to Hospital, provided that Physician remains available to Hospital's service area in the full-time practice of Physician's specialty for a period of at least two (2) years following the effective date of this Agreement.

- Every hospital should include language stipulating pro rata repayment of signing bonus monies advanced should a physician leave the service area prematurely.

Sample Contract Language

If Physician leaves the Hospital's service area or ceases the full-time practice of medicine in Physician's specialty prior to the passage of two (2) years after the effective date of this Agreement, Physician shall repay Hospital on a pro rata basis for money advanced to Physician for the Recruitment Incentive Bonus. If, for example, Physician ceases the full-time practice of Physician's specialty after one (1) year, Physician shall repay Hospital one half of the Recruitment Incentive Bonus.

Purchase of "Tail" Medical Liability Coverage

With many physicians being forced to purchase "claims made" (versus "occurrence") medical liability insurance policies, it is essential that there be no gaps in insurance coverage resulting from their relocation from one state to another. Often continued coverage may not be available, as the recruited physician's malpractice carrier may not be licensed to provide coverage in the state to which the physician is relocating.

In selected instances, it may be necessary for a hospital to pay for the cost of an extended reporting period medical liability insurance policy (commonly referred to as a "tail insurance" policy) to allow a physician to relocate from another state; however, there does not appear to be any safe harbor for this activity. The November 19, 1999, safe harbors do permit a hospital to pay all or part of the malpractice insurance premiums for physicians engaged in obstetrical practice in primary healthcare professional shortage areas. Certified nurse midwives also are included. The safe harbor is limited to malpractice insurance regulated by state laws. Nothing in the safe harbor would authorize payment by the federal healthcare programs to hospitals for costs they may incur in providing malpractice insurance. The safe harbor is intended to facilitate access to obstetrical services for federal healthcare program beneficiaries.

Requirements

Payments for an extended reporting period medical liability insurance policy should be consistent with the following terms and conditions:

- The terms and conditions of any payment for tail insurance should be documented in a written agreement with the physician.
- A maximum dollar amount should be placed on how much a hospital will pay for this medical liability insurance policy (i.e., a cap placed on maximum potential outlay).

- The reasonableness of any payments for professional liability insurance must be considered in combination with other recruitment incentives being extended to a physician (i.e., the overall reasonableness doctrine).

Legal Documentation

- The specific reason for a hospital's payment for tail liability coverage should be listed.
- The payment of the tail liability insurance premium should be subject to a prospective approval by the hospital's chief financial officer.
- The total maximum dollar outlay (cap) should be defined.

Sample Contract Language

The Hospital shall pay a one-time premium for Physician's medical liability policy insuring against any gaps in coverage because of his or her relocation from [Present Location] to [Location of Hospital]. (This insurance is sometimes referred to as "tail insurance.") The insurance carrier and the amount of the premium shall be subject to the approval of the Hospital's Chief Financial Officer before payment. However, the maximum amount Hospital shall pay for such coverage will be [Amount of Maximum Payment] dollars, and Physician shall be required to pay the balance if this amount is not sufficient to purchase such coverage.

Professional Liability Insurance

A hospital may be requested to make payment for part or all of a recruited physician's medical liability insurance premiums to ensure that needed services are available to a hospital's patient population. In light of the Hermann Hospital Closing Agreement, hospitals should try to avoid payments for such insurance (except for hospital-employed physicians).

Physician recruitment incentives are a rapidly evolving, legally gray area. Except for the Hermann Hospital Closing Agreement, no cases or published rulings have addressed whether a tax-exempt hospital's subsidization of the professional liability (malpractice) insurance premiums of its staff physicians violates the prohibitions against private inurement and benefit. As discussed, the November 19, 1999, safe harbors address only payment for obstetrical insurance premiums in primary healthcare professional shortage areas.

In the comments to these safe harbors, the OIG noted that the safe harbors do not call into question the legality of all other types of practitioner malpractice insurance subsidies. Moreover, the fact that a payment practice does not fall within the scope of a safe harbor does not necessarily mean that the practice violates the Anti-Kickback Statute. The OIG, however, went on to comment that malpractice insurance subsidies paid to or on behalf of potential referral sources might be suspect under the statutes. These arrangements are subject to a case-by-case evaluation. The advisory opinion process is available for parties seeking OIG guidance on the anti-kickback implications of particular insurance subsidy arrangements.

Accordingly, great care should be taken in structuring any professional liability insurance subsidy for a recruited physician, including obtaining an advisory opinion from the OIG concerning a particular insurance subsidy arrangement.

The following are some suggested standards to consider if a hospital feels compelled to pay for a physician's medical liability insurance premiums.

Requirements

If a hospital wishes to pay for insurance despite the risks, payments for professional liability insurance should be consistent with the following terms and conditions:

- The private benefit conferred to a physician through the provision of professional liability insurance must not be more than incidental.
- The cost of providing the professional liability insurance to a physician must be insubstantial in light of total hospital revenues, expenses, and activities.
- Significant community benefit should be specifically documented. Examples include improvement in quality of care, reduction in malpractice insurance, and liability costs.
- The reasonableness of any payments for professional liability insurance must be considered in combination with all other recruitment incentives being extended to a physician (i.e., overall reasonableness doctrine).
- The contract to provide malpractice insurance must not restrict a recruited physician from referring patients to other institutions.
- The contract cannot vary the amount of payment for malpractice insurance based on the level or number of referrals a physician makes to a hospital.
- A bona fide insurance policy must be issued to ensure that this provision is not used as a mechanism to disguise an improper financial inducement to a physician.

Legal Documentation

- The terms and conditions of any payment to a physician for professional liability insurance should be documented in a written agreement with the physician.
- Upon termination of any recruitment arrangement involving professional liability insurance, the recruited physician should be required to purchase tail insurance or reimburse the hospital for its purchase of such insurance.
- A maximum dollar amount should be placed on how much a hospital will pay for professional liability insurance.

Sample Contract Language

Hospital shall provide Physician, at Hospital's cost and expense, professional liability insurance with minimum limits of [Amount of Liability Limit] Dollars per occurrence and [Amount of Liability Limit] Dollars annual aggregate. Hospital's actual cost for providing this insurance coverage shall not exceed [Dollar Amount of Annual Premium] per year.

Hospital shall have the right, but not the obligation, to purchase "tail coverage" if Physician terminates this Agreement at any time prior to the expiration of its term. Physician shall immediately reimburse Hospital for the premium Hospital pays for such tail coverage.

Hospital shall also have the right to withhold from any payment remaining to be made to Physician any amounts Physician is hereby required to pay for such tail coverage.

Continuing Medical Education (CME) Grants

Consistent with its educational mission, a hospital may wish to consider medical education grants to a qualified physician to encourage further training and education in his or her area of specialization (i.e., medical education grants), or to provide an additional incentive for relocating and establishing a practice in the community upon completing undergraduate and residency training (i.e., educational stipend grants). The intent of such grants is to enhance the equality of medicine practiced by local physicians, thus additionally benefiting the community.

Payment of grant monies to qualified physicians for continuing education must be linked to an agreement by the physician to convey the skills or knowledge learned to other physicians and patients in the local community, thus enhancing the overall quality of care. The agreement should encourage the physician to use and convey the new knowledge or skills anywhere in the community, not just at the sponsoring hospital (i.e., to benefit the community and not just the hospital).

The provision of educational grants for continuing medical education is an area of close governmental scrutiny. The May 1992 OIG Special Fraud Alert listed "payment for a physician's continuing education courses" and "payment of the cost of a physician's travel and expenses for conferences" as 2 of 10 "suspect" incentive arrangements. (See Exhibit 2-1, *Federal Register/* Vol. 56, No. 145/Monday, July 29, 1991/Rules and Regulations.) Furthermore, the Hermann Hospital Closing Agreement indicated that educational and related expense reimbursements should not be paid when such expenses are primarily related to the physician's private practice of medicine. Moreover, the November 19, 1999, safe harbors do not cover such payments. If a hospital wishes to proceed with such payments, it should consider the following procedures to help reduce legal risk.

Requirements

Payments for continuing education and conferences by a hospital should be consistent with the following terms and conditions:

- In the context of retention activities, such grants should be paid to established physicians only if it can be shown that the community will benefit to a significantly greater degree than the expense of the payments by the hospital.

- It should also be documented why a hospital (instead of the physician) should pay the expense; for example, attendance at conferences pertaining to their hospital duties can increase the skills and knowledge levels for physician members of a hospital's governing board, medical executive committee, and peer review committee, thus allowing them to better serve the particular hospital and its community.
- It is best if a hospital pays only a portion of the total expenses and requires the physician to shoulder a portion of the total CME conference expense (e.g., the hospital pays for transportation and tuition expenses, and the physician pays for room and board). *An exception to this policy occurs when the physician attendee is also a board member and the conference directly relates to his or her board duties. In this case, the educational grant pays all expenses, because the physician receives no personal benefit, and any educational benefits are conveyed directly to the hospital and its community.*
- As a general rule, a hospital should not limit eligibility for participation in education grants to "active admitters" only. Eligibility should rather be based on community need and benefit considerations and not on volume of admissions to a particular hospital.
- In the context of recruitment activities, the reasonableness of any grant payments to a recently recruited physician for continuing education or other educational conferences must be considered in combination with any other recruitment incentives being extended to that physician (i.e., overall reasonableness doctrine).
- Each physician participating in an educational grant program should be required to submit a written summary report on the training received or required to make an oral didactic presentation for both house staff and practicing physicians on any new information or skills acquired. Written reports and oral presentations should be made available to all physicians in the community, regardless of whether they are members of the sponsoring hospital's medical staff.

Legal Documentation

- There should be a cap on the total number of courses attended or total days allowed for attendance at these conferences.
- There should be a requirement that a hospital approve the specific conference in advance.
- Except for unique circumstances when similar training is not available, grants should be restricted to educational conferences taking place in the United States.
- Any CME conference should be sponsored by a legitimate postgraduate medical accrediting body (e.g., AMA, AAFP, AOA). Other nonclinical educational conferences should be sponsored by legitimate, widely recognized organizations.

Agreements relating to educational grants should specify the particular types of CME or educational conferences the physician is to attend. This is especially important if an educational grant is included as part of a recruitment arrangement.

Sample Contract Language

During the term of this Agreement, Physician shall be entitled to attend two (2) continuing education courses within the United States. These courses must be approved for credit by the American Medical Association or other widely recognized accrediting agency and must relate to subject matter pertinent to the practice of [Name of Physician's Field of Specialization]. These courses must be approved in advance by Hospital.

- Each agreement should specify what kinds of expenses are to be covered, as well as specifically excluded.

Sample Contract Language

Expenses eligible for reimbursement by Hospital shall include the following:

- Transportation to and from the meeting as well as local transportation to the meeting site
- Tuition expenses and any course materials or books

Physician shall be responsible for lodging and meal expenses related to these conferences. Any spousal expenses incurred in connection with these conferences shall not be reimbursed.

- Recruitment agreements should place a cap on what a hospital will pay. Each hospital should retain the right to approve expenditures in advance.

Sample Contract Language

Hospital shall reimburse Physician up to [Amount of Maximum Dollar Limit] Dollars during the term of this Agreement for specific expenses relating to attendance at these educational courses, but only to the extent such expenses have been approved in advance by Hospital.

- Each physician should be required to give the sponsoring hospital sufficient proof of participation in and completion of the educational conference or CME course (i.e., a certificate of participation or completion). Each hospital should keep these certificates on file for future documentation.

Sample Contract Language

After each educational course, Physician shall be required to supply Hospital with written certification of attendance or completion.

- Each physician should be required to share what he or she learned with physicians in the community or hospital support staff.

Sample Contract Language

Within sixty (60) days of completing each educational course, Physician shall be required to make a formal presentation or prepare a written report sharing the information gained from the educational course. Initially, this information shall be presented to an appropriate group of physicians on Hospital's staff. This information shall also be made available to any interested physician in the community.

- As a general rule, educational grants should be subject to repayment if a physician fails to meet the terms of the educational grant, thereby depriving a hospital and community of the additional expertise gained through this training.

Sample Contract Language

If Physician shall fail to comply with any of the above requirements or refuse to perform any of the above obligations, Hospital shall have the right to terminate its obligations under this section of the Agreement. In the event of termination, no further payments for educational courses shall be advanced, and Physician shall be required to pay back all sums of money previously advanced for educational courses.

Education Loans and Payment of Student Loans

Payment of student loans presently is an area receiving a high degree of scrutiny. Moreover, the November 19, 1999, safe harbors do not cover this activity. Thus, as a general policy, hospitals should avoid helping recruited physicians repay their student loans, if possible.

Most hospitals recognize, however, that there is intense competition for recruiting certain specialists or certain highly qualified physicians, and hospitals across the country are increasingly offering assistance with student loans. Consequently, assisting with student loans should not be rejected automatically if there is a unique situation or when there is an extraordinary, compelling, and well-documented community need or benefit.

Requirements

- A hospital's payment of a physician's student loan should be considered only in the context of recruiting that physician into the community.
- The reasonableness of any payments for a physician's student loans must be considered in combination with any other recruitment incentives being extended to the physician (i.e., overall reasonableness doctrine).
- A hospital's extension of other types of educational loans to physicians (e.g., loans covering costs of continuing medical education, clinical fellowships, and other education or training) will usually be considered only in the recruitment context. *An exception would typically require an unusual circumstance, for example, when a compelling community need can be demonstrated for extending a loan to a physician already established in the community served by a hospital (e.g., a loan to the only surgeon in a rural area to enable that surgeon to learn how to perform laparoscopic cholecystectomies).*

Legal Documentation

- Any payment made by a hospital for a physician's student loans should be clearly identified and documented in the recruitment agreement.
- Payment on the physician's existing student loans should ideally be made a part of any other loan a hospital is extending and should be subject to all applicable provisions affecting repayment (e.g., immediate repayment upon early termination of the agreement).
- Any educational loan extended by a hospital should be subject to all the requirements discussed in the section on loans and should be incorporated into the legal documentation needed to substantiate the offering of any loan.
- As with all loans, a hospital should attempt to secure all educational loans. Because students and physicians not yet in practice typically have few assets, a hospital may need to purchase a term life insurance policy to secure the unpaid loan balance.

Sample Contract Language

To assist Physician with his or her educational expenses during his or her final year of [Name of Specialty] residency training, the Hospital shall lend Physician the sum of [Dollar Amount] on the first day of [Month, Year] and [Dollar Amount] on the first day of each month thereafter through the _____ day of [Month and Year]. The loan shall accrue interest from the date the funds are advanced at the rate of two (2) points above the Prime Rate as published in the *Wall Street Journal* on [Day, Month, and Year], and adjusted annually. Until [Date], there shall be no payments of principal or interest due. From [Date] until [Date], payments shall be made for interest only on the first day of each month. Beginning [Date] repayment of principal and interest shall be made in equal monthly installments, amortized over three (3) years.

Use of Hospital Property and Services

Use of hospital equipment and services will likely be considered a high-profile incentive by the OIG, as "use of free or discounted . . . equipment" and "provision of free or significantly discounted . . . staff services" were both listed as suspect incentive arrangements in the May 5, 1992, Special Fraud Alert.

The November 19, 1999, safe harbors clarified that space and equipment rental and personal services and management contracts are considered to be safe harbors. First, the safe harbors preclude schemes involving the use of multiple overlapping contracts to circumvent the safe harbor requirement that space and equipment rental and personal services and management contracts be for a term of at least 1 year. This requirement is intended to prevent regular renegotiation of contracts based on the volume of referrals or business generated between the parties. Second, the safe harbors were clarified to provide protection for healthcare providers who rent more space or equipment or purchase more services than they actually need as a means of paying for referrals. Note that the safe harbors do not protect free or discounted equipment or lease incentives. If a hospital nevertheless wishes to consider such incentives, it should follow the suggested procedures below to help reduce legal risk.

Requirements

The use of a hospital's property (facilities, space, and equipment) or services by physicians in their private practice should be consistent with the following terms and conditions:

- A hospital's property or services should be made available on terms and conditions consistent with commercially reasonable fair market value arrangements.
- The arrangement should not exceed 2 years and should not be renegotiated within the first year.
- In exceptional cases, or to the extent that hospital property or services are made available on terms and conditions that are not consistent with commercially reasonable terms, there must be a clear demonstration and documentation of significant community need or benefits.
- The arrangement should not be used if the physician is already receiving an income guarantee or loan to assist in starting up a practice.
- To the extent applicable, the arrangement should be structured to fit the Medicare Fraud and Abuse Safe Harbor Regulations. For example, the components for a lease of a hospital's equipment should include the following:
  - A written and signed lease agreement
  - Specification of the equipment covered by the lease
  - A lease term of at least 1 year in duration
  - The aggregate rental charge set in advance
  - The agreement consistent with fair market value
  - Avoidance of language indicating that the charges are based on the value or volume of patient referrals

Legal Documentation

There should be a written agreement setting forth the terms and conditions of a physician's use of a hospital's property or services. Legal documentation should consist of a lease or service agreement with the following conditions:

- A description of the products or services

Sample Contract Language

The Hospital will provide Physician with [Value of Services] dollars worth of services from the Hospital's Chief Financial Officer to set up office accounting procedures within Physician's practice and to render ongoing accounting assistance.

- The rental or use rate and terms for payment of the same

Sample Contract Language_____

From [Month and Year of Initial Payment] until [Month and Year of Final Payment], Physician shall pay Hospital [Amount of Monthly Payment] per month to reimburse Hospital for the accounting services provided to Physician. Each monthly payment shall be due by the tenth (10th) day of each month.

- The duration of the agreement

Sample Contract Language_____

The term of this Agreement shall commence on [Starting Date] and end on [Ending Date] unless sooner terminated, as herein provided.

- Any restrictions on the use of the products and services

Sample Contract Language_____

None of the accounting services described in Section [Number of Pertinent Section] above may be utilized for purposes other than office accounting setup and assistance. Physician shall not utilize the Hospital's accounting services for personal or business purposes other than those described in Section [Number of Pertinent Section] above.

- The events of triggering default (See "Element VI, Conditions of Termination or Default" on page XX for sample contractual language specifying events that would trigger default.)

Use of Hospital Support Staff

The OIG is likely to consider use of hospital support staff to be a high-profile incentive because the May 1992 Special Fraud Alert listed "hospital's provision of free support staff" as 1 of 10 "suspect" arrangements and because of the overall thrust of the Hermann Hospital Closing Agreement. The November 19, 1999, safe harbors clarified use of support staff safe harbors. If a hospital nevertheless wishes to consider such incentives, it should follow the suggested procedures below to help reduce legal risk.

Requirements

A physician's use of a hospital's support staff in his or her private practice must be consistent with the following terms and conditions:

- Generally, a hospital can provide its support staff to physicians in their private practices at reasonable rates. The reasonableness of such rates can be determined by considering various factors, including local market conditions, local market data, and actual staffing costs for similar physician offices in the area.

- When there is dual use of a hospital's support staff by a physician for both his or her hospital duties and private practice activities, there must be an apportionment between these activities. There must then be a reasonable charge for use attributable to the physician's private practice activities.
- To the extent that a hospital's support staff is made available to physicians in their private practices on terms and conditions that are not consistent with commercially reasonable market rates (e.g., providing hospital support staff at discounted rates or at no cost to a physician), there must be a clear demonstration and documentation of community need or benefit. For example, a hospital may provide support staff at discounted rates if it can demonstrate a community benefit, such as enhancing a physician's access and availability to patients or improving patient convenience.

Legal Documentation

There should be a written agreement setting forth the terms and conditions under which a hospital's support staff will be made available to a physician. Legal documentation should consist of an agreement that includes, at a minimum, the following conditions:

- Duration of agreement
- Description of hospital support staff and what their responsibilities will be to the physician's practice.

Sample Contract Language

The term of this Agreement shall be [Number of Weeks] weeks from the effective date of [Starting Date of Agreement].

During this time, Hospital shall provide Physician with a registered nurse ("Nurse"), currently employed by Hospital, possessing demonstrated experience and expertise in the care of [Specialty] patients. Nurse shall be available to assist Physician at Clinic during Physician's regular office hours from [Starting Date of Agreement] until [Ending Date of Agreement].

- The person who will have ultimate responsibility for supervising personnel

Sample Contract Language

During the time Nurse is working at Clinic, Nurse will report to Physician and be under the direct supervision of Physician.

- Statement of the commercially reasonable compensation that a hospital will be paid for the use of its personnel

Sample Contract Language

Physician shall compensate Hospital for loss of Nurse's services to Hospital during the duration of this Agreement, at the same rate as Nurse's present base wages at Hospital, [Dollar Amount of Hourly Wage] per hour. Physician shall reimburse Hospital [Dollar Amount of Hourly Wage] for each hour or portion thereof that Nurse is working in Clinic.

- Restrictions on how hospital personnel are to be utilized

Sample Contract Language_____

Physician shall utilize Nurse only for duties as normally performed by a registered nurse in an [Specialty] office setting.

During the entire term of this Agreement, Nurse shall remain an employee of Hospital.

- Prohibition against assignment of the agreement without prior written consent. This would include the use of "hospital-paid" consultants providing training for physician support staff and office personnel.

Sample Contract Language_____

Physician shall not assign any rights nor delegate any duty under this Agreement. Physician, however, may at any time form a professional corporation of which Physician retains controlling interest and to which Physician may assign rights and delegate all duties under this Agreement. If a professional corporation is formed, Physician shall remain personally responsible and obligated as a guarantor of the obligations of the corporation to the Hospital. In the event of any such assignment, Hospital shall be notified in advance in writing, and this Agreement shall be amended to the extent necessary to reflect the formulation of the professional corporation as a party to this Agreement.

- Termination provisions

Sample Contract Language_____

This Agreement may be terminated at any time by either Physician or Hospital without cause.

Upon such termination, no further obligations from Hospital shall be due to Physician; however, any remaining unpaid fees due Hospital shall still be paid to Hospital in full in accordance with the terms of this Agreement.

Hospital's Training of Physician's Support Staff

The government is carefully scrutinizing the provision of hospital personnel for training physician support staff, including the use of hospital-paid consultants providing training for physician support staff and office personnel. The May 1992 Special Fraud Alert listed "free training for a physician's office staff" as 1 of 10 suspect incentive arrangements. If a hospital nevertheless wishes to consider such incentives, the following suggested procedures should be considered to help reduce legal risk.

While the May 1992 Special Fraud Alert (Exhibit 2-3) applies to both training of practice support staff through one-time group educational programs and longer-term concentrated training for a single practice, this section will focus only on the latter category of training. One-time, multipractice educational programs are conducted chiefly for established practices and, thus, fall into the category of "retention" activities rather "recruitment" incentives.

Requirements

- Fair market (commercially reasonable) compensation should be paid by a physician to a hospital for training the physician's support staff. The reasonableness of such compensation can be determined by consideration of various factors, including local market conditions, availability of trained personnel, and actual costs for similar services by other organizations.
- A hospital should be able to document that the community it serves will benefit from the training. For example, by improving the management of his or her practice, a physician will be able to spend more time treating patients and less on administrative matters, thereby improving access to health care in the community.
- To the extent that hospital personnel are made available to train a physician's support staff on terms and conditions that are not consistent with commercially reasonable rates, there must be a clear demonstration and documentation of community need or benefit. For example, a hospital could provide discounted training for a physician's office staff if it could demonstrate a community benefit such as enhancing a physician's access and availability to patients, which would improve patient convenience.

Legal Documentation

There should be a written agreement setting forth the terms and conditions under which hospital personnel will be made available to a physician's support staff. Legal documentation should consist of an agreement that includes, at a minimum, the following conditions:

- Description of the training and its benefits to the community

Sample Contract Language_____

To increase the quality of care delivered to obstetrical patients in [Location of Physician's Medical Practice], Physician has purchased a diagnostic ultrasound machine. Physician has requested use of a certified ultrasound technician ("Technician") from Hospital for training Physician's support staff.

- Statement of the commercially reasonable compensation a hospital will be paid for the use of its personnel

Sample Contract Language_____

Physician shall compensate Hospital for loss of Technician's services to Hospital at the same rate as Technician's present hourly wages. Physician shall reimburse Hospital [Amount of Hourly Reimbursement] for each hour or portion thereof that Technician is performing training services in Physician's office.

- Duration of the agreement

*Sample Contract Language*_____

Hospital agrees to make Technician available to Physician for training of Physician's support staff. Beginning on [Initial Date of Training], Technician will be physically present for training purposes in Physician's office every Friday from the hours of nine o'clock in the morning to twelve o'clock noon, up to [Maximum Number of Training Hours] total training hours.

- Description of hospital personnel and what their training responsibilities will be with physician support staff
- Delineation of who will have ultimate responsibility for supervising the personnel

*Sample Contract Language*_____

Technician shall instruct and train Physician's support staff in the proper and safe operation of the diagnostic ultrasound machine and shall supervise their use of said machine on Physician's patients.

While providing training in Physician's office, Technician shall be under the direct supervision of Physician and shall report to Physician in the performance of the above duties.

Office Leases and Leasehold Improvements

Stark I and Stark II address the issues of office leases and leasehold improvements. The provision of free or discounted office leases or leasehold improvements is an area of close governmental scrutiny. The OIG's May 1992 Special Fraud Alert (Exhibit 2-3) listed "discounted or free office rent" as 1 of its 10 suspect incentive arrangements.

Nevertheless, given the competitive environment for needed physicians, a hospital may wish to consider providing discounted or free office leases and leasehold improvements to certain physicians who are relocating to the area. Such incentives should be offered only when a hospital can document that providing them mirrors "fair market value" (i.e., other landlords in the area offer similar incentives to new tenants). It is important that the term (time limit) on the discounted or free portion of the lease corresponds to, and is no greater than, that offered by other landlords in the area for similar lease space. *If a hospital is considering offering free or discounted office space to newly recruited physicians, it must acquire and retain local advertisements and other documentation that other landlords in the area are offering free or discounted commercial office space. Be sure to note the date and title of the publication in which the documentation appeared.*

Requirements

The use of hospital office space through lease or sublease by physicians in private practice should conform to the following conditions:

- Lease rental rates, terms, and conditions should be consistent with commercially reasonable fair market rates, terms, and conditions.
- The reasonableness of rates, terms, and conditions should be determined by considering factors such as market conditions and actual rental charges to other tenants in the same or similar facilities. *In determining commercially fair market rates, a hospital should obtain an opinion letter from a local real estate agent or commercial real estate appraiser. This letter should provide a formula for determining reasonable lease rates or range of current lease rates in similar buildings in the area. This documentation should be updated periodically.*
- When there is dual use of the leased space by a physician for both hospital duties and his or her private practice, there must be an apportionment of the rent between the hospital activities and the physician's private practice activities. Rent at fair market rates should then be charged for use in connection with the physician's private practice activities.
- The hospital agreement regarding a lease or leasehold improvement must be an arms-length transaction.
- Even if a portion of a lease involves free or discounted rent, a hospital should structure the lease so that it ultimately expects to derive a commercially reasonable rate of return from the lease agreement, given local market conditions.

PRACTICE ACQUISITION AND PHYSICIAN EMPLOYMENT

Practice Acquisitions: Usual Circumstances

The acquisition of medical practices by hospitals is currently undergoing extreme regulatory examination by both the IRS and the OIG. As a general policy matter, a hospital should be involved in the purchase of a medical practice only when there is an unusually compelling reason for doing so, based upon clear and significant community need or extraordinary community benefits.

A December 1992 letter from the OIG's chief counsel to the IRS highlights the degree of scrutiny by both agencies. In this letter, the OIG mentions that it has "significant concerns about physician practices purchased by hospitals." In addition, the letter states that any amount paid beyond the "fair-market value of the hard assets of a physician practice would be open to question." Payments to physicians for several types of nontangible practice assets were specifically mentioned as being "highly questionable."

The following is a brief overview of the major issues, should a hospital choose to engage in practice acquisitions:

- **Fair market value standard**—Private benefit and inurement concerns arise if a hospital acquires a practice for a purchase price that is more than its fair market value.
- **Entity through which hospital operates the medical practice after acquisition—**
  - The organizational form or ability to operate a medical practice after acquisition may be determined by nontax considerations (e.g., state law prohibition against corporate practice of medicine or state law governing ownership of stock in medical corporations and professional service corporations).
  - The medical practice may be operated by a hospital or through an exempt affiliate of a hospital (e.g., ambulatory care facility or medical staff foundation).
  - Operation through a taxable affiliate of a hospital offers greater flexibility in compensation arrangements (e.g., incentive compensation arrangement based on percentage of net revenues is possible). Also, a physician can have an equity interest in a taxable affiliate arrangement.
- **Purchase of a practice's intangible assets**—If purchase of intangible assets does occur, both the IRS and the OIG have indicated two circumstances as critical to potential private inurement, private benefit, and anti-kickback violations:
  - Was the purchase price for the practice (and especially the intangible assets) reached via "arm's-length negotiations"?
  - Was the purchase price for the practice established based on an "independent practice appraisal" by an outside entity?

Requirements

The purchase of a physician's practice should adhere to the following requirements:

- A hospital should always obtain an independent appraisal of the practice's value.
- The purchase price paid by a hospital must not exceed fair market value. The concept of arms-length negotiation to reach a value for the practice is especially important.
- Any postacquisition employment of the selling physician must involve total compensation to the physician that is reasonable. Also, this compensation should not significantly increase the physician's annual net income (see last item under "Legal Documentation," below).
- Any hospital should avoid payment for nontangible assets of the practice, if at all possible. In particular, the hospital should attempt to avoid payments for those assets specifically cited in the OIG's December 1992 letter to the IRS. The following payments were cited:
  - Payment for goodwill (See page XX for a full explanation of the evolving status of payment for practice goodwill.)
  - Payment for the value of the ongoing business unit

- ○ Payment for a covenant not to compete
- ○ Payment for patient charts, lists, and records

Legal Documentation

All transactions should be documented by a purchase or sale agreement. Additional documentation should be provided if part or all of a transaction is being financed, including the following:

- A purchase or sale agreement must set forth, at a minimum:
  - ○ What is being purchased or sold (e.g., personal property, real property, accounts receivable)
  - ○ The fair market value price being paid
  - ○ Any condition that must be satisfied before a purchase or sale is finalized (e.g., execution of an employment agreement or assignment of all managed care provider agreements)
  - ○ Representations and warranties of the involved physicians
- There should be a promissory note. (See Exhibit 3-3 for an example of a promissory note.)
- There should be a separate bill of sale for all furniture, fixtures, equipment, and other property.
- Any deeds should be conveyed to the purchasing hospital at the time of the purchase.
- Any personal guarantees should be documented.
- A security agreement or mortgage should be drafted. *When the physician is financing a transaction through a commercial loan being guaranteed by a hospital, documents will exist between the bank extending the loan and the physician. A bank and a hospital will then enter into a guarantee agreement. To the extent the guarantee agreement is secured, there will be a separate security agreement between a hospital and a physician, subordinated to the security interest granted the bank and the appropriate UCC forms.*

  The agreement or mortgage must set forth the following, at a minimum:

  - ○ A grant of security interest
  - ○ A description of any collateral in which security interest is granted
  - ○ A specification of obligations secured
  - ○ The borrower's representations and warranties
  - ○ The events of default and rights of parties upon default
  - ○ Filing of appropriate UCC forms (See Exhibit 3-4, Form UCC-1).

- Every hospital should perform an adequate level of due diligence work before purchasing any practice. At a minimum, this due diligence should include the following items:
  - ○ An "environment assessment" of a practice (for example, there should be no underground storage tanks or groundwater contamination)
  - ○ Confirmation of clear title (UCC and title search, practice is free and clear of liens, etc.)

   ◦ Status of any pending malpractice or other lawsuits against a practice
   ◦ Status of any governmental inspections or audits
   ◦ A formal installment contract

Sample Contract Language

Effective [Date of Agreement], Hospital hereby agrees to purchase from Physician all of the personal and moveable assets found at the medical office at [Street Address of Clinic] in the City of [City and State] including all equipment, machinery, furniture, fixtures, desks, inventory, medical supplies, and other property, all as more particularly described in Exhibit [Number of Exhibit] attached hereto, for the sum of [Amount of Purchase].

In consideration for the conveyance of these assets by the Physician, Hospital promises to pay to the Physician the sum of [Amount of Purchase] on an installment basis. Interest on the unpaid principal shall accrue from [Date of Agreement] at two (2) percent above the prime interest rate as published in the *Wall Street Journal*, as of that date, adjusted annually on the 1st day of [Name of Month] of each year until all sums under this Agreement are paid in full.

This paragraph and the Agreements set forth herein shall constitute a promissory note from Hospital to Physician; however, Hospital shall sign a separate promissory note evidencing the indebtedness to Physician under this paragraph. Hospital shall also execute Uniform Commercial Code filings to help secure this indebtedness.

Hospital has had an opportunity to inspect the subject property. Hospital takes the subject property "as is" with no warranties from Physician except as to merchantable title.

- Any installment contract should contain a forfeiture clause.

The OIG has specifically mentioned that in the course of determining whether a hospital's purchase of a practice constitutes payment for referral (i.e., violation of the anti-kickback statute), it will specifically audit two items:

- The physician's degree of loyalty to a hospital before and after a practice purchase
- The "financial welfare of the physicians involved before and after the acquisition"

Therefore, in practice purchases a hospital should be prepared to document the following:

- There has been no significant increase in the financial welfare (i.e., significant increase in annual income) of the involved physician after the practice purchase, even if a hospital is employing the physician after the acquisition. *The standard exemptions to the safe harbor regulations for employed physicians are not in effect when it can be assumed that a portion of a physician's salary is payment to induce referrals to a particular hospital.*

- There has been no significant shift in a physician's loyalty to a hospital following the purchase. "Loyalty" can be measured by use of hospital ancillary services (e.g., reference lab services), volume of hospital outpatient encounters, inpatient admissions, and other activities.

Also important is documentation proving the following:

- An outside party established the value of the practice via an independent appraisal.
- The purchase price was established via arm's-length negotiations.

Medical Practice Valuation—IRS Update

In its technical instruction text for the 1996 fiscal year, released August 24, 1995, the IRS included practical guidance on medical practice valuation issues. The valuation article provides a great amount of detail that can be applied to real-life transactions, as opposed to global generalizations.

The article, contained in Chapter Q of *Continuing Professional Education, Exempt Organizations, Technical Instruction Program for FY 1996*, recognized that, as hospital acquisitions of medical practices raise questions about arm's-length negotiation, the "best determinant of fair market value is a properly performed, unbiased valuation appraisal of the medical practice."

The article outlines valuation methodology principles for determining business enterprise value (BEV) under the cost approach, market approach, and income approach and states that a valuation appraisal should include all three approaches.

The article also suggests which of the three approaches should be used to value specific types of tangible and intangible practice assets. In a section discussing the income approach and the pitfalls of revenue growth projections, the article outlines several factors that may be used to verify assumptions, including adjustments that may be necessary because of certain federal regulatory requirements.

Finally, the article explains how to apply the valuation methodologies to any tangible assets and validate the bottom line using the allocation technique. It discusses methods for valuing specific intangibles present in medical practices, including business goodwill, medical records, assembled work force, going concern value, noncompete covenants, managed care contracts, and trade name. The article includes examples of discounted cash flow techniques and the allocation technique.

Practice Acquisitions: Integrated Delivery Systems

For some physicians, the private practice of medicine today is more burdensome than ever before. The causes for this shift in thinking include declining fee-for-service reimbursement, increased managed care activity, decreased Medicare and Medicaid reimbursement, loss of patients to health maintenance organizations (HMOs), healthcare reform proposals of federal and state governments, medical malpractice concerns, and increased overhead expenses. At the same time, some hospitals are experiencing a significant decline in revenue, increased competition, and demand for cost containment.

As a result of these pressures, there has recently been a move in many areas of the country to create integrated delivery systems (IDSs), including the acquisition of physician practices by hospitals, in an effort to eliminate duplicative services and become more efficient and coordinated in delivering health care.

Integrated Delivery System Models

For the purposes of this discussion, an IDS is defined as an organization or system that integrates the delivery of hospital health care with the delivery of health care by physicians. An IDS can take a number of forms, or models, including the following.

Management Service Organizations. Management service organizations (MSOs) are separate entities or affiliations created to provide services to physicians in a vertically integrated system, including management, billing, medical equipment, nursing, and support staff. An MSO also might acquire the practice assets of the physician and lease office space back to him or her.

An MSO is often a subsidiary or related corporation of a hospital. It also may be owned either independently by a hospital or jointly by a hospital and physicians. It may be either a nonprofit or a for-profit corporation.

Note, however, that an MSO is not itself a provider of health care. Instead, it provides support for the delivery of health care in the form of services for physicians.

In part, MSOs are service bureau operations (billing, collection, and other management and administrative services), but in the IDS context, they can be much more. A comprehensive MSO might purchase some or all of the hard assets of the medical practices; provide the practice facilities, information systems, and personnel through a management service agreement (MSA); and otherwise serve as a catalyst for bringing together previously independent practices. The medical practices remain the providers of medical care and retain the patient relationships, the managed care contracts, and the provider numbers, while the MSO bills, as agent, in the name of the medical practice. Because the MSO is not a provider of medical care, and given the restrictions imposed by the corporate practices of medicine doctrine in some states (e.g., a business corporation would thus be prohibited from rendering professional medical services), an MSO usually will not purchase intangible assets such as goodwill, covenants not to compete, HMO contracts, or patient records.

Hospital-Owned Clinical Networks. In those states where the corporate practice of medicine is not prohibited, hospitals may acquire the medical practice assets of physicians and operate those assets as a vertically integrated outpatient clinic of the hospital. The physicians become employees or independent contractors of the hospital. Typically, the physicians are paid a base salary plus a productivity bonus. The office, staff, medical equipment, and medical malpractice coverage are provided by the hospital. The hospital itself (or through an independent company) manages the business of the practice, including billings. All revenue generated by the clinic belongs to the hospital.

The Foundation Model. Some hospitals and physicians have been involved in the creation of nonprofit, tax-exempt entities to purchase and operate physician clinics fully integrated with hospitals in the delivery of health care. These entities may be created by hospitals independently or by hospitals jointly with physicians and other organizations and are sometimes referred to as the foundation model. Because the foundation model represents a fully integrated system, it merits further review.

In the foundation model, the physicians contract with the separate entity (the foundation) to provide physician services. Compensation might be a fixed salary, a fixed salary plus a productivity bonus, or a capitated compensation arrangement combined with a salary. Likewise, hospitals contract with the foundation to provide services. Governance might be shared among the hospital, physicians, consumers, and members of the public.

The general pattern is that the foundation provides capital equipment, office space, and management expertise. Depending on state law regarding the corporate practice of medicine, the foundation either employs the physicians or independently contracts with a medical group to render service to the foundation's patients. In any event, the foundation, unlike an MSO, is the direct provider of care. It holds managed care contracts, bills, and other collections in its own name for services and owns patient medical records and accounts receivable.

The advantages of the foundation model lie mostly in a large degree of economic and operational integration and efficiencies, both among the participating providers and between the foundation and its related hospitals. This permits coordinated dealings with managed care plans and minimization of antitrust risk. The foundation can qualify as a tax-exempt organization under the Internal Revenue Code, which will exempt it from many federal, state, and local taxes, and potentially allow access to tax-exempt bond financing.

Two IRS rulings during 1993 shed some light on the IRS's position in forming a tax-exempt foundation. (See Friendly Hills Health Care Network Ruling Letter issued on February 8, 1993, and Facey Medical Foundation Ruling issued on March 31, 1993.) In both rulings, the IRS gave a favorable tax-exemption determination. Note that one of the most important attractions of a tax-exempt foundation is the potential for obtaining financing through the issuance of tax-exempt bonds, thus realizing a significant savings through lower interest rates.

The IRS has also established a 20% safe harbor regulation concerning foundations seeking tax-exempt status. The IRS will expedite tax exemption proceedings for foundations that limit physician representation on the governing board to 20% or less. The Deaconess-Billings Clinic Health System in Montana, for example, has reportedly taken advantage of the 20% rule to expedite the tax-exemption proceedings. In addition to Friendly Hills and Facey, Deaconess-Billings Health System received a favorable IRS determination ruling.

See also the Harriman Jones Medical Foundation Determination Letter released on February 3, 1994, and the Rockford Memorial Health Services

Corporation Determination Letter, released April 4, 1994. Taken together, these five rulings provide some general principles that may serve as guidelines for future attempts to gain tax-exempt status for IDSs.

In addition to the guidelines set forth in these determination letters, the IRS also has published an instructional booklet for IRS agents entitled *Continuing Professional Education Exempt Organizations Technical Instruction Program for FY 1994* that, on pages 212–243 of Chapter N, includes a list of some of the issues presented by a foundation seeking tax-exempt status. As has been previously indicated, Chapter P of the 1996 CPE textbook updates and supplements Chapter N with an expanded level of detail and analysis.

Requirements

Acquiring medical practices and establishing an IDS involves many of the same legal considerations as discussed elsewhere regarding physician recruitment, including antitrust and anticompetition statutes, private inurement and private benefit considerations regarding tax-exempt Section 501(c)(3) corporations, employment law issues, the Medicare antifraud and abuse statute, Stark I and Stark II anti-self-referral legislation, corporate practice of medicine issues, reimbursement and payment issues, and insurance and HMO licensure issues. All these areas should be carefully reviewed with legal counsel before considering forming or participating in an IDS.

In addition, special attention should be paid to the purchase price of any assets. If, for example, a physician is paid more than the fair market value for his or her assets, the excessive amount paid might be considered by the IRS as private inurement or private benefit that could result in the hospital losing its tax-exempt Section 501(c)(3) status, which in turn could lead to the IDS failing to qualify for tax-exempt status. This could trigger a default under any tax-exempt bond financing that might exist.

Along these same lines, excessive payments for acquiring a physician's assets could violate the anti-fraud and abuse statute. By a letter dated December 22, 1992, the OIG made its views known to the IRS concerning the application of the anti-fraud and abuse statute to physician practice acquisitions. (See December 1992, Thornton Letter to IRS, Exhibit 2-4.) Although the comments were informal, they provide a guide to hospitals regarding practice acquisitions. One of the OIG's primary concerns as stated in the 1992 letter was that hospitals may be paying large sums of money for practice acquisitions that are tantamount (in the OIG's opinion) to payments to retain existing referrals or to attract new referrals of patients to a hospital. The OIG's letter observed that it may be appropriate to exclude certain items in determining the fair market value of a physician's practice, as follows:

- Goodwill and going concern value
- Covenants not to compete
- Exclusive dealing arrangements
- Patient list and patient records

Taken at face value, the OIG's informal comments could present significant concerns to hospitals or IDSs when acquiring physician practices; however, the OIG is quoted in *Medicare Compliance Alert*, Volume 6, No. 9, January 17, 1994, as stating that the issue of payments for intangibles such as goodwill "is not a yes or no answer." Furthermore, a letter dated November 2, 1993, from the OIG to the American Hospital Association states that payment for intangibles would not be a "per se" violation of law.

EXHIBIT 3-1   ACCESS TO RECORDS

[Social Security Act: 42 USCS 1395(X)(V), Subparagraph (I)]

(1) In determining such reasonable cost, the Secretary may not include any costs incurred by a provider with respect to any services furnished in connection with matters for which payment may be made under this title [42 USCS 1395 et seq.] and furnished pursuant to a contract between the provider and any of its subcontractors which is entered into after the date of the enactment of this subparagraph [enacted Dec. 5, 1980] and the value or cost of which is $10,000 or more over a twelve-month period unless the contract contains a clause to the effect that:

    i.   Until the expiration of four years after the furnishing of such services pursuant to such contract, the subcontractor shall make available, upon written request by the Secretary, or upon request by the Comptroller General, or any of their duly authorized representatives, the contract, and books, documents, and records of such subcontractor that are necessary to certify the nature and extent of such costs, and

    ii.   If the subcontractor carries out any of the duties of the contract through a subcontract, with a value or cost of $10,000 or more over a twelve-month period, with a related organization, such subcontract shall contain a clause to the effect that until the expiration of four years after the furnishing of such services pursuant to such subcontract, the related organization shall make available, upon written request by the Secretary, or upon request by the Comptroller General, or any of their duly authorized representatives, the subcontract, and books, documents and records of such organization that are necessary to verify the nature and extent of such costs.

The Secretary shall prescribe in regulation [regulations] criteria and procedures which the Secretary shall use in obtaining access to books, documents, and records under clauses required in contracts and subcontracts under this subparagraph.

EXHIBIT 3-2 SAMPLE PHYSICIAN RECRUITMENT AGREEMENT

Please Note: This is an *example* of a physician recruitment contract and is not intended as a "model" contract, nor is it intended for use by any organization in actual recruitment contracting activities.

PHYSICIAN RECRUITMENT AGREEMENT

This Physician Recruitment Agreement ("Agreement") is entered into this [Day of Month] day of [Name of Month], [Year] by [Name of Hospital], a [Name of State] not-for-profit corporation ("Hospital") and [Full Name and Degree of Physician].

RECITALS

WHEREAS, Hospital is a [Name of State] not-for-profit corporation recognized as exempt from income tax pursuant to Section 501(c)(3) of the Internal Revenue Code and Hospital is organized and operated for the purpose of promoting and providing health care services to the public.

WHEREAS, Hospital has documented in attached Exhibit A that the [Name of Service Area or Community] area is medically underserved with respect to the presence and availability of physicians specializing in [Name of Recruited Physician's Specialty]. In addition, Hospital's Medical Staff Development Plan calls for the recruitment of physicians to serve the public within the [Name of Service Area] area.

WHEREAS, Physician presently maintains a private medical practice in [City and State], which is outside of Hospital's service area and Hospital has determined that it is in the public interest and consistent with Hospital's charitable, scientific, and educational purposes for it to encourage and assist qualified physicians to practice in the [Name of Service Area] area.

WHEREAS, Physician has expressed an interest and desire to establish a private practice and provide medical services to persons residing in Hospital's service area, and has requested assistance from Hospital in relocating to this service area.

WHEREAS, Physician has agreed to relocate his practice of [Name of Specialty] from [Location of Present Practice] to [Location of Service Area]; Hospital and Physician now wish to set forth their respective rights and responsibilities.

OBLIGATIONS OF HOSPITAL

1. **Relocation expenses.** In consideration for Physician relocating practice to [Name of Hospital's Service Area], Hospital agrees to reimburse Physician for the actual and reasonable costs of a professional mover to transfer Physician's furniture and personal belongings from [Present Location] to [Name of Hospital's Service Area]. These moving expenses shall be subject to the prior review and written approval of Hospital's Chief Financial Officer before Hospital shall be obligated to make actual payment. In no event shall the total moving expenses reimbursed and paid by Hospital under this paragraph exceed the sum of [Amount of Payment Cap].

   In addition, Hospital shall pay Physician for reasonable expenses incurred in connection with house-hunting trips between [Present Location] and [Hospital's Service Area]. These expenses, however, shall be subject to the prior review and written approval of Hospital's Chief Financial Officer before Hospital is obligated to make payment. In no event shall the total expenses reimbursed and paid by Hospital under this paragraph exceed the sum of [Amount of Payment Cap].

   If temporary housing is needed to complete relocation of Physician and Physician's immediate family to [Name of Service Area], then Hospital shall pay up to [Financial Cap in Dollars] per month for temporary housing, but not to exceed [Time Cap in Months] months.

   Implementation of disbursements for relocation expenses shall be the responsibility of Hospital's Chief Financial Officer, who shall be responsible for establishing all procedures and documentation necessary to carry out the intent of this Agreement.

2. **Loan to guarantee income.** Hospital shall lend Physician sums of money to guarantee that for the first year of practice, Physician shall receive actual net compensation, before payment or withholding of taxes, equal to [Amount of Monthly Net Income Guarantee] per year after payment of the Overhead Expenses, computed on a monthly basis.

For example, if Physician has an annual Income Guarantee in the amount of eighty thousand dollars ($80,000), had monthly Gross Receipts from Physician's practice of five thousand dollars ($5000), and monthly Overhead Expenses of thirty-four hundred dollars ($3400), the income guaranty would be computed as follows:

$5000   Monthly Gross Receipts
−3400   Monthly Overhead Expenses
$1600   Actual Net Compensation from Practice

$6666   Monthly Income Guaranty
−1600   Actual Net Compensation from Practice
$5066   Amount of Loan Funds Advanced by Hospital

Beginning on [First Day of Loan] and each month thereafter for one (1) year, Physician shall verify in writing to Hospital, Physician's reasonable Overhead Expenses in a "Verification of Receipts and Overhead Expenses" report of the Hospital's design. This report shall be received by Hospital on or before the fifteenth (15th) day of each month.

Payment of any loan monies to be advanced by Hospital to Physician shall occur on or before the fifteenth (15th) day of each month provided Physician's monthly "Verification of Receipts and Overhead Expenses" report has been received by Hospital.

Overhead Expenses shall mean those reasonable costs and expenses directly related to operation of the practice. These costs and expenses include:
i.   Office rent and utilities
ii. Property insurance
iii. Professional liability insurance premiums or other insurance required by this contract
iv. Health and accidental disability insurance
v.   Employee salaries, payroll taxes, and reasonable fringe benefits
vi. Office and clinical supplies
vii. Telephone costs

Reasonable Overhead Expenses shall not include any personal expenses such as a personal automobile, personal debts or loans, and payments to Physician's deferred compensation plan.

Implementation of the loan to guarantee income shall be the responsibility of Hospital's Chief Financial Officer, who shall be responsible for establishing all procedures and documentation necessary to carry out the intent of this Agreement.

OBLIGATIONS OF PHYSICIAN

1. **General obligations.** Physician shall practice medicine on a full-time basis excluding any other employment or professional duties and shall maintain regular office hours for the public as are usual and customary in the [Name of Service Area or Community] area for physicians in the specialty of [Name of Physician's Specialty].

Physician shall maintain a medical license in the State of [Name of State] in good standing throughout the term of this Agreement with such licensure not containing any restrictions or conditions that affect Physician's ability to practice medicine.

Physician shall maintain Active Status on the Medical Staff of Hospital in good standing throughout the term of this agreement.

Physician shall take affirmative action to ensure that Medicare and Medicaid patients have full access to his office, and Physician shall in no way restrict the number of Medicare and Medicaid patients who are seen or treated by Physician.

Physician shall not limit or restrict the number or type of indigent or charitable patients that Physician sees and treats. Physician shall keep a record of all such patients and make those records available to the Hospital upon request to ensure that such patients do have access to the health care system in [Name of Community or Service Area].

Physician shall at all times engage in his or her profession in accordance with the generally accepted standards of Physician's profession and shall faithfully adhere to the standards and principles of medical ethics of the American Medical Association and all other associations or boards concerned with Physician's area of medical expertise.

2. **Relocation Expenses.** Relocation expenses need not be repaid to Hospital by Physician, provided that Physician remains available to Hospital's service area in the full-time practice of Physician's specialty for a period of at least two (2) years after [Effective Date of this Agreement].

If Physician leaves the Hospital's service area or ceases the full-time practice of medicine in Physician's specialty prior to the passage of two (2) years after the effective date of this Agreement, Physician shall repay the Hospital on a pro rata basis for all sums of money advanced to Physician for relocation and moving. If, for example, Physician ceases the full-time practice of Physician's specialty after one (1) year, Physician shall repay the Hospital one half of the moving and other relocation expenses.

There shall be no obligation to repay the relocation expenses in case of Physician's death or disability.

3. **Medical liability insurance.** Physician shall obtain and maintain malpractice insurance with the minimum limits of _____ Dollars ($_____) per occurrence and _____ Dollars ($_____) in aggregate, or in such other amounts as required by Hospital throughout the term of this Agreement. Upon request of Hospital from time to time, Physician shall furnish adequate proof of such insurance coverage to Hospital.

4. **Third-party reporting.** Physician recognizes that Hospital is a participant in various third-party payment programs including, without limitation, Medicare and Medicaid, as well as various managed care programs, in which participation is essential to the ability of Hospital to serve the community and improve the community's access and availability to health care. Physician agrees to cooperate fully with Hospital and provide assistance for participation in payment associated with such programs. Such cooperation shall include, but not be limited to, the following:

   a. Physician agrees that, if this Agreement is subject to Social Security Act §1395(x)(V)(I), as it may be amended from time to time, Physician shall perform the obligations as may be from time to time specified for subcontractors in the Social Security Act, and the regulations promulgated pursuant thereto; and

   b. Physician agrees to make available at the Hospital such information and records as Hospital may reasonably request to facilitate Hospital's compliance with the requirement of the Medicare Conditions of Participation and the Medicaid Provider Agreement and, if applicable, to facilitate Hospital's substantiation of its reasonable costs in accordance with the requirements applicable to Hospitals pursuant to the Medicare and Medicaid programs.

5. **Qualification for advancement of funds.** Prior to the advancement of any loan funds under this Agreement, Physician shall agree to allow Hospital to demonstrate a satisfactory credit risk profile by Physician through a credit search by a professional credit agency.

Physician also agrees to submit a Net Worth Statement to Hospital prior to advancement of any loan funds.

6. **Access.** Physician shall provide Hospital with reasonable access to Physician's financial records and reports during normal business hours to verify the Overhead Expenses and the amount of loan funds advanced to guarantee income.

7. **Security for loan to guarantee income.** Until all loans described in this Agreement are either repaid or forgiven in whole, Physician shall obtain and keep in force a decreasing term life insurance policy on Physician's life in an amount at least equal to the unpaid principal and accrued interest on the loan from Hospital. This policy shall name Hospital as primary beneficiary.

Within thirty (30) days of the effective date of this Agreement, Physician shall furnish Hospital with a Certificate of Insurance or other evidence that the policy is in effect and that the beneficiary cannot be changed, nor can the policy be terminated or cancelled without prior notice to and approval of Hospital. If Physician should die before full payment of the loan or before it becomes fully forgiven by Hospital, the insurance proceeds shall be considered as liquidated damages and shall be paid to the Hospital to fully discharge Physician's indebtedness to the Hospital, and the balance, if any, shall be paid to the contingent beneficiary under the policy.

In addition, Physician shall execute necessary Promissory Notes and grant a security interest in all accounts receivable, inventory, furniture, fixtures and equipment, and grant mortgages on any real estate owned by Physician or Physician's spouse.

8. **Repayment of excess funds advanced.** If, in any month during the first twelve (12) months following Physician's commencement of his Practice in accordance with the "Loan to Guarantee Income" section of this Agreement, Net Income of Physician exceeds [Amount of Monthly Income Guarantee], Physician shall repay outstanding amounts previously paid by Hospital pursuant to the "Loan to Guarantee Income" section of this Agreement to the extent of such excess. Physician shall make such repayment to Hospital no later than the twentieth (20th) day of the following month.

9. **Standard repayment of loan to guarantee income.** All income guarantee loan amounts owing to Hospital by Physician shall accrue interest from the date the funds are advanced, at the rate of two (2) points above the prime rate as published in the *Wall Street Journal*, on January 1, 20_____, and adjusted annually.

   Interest and principal shall be paid by Physician according to the following schedule:
   a. From [Starting Date of Loan] until [12th Month of Loan], there shall be no payments of principal or interest due.
   b. From [13th Month of Loan] until [24th Month of Loan], payment shall be made for interest only on the first day of each month.
   c. From [25th Month of the Loan] until [Last Month of the Loan], repayment of principal and interest shall be made in equal monthly installments amortized over [Number of Years] years.

10. **Alternative repayment of loan to guarantee income.** As an alternative means of repayment of loans, the Hospital shall acknowledge that one fourth (1/4) of the principal balance and accrued interest due from Physician to Hospital has been paid beginning on [Second Anniversary of Effective Date of this Agreement] and one fourth (1/4) of the principal balance and accrued interest on [Subsequent Anniversaries of Effective Date of this Agreement] of each year thereafter if Physician has met all of the following requirements:
    a. Physician shall be in the full-time practice of medicine in [City and State], and Physician's services are available to the public as described in this agreement.
    b. Physician shall work a normal work week as may be required of other physicians in the area who practice in Physician's specialty.
    c. Physician shall accept patients referred by the Hospital's referral service regardless of the patient's ability to pay.
    d. Physician shall not limit the number of indigent or charitable patients seen or treated. Physician shall keep a record of all such patients and make those records available to the Hospital upon request.
    e. Physician shall assist the Hospital in its educational program regarding resident physicians so as to enhance the Hospital's position as a teaching institution. The educational duties of Physician shall be mutually agreed upon in writing by Physician and the Hospital's Director of Medical Education.
    f. Physician shall be placed on the on-call list of the Hospital's emergency room and, when called and when available, shall see and treat patients in the emergency room regardless of the patient's ability or inability to pay for service.
    g. Physician, if requested, shall assist in fundraising efforts for the Foundation to promote the charitable and educational purposes of the Foundation and the Hospital.
    h. Physician shall provide reasonable assistance to the Hospital in its physician recruitment programs.

i.   Physician shall maintain active professional staff privileges in Physician's specialty at Hospital and fulfill the obligations of a staff member as defined by the Professional Staff Bylaws.

PROHIBITIONS AGAINST RESTRICTIONS

Hospital and Physician understand and agree that nothing contained in this Agreement shall in any way require or suggest that Physician refer patients or admit patients to the Hospital at any time whatsoever. Physician shall be absolutely free to refer or admit patients to any hospital or other healthcare facility that Physician, in consultation with Physician's patients, deems appropriate without loss of any benefits whatsoever under this Agreement.

Although Physician shall be required to maintain active professional staff privileges in his or her specialty at the Hospital and fulfill the obligations of a staff member as defined by the Professional Staff Bylaws, Physician shall be completely free to maintain professional staff privileges at any other area hospital or healthcare facility of his or her choosing.

DEFAULT AND TERMINATION

1. **Standard default and termination.** If Physician shall fail or refuse to perform all of his or her obligations or meet his or her duties under this Agreement, Hospital shall give Physician written notice specifying the nature of such failure or refusal. If Physician does not substantially cure such failure or refusal within thirty (30) days after receipt of the notice, Hospital shall have the right, upon further written notice to Physician, to declare Physician in default and to terminate this Agreement immediately.

    However, if Physician's license to practice medicine in the State of [Name of State] is restricted, revoked, canceled, surrendered, or suspended so that Physician does not maintain the ability to practice medicine in a full and unrestricted manner, and such condition continues for more than a thirty- (30) day continuous period, this Agreement may, at the option of the Hospital, be summarily terminated by giving notice of the termination to Physician.

    Upon such termination, no further forgiveness of the loans shall accrue, and thereafter the then-remaining unpaid and unforgiven portions thereof shall be paid in full in accordance with their terms, and the payment of any other sums by Hospital hereunder shall also terminate.

2. **Violation of existing regulations.** If any provision of this Agreement shall be deemed to be invalid or in violation of any of the laws of the State of [Name of State] or any laws, rules, or regulations of the United States, or interpretations thereof as they now exist, this Agreement may be terminated immediately by either party, or, at the Hospital's option, the offending portion of the Agreement may be deemed severed and the remaining portion of the Agreement continue in full force and effect.

    In the event of such termination, neither Hospital nor Physician shall have any further duties or obligations under this Agreement except that Physician shall be required to pay back all loans advanced by the Hospital, including interest, pursuant to this Agreement, and said loans shall be repaid in full within ninety (90) days of termination, unless other means of repayment are approved by the Hospital.

3. **Future legislation and interpretations.** In the event of future legislation, government rule or regulation, policy or governmental interpretation thereof that applies to this Agreement and prohibits or invalidates any of its provisions, or causes either the Hospital or Physician not to qualify under or otherwise be in violation of any Medicare or Medicaid reimbursement regulations, or if the Hospital's continuing ability to qualify as a tax-exempt 501(c)(3) corporation is in jeopardy at any time as determined by the Hospital, then the parties hereto shall either forthwith cause to be made to this Agreement such amendments as may be reasonably required to bring its terms back into compliance or, in the alternative, terminate this Agreement.

    In the event of such termination, neither Hospital nor Physician shall have any further duties or obligations under this Agreement except that Physician shall be required to pay back all loans advanced by the Hospital, including interest, pursuant to this Agreement, and said loans shall be repaid in full within ninety (90) days of termination, unless other means of repayment are approved by the Hospital.

CONCLUDING STATEMENTS

1. **Entire agreement.** This Agreement constitutes the entire understanding between the parties, and all prior negotiations and understandings between the parties have been merged into this Agreement. There are no understandings, representations, or agreements, either oral, written, or implied other than those set forth herein; and all prior agreements are expressly terminated as of the effective date of this Agreement. Waiver of any provision of this Agreement shall not be deemed a waiver of future compliance therewith, and such provisions shall remain in full force and effect.
2. **Changes in agreement.** No amendment, waiver, change, modification, or termination of any of the terms, provisions, or conditions of this Agreement shall be effective unless made in writing and signed or initialed by all parties.
3. **Notices.** Until changed by a similar notice in writing, written notices given or required to be given under this Agreement shall be deemed duly served when personally received by one of the parties set forth below; or in lieu of such personal service, when deposited in the U.S mail, by certified mail, postage prepaid, return receipt requested, and addresses as follows:
   If sent to Hospital:
   [Name, Title, and Business Address of Hospital's Representative]
   If sent to Physician:
   [Name, Degree, and Business Address of Physician]
4. **Assignment.** Physician shall not assign any rights nor delegate any duty under this Agreement. Physician may, however, at any time form a professional corporation of which Physician retains controlling interest and to which Physician may assign rights and delegate all duties under this Agreement. If a professional corporation is formed, Physician shall remain personally responsible and obligated as a guarantor of the obligations of the corporation to the Hospital. In the event of any such assignment, Hospital shall be notified in advance in writing, and this Agreement shall be amended to the extent necessary to reflect the formulation of the professional corporation as a party to this Agreement.

IN WITNESS WHEREOF, both Physician and Hospital have caused this Agreement to be duly executed and delivered as of the date and year first above written.

FOR HOSPITAL:

_____

[Name of Hospital Officer]

_____

[Title of Hospital Officer]

FOR PHYSICIAN:

_____

[Name of Physician]

_____

[Degree of Physician]

EXHIBIT 3-3   EXAMPLE OF PRACTICE SUPPORT PROMISSORY NOTE

_____, 20___

On or before _____, 20____ (or if such day is not a business day, on the next following business day), the undersigned Physician, for value received, hereby promises to pay to the order of _____ ("Hospital"), at such place as Hospital may from time to time designate in writing, the principal sum ("principal") of _____ Dollars ($_____) or, if less, the aggregate unpaid principal amount of all loans made by Hospital to Physician as such unpaid principal amount is shown either on the schedule attached hereto (and any continuation thereof) or in Hospital's records, pursuant to that certain Income Guarantee Agreement of even date herewith ("Agreement"), as the same may be amended, modified, or supplemented from time to time. The undersigned further promises to pay per annum interest on the outstanding unpaid principal amount at a rate equal to one percent (1%) over the prime rate as stated by the _____ on the date herewith, and then at the level of such per annum rate calculated annually hereafter.

Manner of Repayment

Payment of both principal and interest is to be made in lawful money of the United States of America. Physician shall have the right to prepay the principal amount outstanding in whole or in part without penalty.

This Note evidences indebtedness incurred under, and is subject to, the terms and provisions of the Agreement, including those under which this Note may or must be paid. Terms used, but not otherwise defined herein, are used herein as defined in the Agreement.

If the Agreement terminates pursuant to any of the reasons stated in Section _____ of the Agreement, then this Note will become immediately due and payable and Physician shall pay to the order of _____ the unpaid principal amount and interest.

Forgiveness

If the principal and interest due and payable under this Note on _____, 20_____, is less than or equal to _____ Dollars ($_____), then such principal amount and interest shall be forgiven and no longer due and payable under this Note if Physician agrees to extend the Agreement for an additional one- (1) year period beyond the Subsidy Period and if during the entire period of extension Physician complies with all his obligations under the Agreement as stated in Sections _____ through_____ of the Agreement.

If the principal and interest due and payable under this Note on _____, 20_____, exceed _____ Dollars ($_____), then such principal and interest shall be forgiven and extend the Agreement for an additional two- (2) year period beyond the Subsidy Period if during the entire period of extension Physician complies with all his obligations under the Agreement as stated in Sections _____ through _____ of the Agreement.

Assignment

The rights of Hospital hereunder shall inure to the benefit of Hospital's legal representatives, successors, and assigns. This Note is not assignable by Physician.

Costs of Collection

In addition to, and not in limitation of, the foregoing and the provisions of the Agreement herein above referred to, the undersigned further agrees, subject only to any limitation imposed by applicable law, to pay all expenses, including reasonable attorneys' fees and expenses, incurred by the holder of this Note in seeking to collect any amounts payable hereunder that are not paid when due, whether by acceleration or otherwise.

Severability

If any provision of this Note or the application thereof to any party or circumstances is held invalid or unenforceable, the remainder of this Note and the application of such provision to other parties or circumstances will not be affected thereby, and the provisions of this Note shall be severable in any such instance.

Governing Law

This instrument shall be governed by and interpreted in accordance with the laws of the State of _____. Physician and Hospital hereby consent to the exclusive jurisdiction of any local, state, or federal courts located within _____ County, _____, and waive any objection that they may have based on improper venue of *forum non conveniens* to the conduct of any proceeding in any such court. Nothing contained in this Note shall affect the right of Hospital to serve legal process in any manner permitted by law.

Waiver of Breach

Waiver of a breach of any provision, term, or condition of this Note shall not operate or be construed as a waiver of any subsequent breach, and the acceptance of a past due payment shall not be construed as a waiver of Hospital's rights to require strict compliance with all terms and conditions herein.

_____
Physician

_____
Date

EXHIBIT 3-4 EXAMPLE OF UCC FINANCING STATEMENT

UCC FINANCING STATEMENT

FOLLOW INSTRUCTIONS (front and back) CAREFULLY

A. NAME & PHONE OF CONTACT AT FILER [optional]

B. SEND ACKNOWLEDGMENT TO: (Name and Address)

THE ABOVE SPACE IS FOR FILING OFFICE USE ONLY

1. DEBTOR'S EXACT FULL LEGAL NAME - insert only one debtor name (1a or 1b) - do not abbreviate or combine names

1a. ORGANIZATION'S NAME			

OR

1b. INDIVIDUAL'S LAST NAME	FIRST NAME	MIDDLE NAME	SUFFIX

1c. MAILING ADDRESS	CITY	STATE	POSTAL CODE	COUNTRY

1d. TAX ID #: SSN OR EIN	ADD'L INFO RE: ORGANIZATION DEBTOR	1e. TYPE OF ORGANIZATION	1f. JURISDICTION OF ORGANIZATION	1g. ORGANIZATIONAL ID #, if any
				☐ NONE

2. ADDITIONAL DEBTOR'S EXACT FULL LEGAL NAME - insert only one debtor name (2a or 2b) - do not abbreviate or combine names

2a. ORGANIZATION'S NAME			

OR

2b. INDIVIDUAL'S LAST NAME	FIRST NAME	MIDDLE NAME	SUFFIX

2c. MAILING ADDRESS	CITY	STATE	POSTAL CODE	COUNTRY

2d. TAX ID #: SSN OR EIN	ADD'L INFO RE: ORGANIZATION DEBTOR	2e. TYPE OF ORGANIZATION	2f. JURISDICTION OF ORGANIZATION	2g. ORGANIZATIONAL ID #, if any
				☐ NONE

3. SECURED PARTY'S NAME (or NAME of TOTAL ASSIGNEE of ASSIGNOR S/P) - insert only one secured party name (3a or 3b)

3a. ORGANIZATION'S NAME			

OR

3b. INDIVIDUAL'S LAST NAME	FIRST NAME	MIDDLE NAME	SUFFIX

3c. MAILING ADDRESS	CITY	STATE	POSTAL CODE	COUNTRY

4. This FINANCING STATEMENT covers the following collateral:

8. OPTIONAL FILER REFERENCE DATA

FILING OFFICE COPY ó NATIONAL UCC FINANCING STATEMENT (FORM UCC1) (REV. 07/29/98)

Instructions for National UCC Financing Statement (Form UCC1)

Please type or laser-print this form. Be sure it is completely legible. Read all Instructions, especially Instruction 1; correct Debtor name is crucial. Follow Instructions completely. Fill in form very carefully; mistakes may have important legal consequences. If you have questions, consult your attorney. Filing office cannot give legal advice. Do not insert anything in the open space in the upper portion of this form; it is reserved for filing office use.

When properly completed, send Filing Office Copy, with required fee, to filing office. If you want an acknowledgment, complete item B and, if filing in a filing office that returns an acknowledgment copy furnished by filer, you may also send Acknowledgment Copy; otherwise detach. If you want to make a search request, complete item 7 (after reading instruction 7 below) and send Search Report Copy, otherwise detach. Always detach Debtor and Secured Party Copies.

If you need to use attachments, use 8-1/2 × 11-inch sheets and put at the top of each sheet the name of the first Debtor, formatted exactly as it appears in item 1 of this form; you are encouraged to use Addendum (Form UCC1Ad).

A. To assist filing offices that may want to communicate with filer, filer may provide information in item A. This item is optional.

B. Complete item B if you want an acknowledgment sent to you. If filing in a filing office that returns an acknowledgment copy furnished by filer, present simultaneously with this form a carbon or other copy of this form for use as an acknowledgment copy.

Instructions for National UCC Financing Statement AMENDMENT Addendum (Form UCC3Ad)

1. Enter information exactly as given in item 1a on Amendment form.
2. Enter information exactly as given in item 9 on Amendment form.
3. If space on Amendment form is insufficient or you must provide additional information, enter additional information in item 13.

Part IV

Templates and Tools

The agreements, contracts, tools, and resources making up this section are assembled from a variety of sources and for various purposes in the recruitment initiative. They serve as examples in constructing recruiting arrangements. The sample agreements, which represent various scenarios, relationships, and concepts, include the following:

1. Physician recruitment agreement—forgivable loan
2. Agreement for professional services—primary care clinic, employee status
3. Medical director agreement for a department within a hospital—employment relationship
4. Professional services agreement for director and trainer at a family practice residency program—employee relationship, arbitration provision included
5. Agreement for professional services (Emergency Department)—independent contractor
6. Agreement for professional services (Emergency Department)—employee relationship
7. Physician recruitment agreement—independent contractor
8. Nurse practitioner recruitment agreement—forgivable loan
9. Medical office lease agreement—hospital and physician (hospital-owned space)

These templates are somewhat generic and will not fit every situation—no document is applicable for every circumstance. They are merely examples of contracts in the physician recruitment and employment areas that may be cited when developing specific agreement language. Furthermore, the financial terms used in the templates are hypothetical and should not be used as standards for agreements.

Likewise, this section provides sample tools, forms, questionnaires, and training documents to help complete the essential steps in the process of recruitment, orientation, and retention, namely:

1. Physician recruitment guidelines
2. Position postings
3. Contingency search agreement—primary care
4. Contingency search agreement—specialty and subspecialty
5. Physician recruitment questionnaire—preinterview
6. Professional questions and attestation
7. Defining the position—getting a feel for the opportunity
8. Candidate screening—initial interview
9. Candidate interview checklist
10. Candidate interview questionnaire
11. Candidate peer interview evaluation grid
12. Candidate evaluation checklist
13. Letter to reviewers
14. Physician orientation and development
15. Physician retention plan
16. Checklist for initiating hospital-employed physician practice

These tools have been developed and are actually used by people whose job is to recruit physicians and other providers in an effort to cover all the bases in the recruitment and retention initiative.

PHYSICIAN RECRUITMENT AGREEMENT—FORGIVABLE LOAN

This Physician Recruitment Agreement is entered into this _____ day of _____, 20____, by and among _____, a not-for-profit corporation ("Hospital"); _____ ("P.C."); and _____ ("Physician").

Recitals

A. The Hospital is a not-for-profit corporation as described under Section 501(c)(3) of the Internal Revenue Code. The Hospital is organized and operated for the purposes of promoting and providing healthcare services to the public and is also organized for charitable, scientific, and educational purposes.

B. The Hospital through its Board of Trustees has determined that it is consistent with the Hospital's charitable, scientific, and educational purposes to encourage and assist physicians to practice medicine within the community and surrounding areas.

C. Physician is completing a residency program in his specialty of family practice medicine, and in contemplation of completing his training, he is attempting to establish a medical practice in _____ and to make his professional services available to that community and surrounding areas on a full-time basis provided that certain financial incentives are made available to him so that he can establish and maintain the practice of medicine.

D. P.C. is willing to provide space and staff to Physician in P.C.'s existing practice in _____ and is willing to assist him in the start-up of practice.

E. The Board of Trustees of the Hospital has determined that a Physician Recruitment Agreement should be entered into with Physician that will be in the best interest of the community of _____ and surrounding areas. Furthermore, the Board of Trustees of the Hospital has reviewed and approved the terms of the proposed Physician Recruitment Agreement, and all parties wish to set forth their agreement in writing.

NOW, THEREFORE, the Hospital, P.C., and Physician agree as follows:

1. Loan to physician (income guarantee)
    In exchange for Physician's commitment to establish and maintain the practice of medicine to serve the community of _____ and surrounding areas as described in this Agreement, the Hospital hereby agrees and commits to lend Physician sums of money as described below in this paragraph over a one- (1) year period of time, which loan commitment shall commence on the first day of July 20__, and end on the 30th day of June 20__. The loan shall be in the form of an income guarantee for Physician for a one- (1) year period of time, but only if he remains in the full-time practice of medicine in _____.

    If in the one- (1) year period of time during the loan commitment period revenues from Physician's practice of medicine in _____, net of reasonable and customary overhead expenses in the agreed amount of One Hundred Ninety Thousand Dollars ($190,000) per year, does not reach One Hundred Ten Thousand Dollars ($110,000) (as annualized and projected on a monthly basis), the Hospital, upon the request of Physician, shall lend a sum of money to Physician to bring his income, net of the agreed overhead expenses, to the level of One Hundred Ten Thousand Dollars ($110,000) per year; provided, however, that the total amount to be lent by the Hospital shall not exceed Seventy-five Thousand Dollars ($75,000) for the one- (1) year term of the loan commitment. Physician may draw on the loan during the one- (1) year loan commitment period of time on a monthly basis or such other periodic basis as may be mutually agreeable between Hospital and Physician. The loan shall be made to Physician and not P.C. P.C. and Physician, upon request of the Hospital, shall make business and financial records available to the Hospital to verify the income level of Physician and the overhead expenses attributable to him, which records shall be kept confidential by the Hospital to the extent allowed by law. Periodically and at the end of the one- (1) year term of the loan, Physician and the Hospital shall make reconciliations regarding the amounts advanced by the Hospital. A hypothetical example of the loan advances and reconciliations is set forth in the attached Exhibit A.

2. Repayment

Any sums advanced under the loan commitments described above to Physician shall accrue interest at the fixed rate of two (2) percentage points over the prime rate as published in the *Wall Street Journal* as of the first date when any sums are advanced under the loan commitment. No payments of either interest or principal shall be required during the first year following July 1, 20__, if Physician is otherwise in compliance with this Agreement; provided, however, accrued interest at the end of the first year shall be added to the unpaid principal and the loan shall be amortized and repaid as described below in this paragraph. Beginning on July 1, 20__, and for a period of three (3) years thereafter, payment of principal and interest shall be made in equal monthly installments until all sums are paid in full; provided, however, Physician shall not be deemed to be in default in the repayment of the loan if the alternative repayment provisions of paragraph 4 below are being fully met.

3. Promissory note and security

Physician shall execute a Promissory Note for each draw under the loan commitment in a form to be prescribed by the Hospital. If Physician neglects to execute a Promissory Note, however, this Agreement shall constitute a Promissory Note and shall be evidence of his promise to pay all sums advanced by the Hospital pursuant to the terms of this Agreement. This Agreement shall constitute a financing agreement for the purposes of the Uniform Commercial Code and, if requested by the Hospital, Physician shall execute a Uniform Commercial Code Financing Statement in recordable form regarding any medical equipment or other medical personal property that he might own that will help secure the loan described in this Agreement. Physician shall also grant a mortgage to the Hospital on any real estate owned by him to help secure the loan by the Hospital so long as the granting of the mortgage would not violate any preexisting mortgages regarding Physician. Implementation of the loan, as well as the obligation for obtaining necessary Promissory Notes and security for the loan, shall be the responsibility of the Chief Financial Officer of the Hospital.

4. Alternative repayment of loan

As an alternative means of repayment of the loans described in paragraph 1 of this Agreement, the Hospital shall acknowledge that one third (1/3) of the principal balance and accrued interest on loans made under paragraph 1 of this Agreement has been paid beginning on July 1, 20__, and on July 1 of each year thereafter for a total of three (3) years (with a proration being made on a monthly basis) if Physician has met all of the following community service requirements:

    A. Physician shall be in the full-time practice of medicine in the community of _____ in his specialty of family practice.

    B. Physician shall work a normal workweek in the practice of medicine as may be required of other physicians in the community, meaning a forty-(40) hour workweek with customary call coverage and rounds in addition to these hours, subject to customary vacation and leave time for sickness and continuing medical education.

    C. Physician shall not restrict or limit the number of Medicare or Medicaid patients who are seen or treated by him and shall remain eligible to participate in the Medicare and Medicaid programs and shall observe all applicable rules and regulations pertaining to those programs.

    D. Physician shall accept patients referred by the Hospital's referral services regardless of the patient's ability to pay.

    E. Physician shall not limit the number of indigent or charitable patients seen or treated by him. Physician shall keep a record of all such patients and make those records available to the Hospital; provided, however, this report shall not identify patient names or otherwise breach physician–patient confidentiality.

    F. Physician shall assist the Hospital in its medical educational program regarding medical students, interns, and residents so as to enhance the Hospital's position as a duly accredited teaching institution. The educational duties of Physician shall be mutually agreed upon in writing by Physician and the Hospital.

    G. To help carry out the educational duties described above, Physician shall maintain active professional staff privileges in his specialty at the Hospital and shall fulfill the obligations of a staff member as defined by the Hospital's Professional Staff Bylaws; however, Physician also shall be free to join the professional staff of any other hospital without the loss of any benefits under this Agreement.

    H. Physician shall be placed on the on-call list in the Emergency Department of the Hospital and when reasonably available shall see and treat patients in the Hospital's Emergency Department.

If all the above described community service requirements are met at the end of three (3) years, all of the principal balance and accrued interest on the loans made by the Hospital to Physician under paragraph 1 of this Agreement shall be acknowledged by the Hospital as paid in full. Physician acknowledges that for each year the above-described loan is repaid by community service, the Hospital will be obligated under federal law to issue IRS Form 1099, and Physician shall be responsible for all income tax consequences flowing from loan forgiveness. Physician acknowledges that he has had an opportunity to consult with his attorney or tax advisor to plan for payment of income tax resulting from loan forgiveness.

5.   Obligations of P.C.

P.C. agrees to maintain Physician in P.C.'s medical practice in _____ and to provide him with staff, office space, furniture, examination rooms, equipment, and other amenities necessary to maintain the full-time practice of medicine. This commitment shall continue until _____, 200__, or until all sums owed by Physician to the Hospital are paid in full, whichever occurs first; provided, however, if Physician or P.C. ever terminates their relationship, P.C. shall have no obligations or liability to the Hospital under this Agreement, and Physician solely shall be liable to repay any sums under this Agreement to the Hospital. Prior to the Hospital funding the first loan draw, P.C. and Physician shall provide written verification satisfactory to the Hospital that an arrangement is in effect with Physician allowing him to practice in P.C.'s office.

6.   Freedom in referrals

Hospital, P.C., and Physician understand and agree that nothing contained in this Agreement shall in any way require or suggest that either P.C. or Physician, or any other physicians associated with P.C., refer or admit patients to the Hospital at any time whatsoever. Both P.C. and Physician shall be absolutely free to refer or admit patients to any hospital or other health-care facility that they, in consultation with their patients, deem appropriate, in their sole discretion, all without loss of any benefits whatsoever under this Agreement.

7.   Third-party reporting

P.C. and Physician recognize that the Hospital is a participant in various third-party payment programs, including, without limitation, Medicare and Medicaid. P.C. and Physician agree to cooperate fully with the Hospital and provide assistance to the Hospital for participation in such programs, including furnishing, upon request, financial information or other books, records, and documentation concerning this Agreement for a period of up to four (4) years after the termination or expiration of this Agreement to the United States Comptroller General, or designee, pursuant to Section 1861(v)(1)(L) of the Federal Social Security Act.

8.   Default

If any party fails or refuses to perform the obligations under this Agreement, the affected party shall give the defaulting party written notice specifying the nature of the default. If the default is not substantially cured within thirty (30) days after personal delivery or mailing of the notice, the affected party shall have the right to terminate this Agreement immediately. If Physician's license to practice medicine in the State of _____ is restricted, revoked, canceled, surrendered, or suspended so that Physician does not maintain his license to practice medicine in a full and unrestricted manner, and such condition continues for more than thirty (30) continuous days, this Agreement may, at the option of the Hospital, be summarily terminated by giving notice of the termination to the other parties to this Agreement; provided, however, such a termination shall not eliminate the duty to repay any sums of money owed by Physician to the Hospital pursuant to the above-described loan commitment, which repayment shall be immediately due and owing in full to the Hospital.

9. Entire agreement

This Agreement constitutes the entire understanding among the parties, except for an agreement between P.C. and Physician, and all prior negotiations and understandings among the parties have been merged into this Agreement. There are no understandings, representations, or side agreements, either oral, written, or implied, among the parties other than those set forth in this Agreement and in the agreement between P.C. and Physician.

10. Future legislation and interpretations

The parties to this Agreement are of the opinion that all of the terms of this Agreement comply with present law; however, the parties are mindful of continuous discussions regarding possible healthcare legislation at the federal and state levels. Furthermore, the parties are aware that federal and state regulations are subject to periodic interpretations and court decisions that could affect this Agreement. In the event of future legislation, court decision, governmental regulation, policy, or governmental interpretation thereof that applies to this Agreement and prohibits or invalidates any of its provisions, or causes the Hospital, P.C., or Physician not to qualify under or otherwise be in violation of any Medicare or Medicaid reimbursement regulations, or other laws, or if the Hospital's continuing ability to qualify as a tax-exempt Section 501(c)(3) corporation is in jeopardy at any time because of this Agreement, as determined by the Hospital, then the parties shall either forthwith cause to be made to this Agreement such amendments as may reasonably be required to bring its terms back into compliance with the law or, in the alternative, terminate this Agreement. In the event of such termination, no party shall have any further duties or obligations under this Agreement except that Physician shall be required to pay back all loans advanced by the Hospital, including interest, and said loans shall be repaid in full within ninety (90) days of termination unless other acceptable means of repayment are approved by the Hospital in its reasonable discretion consistent with federal and state law.

11. Notices

Written notices required to be given under this Agreement shall be deemed served when personally received or in lieu of personal service when deposited in the United States Mail, by certified mail, postage prepaid, return receipt requested, and addressed as follows:

- **To Hospital:**

  _____

  _____

  _____

  _____

- **To P.C.:**

  _____

  _____

  _____

  _____

- **To Physician:**

  _____

  _____

  _____

  _____

12. Miscellaneous conditions

   The following conditions also apply to this Agreement:

   A. Recitals. The recitals at the beginning of this Agreement are intended to describe the intent of the parties and the circumstances under which this Agreement is executed and, consequently, shall be considered in the interpretation of this Agreement.

   B. Amendment. This Agreement may be amended only by the written consent of the parties.

   C. Waiver. The failure or delay of either party to insist in any one or more instances upon performance of any terms or conditions of this Agreement shall not be construed as a waiver of past or future performance of any such terms, covenants, or condition; but the obligations of such party with respect thereto shall continue in full force and effect.

   D. Severability. If one or more of the provisions contained in this Agreement are declared to be invalid, illegal, or unenforceable in any respect by a court of competent jurisdiction, the validity, legality, and enforceability of the remaining provisions of this Agreement shall not in any way be impaired thereby unless the effect of such declaration of the court would be to materially and substantially impair or diminish either party's rights and benefits hereunder, subject to the rights of the parties to otherwise terminate this Agreement as provided elsewhere in this Agreement.

   E. Governing law. This Agreement shall be interpreted under and governed by the law of the State of _____, without regard to choice of law or conflict of law principles.

IN WITNESS WHEREOF, the parties have caused this Agreement to be duly executed and delivered as of the date and year first above written.

HOSPITAL   PHYSICIAN

By _____   By _____

_____   _____

Title:_____   Title: _____

                                                  P.C. _____

                                                  By:_____

                                                  Title: _____

Hypothetical Examples of Income Guarantee

I. Assumptions
    < Annual income guarantee: $110,000 (net of overhead)
    < Agreed annual overhead: $190,000
    < If physician grossed $300,000 or more in
    one year, the Hospital would have no
    obligation (or the Hospital should be
    repaid for all advances).

II. Examples
    1. Month One
        Receipts $13,000
        Overhead   15,833
        Income net of overhead   -$ 2,833
        Amount of loan: $ 9,166
                                                              + 2,833
                                                              $11,999

    2. Month Two
        Receipts $14,500
        Overhead   15,833
        Income net of overhead   -$1,333
        Amount of loan: $9,166
                                                              + 1,333
                                                              $10,499

    3. Month Three
        Receipts $16,000
        Overhead   15,833
        Income net of overhead $167
        Amount of loan: $9,166
                                                              -167
                                                              $ 8,999

    4. Month Four
        Receipts $17,500
        Overhead   15,833
        Income net of overhead $1,667
        Amount of loan: $9,166
                                                              -1,667
                                                              $7,499

    5. Month Five
        Receipts $18,500
        Overhead   15,833
        Income net of overhead $2,667
        Amount of loan: $9,166
                                                              -2,667
                                                              $6,499

6. Month Six
Receipts		$22,000
Overhead	15,833	
Income net of overhead		$6,167
Amount of loan:		$9,166
		−6,167
		$2,999

7. Month Seven
Receipts		$24,000
Overhead	15,833	
Income net of overhead		$8,167
Amount of loan:		$9,166
		−8,167
		$999

8. Month Eight
Receipts		$25,000
Overhead	15,833	
Income net of overhead		$9,167
Amount of Loan:		$9,166
		−9,167
		$−1

9. Month Nine
Receipts		$26,000
Overhead	15,833	
Income net of overhead		$10,167
Amount of Loan:		−0
Repayment to Hospital:		$10,167
		−9,166
		$1,001

10. Month Ten
Receipts		$27,000
Overhead	15,833	
Income net of overhead		$11,167
Repayment to Hospital:		$11,167
		−9,166
		$2,001

11. Month Eleven
Receipts		$28,000
Overhead	15,833	
Income net of overhead		$12,167
Repayment to Hospital:		$12,167
		−9,166
		$3,001

12. Month Twelve

Receipts		$28,000
Overhead	15,833	
Income net of overhead		$12,167
Repayment to Hospital:		$12,167
		−9,166
		$3,001

Gross Amount of Annual Loan:	$49,493*
Amount of Repayment/Reconciliation	$9,004

Net Amount of Loan: (Principal only) $49,493–$9,004 = $40,489
(Plus accrued interest)
*In no event shall loan exceed $75,000 for the 1-year term.

AGREEMENT FOR PROFESSIONAL SERVICES—EMPLOYEE (PRIMARY CARE CLINIC—EMPLOYEE STATUS)

This Agreement is entered into this ____ day of _____, 200___, by and between _____ ("Hospital") and _____ ("Physician").

Witnesseth:

WHEREAS, Hospital operates a primary care clinic open to the public and located at _____ ("Clinic"); and

WHEREAS, one of the reasons the Hospital operates the Clinic is to help train physicians while in residency at the Hospital; and

WHEREAS, Hospital wishes to retain Physician to provide services to the public and to help train residents at the Clinic and the Hospital;

NOW, THEREFORE, the Hospital and Physician agree as follows:

1. Duties of physician

Physician shall see and treat patients at the Clinic in her specialty of pediatrics and shall assist in performing those duties and responsibilities needed for the proper, efficient, and professional operation of the Clinic. These duties shall include those matters set forth in Exhibit A attached to this Agreement. Physician shall devote her full time to the duties and responsibilities at the Clinic and Hospital with the exclusion of all other professional activities unless the Hospital, in its discretion, allows Physician to engage in such other activities. Physician shall be expected to work a normal week (40 hours, plus every third weekend on call) and in addition perform rounds on her hospitalized patients, and when appropriate and assigned, rounds on resident's and/or other Clinic's hospitalized patients. Physician hereby assigns to the Hospital all rights she may now or hereafter possess to receive income, payment, and/or reimbursement for any and all professional medical services rendered by her under this Agreement. If requested by the Hospital, the Physician shall execute such documents as may be necessary or desirable to effectuate said assignment with respect to public and private third-party reimbursement programs. Physician shall also provide training and supervision for interns and residents assigned to the Clinic and her rotations at the Hospital or other hospitals as required by the Clinic Director and the Hospital's Director of Medical Education, all consistent with applicable accreditation standards. The Physician shall be loyal to the duties, goals, and objectives of the Hospital, all as expressed in the Articles of Incorporation and Bylaws and other policy statements of the Hospital. The Physician shall carefully guard the Hospital's proprietary rights, and Physician shall not disclose any confidential information concerning the Hospital to third parties without the prior written consent of the Hospital.

2. Additional duties of physician

Physician shall have the following additional duties and obligations as an employee of the Hospital:

A. At all times during the term of this Agreement, Physician shall maintain membership in good standing on the active professional staff of the Hospital and maintain admitting privileges and agree to abide by all Hospital and professional Staff Bylaws, rules, and regulations; provided, however, Physician shall not be prohibited from maintaining professional staff privileges at any other hospitals.

B. Physician shall maintain an unrestricted license to practice medicine in the state during the term of this Agreement. Physician shall not permit her license to be revoked, surrendered, or suspended. Physician shall maintain current and unrestricted federal (DEA) and state narcotic registrations.

C. Physician shall become board certified in her specialty of pediatrics within three years of the commencement date of this Agreement pursuant to the standards of the American Board of Pediatrics.

D. Physician shall participate on Hospital professional staff committees to which she is assigned.

E. Upon request, Physician shall supervise any employees working with her.

F. Upon request, Physician shall assist the Hospital in expanding departmental services and formulating institutional long-range plans.

G. Physician shall submit to a postoffer preemployment physical examination, and Hospital shall be entitled to inquire whether or not physician is capable of performing the essential functions of the position with or without reasonable accommodation, and if accommodation is required, the extent and nature of said accommodation.

H. Physician shall assist in the education of interns and residents as directed by the Hospital at the Clinics and the Hospital, including responsibilities as mutually agreed upon.

I. Consistent with the Hospital charitable and nonprofit objectives, Physician shall see and treat patients regardless of their ability or inability to pay for services on the same basis as all other similarly situated patients of the Clinic. Physician shall also see and treat any Medicaid or Medicare patients coming to her at the Clinic and continually remain eligible for Medicare and Medicaid participation.

J. Physician will cooperate fully with the call coverage system established for the Clinic, which will require Physician to participate on an equivalent basis with the other physicians assigned to the Clinic. Physician shall also cooperate with the other physicians of the Clinic in the residency program and associated physicians.

3. Physician to be employee of hospital

In performing the professional services and all duties described in this Agreement, Physician shall be an employee of the Hospital, and Physician understands and agrees that Physician's salary shall be subject to tax withholding pursuant to state and federal tax laws, including federal income tax and taxes under the Federal Insurance Contributions Act (FICA) and Federal Unemployment Tax Act (FUTA). Physician, however, shall exercise her own independent professional judgment in the practice of medicine, and the Hospital shall in no way interfere with this independent professional judgment

or direct Physician as to how to medically treat patients in any way. Nothing in this paragraph, however, shall be deemed to prevent a review of Physician's professional competence by the appropriate physician peer review committees of the Hospital, as well as the duly licensed Director of Medical Education.

4. Contract fees
   A. In exchange for the professional services to be performed by the Physician, Physician shall receive an annual base salary of Eighty Thousand Dollars ($80,000). All revenues generated by Physician through professional activities during this Agreement shall become the property of the Hospital.
   B. In addition to the above-described base salary, Physician shall be entitled to earn a productivity bonus. The productivity bonus for the year beginning July 1, 20__, and ending on June 30, 20__ shall be computed in accordance with this paragraph; however, major capital expenditures by the Hospital, or new or unanticipated expenses of the Hospital may require an adjustment of the productivity bonus, but only after the first year (and assuming the Agreement is extended beyond one year). The Hospital and Physician shall attempt to agree mutually on a reasonable productivity bonus after the first year if this Agreement is extended beyond the initial one-(1) year term. The initial productivity bonus shall be calculated as follows: Once patient revenues attributable to Physician's professional services and actually received by the Hospital reach One Hundred Eighty-five Thousand Dollars ($185,000) for the year (measured from July 1, 200__), Physician shall be paid a productivity bonus equal to twenty percent (20%) of all patient revenues actually received by the Hospital in excess of One Hundred Eighty-five Thousand Dollars ($185,000) and thirty percent (30%) of patient revenue actually received by the Hospital over Two Hundred Sixty-four Thousand Dollars ($264,000). For the purposes of computing the productivity bonus, revenues will be reviewed monthly by the Hospital when accounting information is available, which accounting information shall be made available monthly to Physician upon request. For each month the Physician may be paid an advance on the expected and projected annual productivity bonus at the discretion of the Hospital's Chief Financial Officer, with reconciliations made quarterly and at the end of each year. If the total adjusted gross revenues for the year to date or the trend of that revenue does not justify payment of the productivity bonus, it shall be the prerogative of the Chief Financial Officer of the Hospital not to make such advance payments. At the end of the year under this Agreement (June 30), the balance of the earned productivity bonus, if any, shall be paid within thirty (30) days after the Hospital receives the financial data in order to compute the productivity bonus. In computing the productivity bonus, the revenue received by the Hospital shall relate back to the date services were performed. In no event shall the base salary and the productivity bonus in the aggregate exceed the sum annually of $180,000.

C. During the term of this Agreement and one hundred eighty- (180) day period referred to in Item C(ii) below, the Hospital shall make a reasonable and good-faith effort to collect all accounts receivable in a timely manner. Accounts receivable accumulated from the Physician's professional services at the end of the Agreement shall be credited to the Physician in the following manner:

    i. If Physician continues her agreement with the Hospital, all Physician's accumulated accounts receivable will roll over to the next contracted period, if any. Collections from these accounts receivables, however, will apply to the prior year in determining the productivity bonus.

    ii. If either Physician or Hospital discontinues the Agreement, the collection of the accounts receivable will continue in a normal manner. If Physician has qualified for the productivity bonus for the contract period or additional time period worked, the bonus shall be paid out monthly to the Physician. At the end of one hundred eighty (180) days following expiration or termination of this Agreement, all financial responsibilities of the Hospital to the Physician shall cease.

5. Employee fringe benefits

In addition to the salary described above, Physician shall be entitled to receive the following benefits from the Hospital in connection with her employment:

A. Health and dental insurance. The Hospital shall make health insurance and dental insurance available to Physician and her immediate dependents pursuant to the Hospital's insurance plan for employees existing at the time of Physician's employment and as the insurance plan might be modified from time to time for all employees with the same cost basis as is afforded to other similarly situated Physician employees. The intent of this paragraph is that Physician shall be entitled to the same health insurance benefits during the term of her employment as are afforded to any other similarly situated Hospital employee.

B. Continuing medical education. Physician shall be entitled to forty (40) hours of paid time off per year to attend continuing medical education courses within the United States and Canada. These courses must be approved at least four (4) weeks in advance in writing by the Hospital. Expenses eligible for reimbursement, but not to exceed Two Thousand Dollars ($2,000) in any one year, shall include the following:

    i. Transportation to and from the meeting as well as local transportation to the meeting site

    ii. Tuition expenses

    iii. Lodging while at the meeting

    iv. Direct reimbursement of reasonable food costs, excluding alcoholic beverages, gifts, or other nonessential expenses

    v. Spousal expenses in connection with continuing medical education shall not be reimbursed.

CME time may be carried over for a five- (5) month period of time following the end of each contract year except following any contract termination or expiration date.

C. Professional liability coverage. Professional liability coverage shall be afforded to Physician during the term of her employment, with coverage limits in the amount of Two Million dollars ($2,000,000) for any one occurrence per year and Ten Million Dollars ($10,000,000) for all Hospital occurrences per year under the Hospital's Professional Liability Insurance policy. Following termination or expiration of this Agreement, the Hospital shall have no further obligation to furnish professional liability coverage; provided, however, all covered acts or omissions that occurred during the time Physician was an employee shall remain covered under the Hospital's Professional Liability Loss fund after Physician leaves the employment of the Hospital. If patients need to be admitted to a hospital other than the Hospital, Physician shall still be considered an employee of the Hospital and shall still have professional liability coverage under this paragraph.

D. Vacation, sick leave/personal time. Physician shall be entitled to one hundred twenty (120) hours of paid vacation per year, with the time being approved at least four (4) weeks in advance in writing by the Hospital's Chief Executive Officer or his designee. The vacation time may be carried over for a period of five (5) months in the following year except following any contract termination or expiration date. These hours of vacation are in addition to the above-described paid time off to attend continuing medical education courses. Physician shall also be entitled to forty (40) hours of paid sick leave/personal time per year, which may be carried over for a period of five (5) months in the following year except following any contract termination or expiration date. Physician shall be responsible to provide coverage (or trade with other attendings) if four (4) weeks' advance notice is not given in writing for all vacations or absences from her normally scheduled or committed hours; provided, however, that Hospital will make a diligent effort to assist Physician in locating other physicians to provide coverage in emergency situations.

E. Other benefits. In addition to the above-described fringe benefits, Physician shall be entitled to the following:
  i. Receive such other benefits as are received by other Hospital employees that are not inconsistent with this Agreement.
  ii. The Hospital shall also pay for required medical staff and professional dues.
  iii. The Hospital shall pay for three (3) subscriptions to medical journals not exceeding a total of Two Hundred Fifty Dollars ($250) per year in subscription costs.
  iv. The Hospital shall provide a basic cellular phone and basic air time. Physician shall be afforded the same privileges regarding cellular phones as are afforded to other physicians at the Clinic. All personal calls shall be reimbursed by the Physician promptly after receipt of such bills.

If there is a conflict between the Hospital's employee benefit plan and the terms of this Agreement, this Agreement shall govern.

6. Term of agreement

This Agreement shall commence on the 1st day of July, 20__, and shall expire on June 30, 20__. If Physician has performed satisfactorily under this Agreement, and assuming the Hospital has a continuing need for a pediatrician at the Clinic, Hospital and Physician shall, at least one hundred twenty (120) days prior to the end of this Agreement, begin discussions regarding whether or not to extend this Agreement as well as the terms of Physician's salary, productivity bonus, or any other provision of this Agreement. If a mutual understanding cannot, for whatever reason, be reached regarding an extension, this Agreement shall expire according to its terms.

7. Default; termination

If Physician shall fail or refuse to perform any of her obligations or meet any of her duties under this Agreement, Hospital shall give Physician written notice specifying the nature of her default or breach. If Physician fails to cure the default or breach within ten (10) days after receipt of such notice, Hospital shall have the right, upon further written notice to Physician, to terminate this Agreement immediately; provided, however, that if Physician's license to practice medicine in the state is revoked, canceled, surrendered, or suspended; Hospital medical staff privileges are limited, restricted, or revoked; or if she commits any illegal act in her practice or becomes involved in any immoral act or act involving moral turpitude regarding or adversely reflecting upon her medical practice or the Clinic, this Agreement may be summarily terminated by giving notice of such termination to Physician. Likewise, if Hospital shall fail or refuse to perform any of its obligations or meet any of its duties under this Agreement, Physician shall give Hospital written notice specifying the nature of the default. If Hospital fails to cure such default within ten (10) days after receipt of such notice, Physician shall have the right, upon further written notice to Hospital, to terminate this Agreement immediately. If at any time Physician is unable to perform her normal duties for a period of three (3) consecutive months by reason of illness, accident, disability, or similar causes, Hospital may, at its option, terminate this contract without further liability, except that the Hospital shall pay all salary due the Physician during the three- (3) month period of disability. Notwithstanding any provision of this Agreement to the contrary, however, Physician shall be entitled to all benefits of the Federal Family Leave Act without Hospital terminating this Agreement; provided, however, any leave under the Family Leave Act shall be without pay except for any accrued vacation or accrued sick days.

8. Noncompete

Physician acknowledges that as an employee of the Hospital, she will have access to certain Hospital proprietary information and proprietary documents as well as access to confidential information concerning the Hospital. Furthermore, Hospital has committed to expend substantial sums of money in order to maintain Physician to provide services at the Clinic and to train her through continuing medical education courses. In view of the special employment relationship between the Hospital and Physician and in consideration of the expenses and costs to be paid by the Hospital as described in this Agreement, Physician agrees that she shall be prohibited from entering into any contract or other professional relationship, written or unwritten, expressed or implied, concerning the furnishing of medical services in connection with any other hospital, subsidiary of a hospital, or hospital-related corporation except Hospital, within a radius of five (5) miles measured from the main entrance to the Clinic without first obtaining the prior written consent of the Hospital, which may be withheld in the sole discretion of the Hospital. This covenant shall remain in full force and effect for one (1) year after the last date Physician renders patient care under this Agreement. In the event of any breach, this noncompete provision may be enforced by the Hospital at law or in equity in a court of competent jurisdiction. The Hospital shall not only be entitled to seek money damages for a breach of this covenant, but also to seek injunctive relief as may be deemed appropriate. If any standard, time limit, distance, clause, or condition of this noncompete covenant is ever deemed by a court of competent jurisdiction to be unreasonable, the court is hereby authorized to impose a substitute standard that is deemed by the court to be reasonable in view of the intentions of the Hospital and Physician as set forth in the Agreement. This covenant, however, shall not be enforced by the Hospital if Physician is compelled to terminate this Agreement because of Hospital's material default, following notice and right to cure as described above in paragraph 7.

9. Assignment

Physician shall not assign any right, nor delegate any duty under this Agreement; provided, however, that Physician may, at any time, form a professional corporation or other recognized legal entity of which she retains controlling interest and to which she may assign her rights and delegate all her duties under this Agreement. In the event of any such assignment, Physician shall notify Hospital in advance in writing, and this Agreement shall be amended to the extent necessary to reflect the formulation of the professional corporation or other legal entity as a party to this Agreement.

10. Notices

Notices provided to be given pursuant to this Agreement shall be given either in writing in person, or in writing by certified mail, postage prepaid, return receipt requested, addressed as follows:

- **To Hospital:**

_____

_____

_____

_____

- **To Physician:**

_____

_____

_____

_____

11. Future legislation

In the event of future legislation, safe harbor regulations, government rule or regulation, policy, or governmental interpretation thereof that applies to this Agreement and prohibits or invalidates any of its provisions or causes the Hospital or Physician not to qualify under or otherwise be in violation (actual or potential) of any Medicare, Medicaid, or reimbursement regulations or other law or if the Hospital's continuing ability to qualify as a tax-exempt Section 501(c)(3) corporation is in jeopardy (actual or potential) at any time, as determined by the Hospital, then the parties hereto shall either forthwith cause to be made to this Agreement such amendments as may be reasonably required to bring its terms back into compliance or, in the alternative, the Hospital or Physician may summarily terminate this Agreement without penalty.

12. Confidentiality

To the extent permitted by law, neither Hospital nor Physician shall divulge the salary information contained in this Agreement to any other physicians. Both parties shall make a good-faith effort to keep the salary information confidential.

13. Patient records

Upon expiration or termination of this Agreement as provided above in paragraphs 6, 7, or 11, all patient records and charts shall remain at the Clinic in the possession of the Hospital. The Hospital, however, shall cooperate in furnishing copies of the records and charts to patients who request them.

14. Miscellaneous conditions

The following conditions also apply to this Agreement:

A.   Recitals. The recitals at the beginning of this Agreement are intended to describe the intent of the parties and the circumstances under which this Agreement is executed and, consequently, shall be considered in the interpretation of this Agreement.

B.   Amendment. This Agreement may be amended only by the written consent of the parties.

C.   Waiver. The failure or delay of either party to insist in any one or more instances upon performance of any terms or conditions of this Agreement shall not be construed as a waiver of past or future performance of any such terms, covenants, or condition; but the obligations of such party with respect thereto shall continue in full force and effect.

D. Severability. If one or more of the provisions contained in this Agreement are declared to be invalid, illegal, or unenforceable in any respect by a court of competent jurisdiction, the validity, legality, and enforceability of the remaining provisions of this Agreement shall not in any way be impaired thereby unless the effect of such declaration of the court would be to materially and substantially impair or diminish either party's rights and benefits hereunder.

E. Governing law. This Agreement shall be interpreted under and governed by the law of the State of _____, without regard to choice of law or conflict of law principles.

F. Entire agreement. This Agreement constitutes the entire agreement between the parties and replaces and supersedes all prior written and oral statements and understandings between the parties. Furthermore, there are no side deals, understandings, or other arrangement or agreement between the parties, either express or implied, pertaining to the subject matter of this Agreement.

PHYSICIAN   HOSPITAL

_____   By _____

                                                     Title: _____

Exhibit A—Physician Responsibilities

1. Physician shall make Hospital rounds as appropriate and required. Residents and/or interns will not have sole responsibility for "rounding."
2. Physician shall sign Hospital medical records and dictate discharge summaries on a weekly basis.
3. Physician shall respond to outside supervisory or peer review inquiries within the designated time frame and inform Hospital Administration of such letters.
4. Physician shall encourage patients to return by requesting follow-up appointments where appropriate on a day that the Physician is in the Clinic. Physician shall distribute business cards to patients as appropriate.
5. Physician shall treat walk-in patients.
6. The physician will foster a family care relationship with patients.
7. Physician shall practice pediatric medicine at the Clinic and will make referrals to other physicians where medically necessary or appropriate for the patient's well-being.
8. Physician shall either handwrite or dictate progress notes on all patients treated in the clinic. In addition, all medications dispensed (sample or prescriptions to be filled) will be noted in the chart. If progress notes are dictated, simple handwritten notes will be made in the chart for reference on an interim basis.
9. Physician shall keep the Clinic Director informed of personnel, equipment, or patient care problems.
10. Physician shall work closely with the Clinic Director on those issues pertaining to staffing, revenue, and other related Clinic issues.
11. Physician shall perform in a professional manner at all times, setting an example for all Clinic staff.
12. Physician shall work closely with all physicians within the Clinic to ensure that information is openly shared with affected individuals.
13. Consistent with the Hospital's charitable and nonprofit objectives, Physician shall see and treat patients regardless of their ability or inability to pay for services. Physician shall also see and treat all Medicaid or Medicare patients coming to her at the Clinic.

MEDICAL DIRECTOR AGREEMENT—EMPLOYEE

**Medical Director Agreement
(Department of _____)**

This Agreement is entered into this _____ day of _____, 200__, by and between _____, a nonprofit corporation ("Hospital"), and _____ ("Physician").

Recitals

A. The Hospital is a not-for-profit corporation as described under Section 501(c)(3) of the Internal Revenue Code.

B. The Hospital desires to retain the services of a Physician to be a Medical Director within the Hospital.

C. Physician is a duly licensed physician in the state and is qualified and willing to provide Medical Director services in accordance with the terms of this Agreement.

NOW, THEREFORE, Hospital and Physician agree as follows:

1. Scope of services
    Physician shall provide the following services to the Hospital
    a. Accreditation and licensure. Assist Hospital in the operation and management of the Department of _____ ("Department") to help ensure continued licensure, certification, and accreditation, as well as participation in the Medicare and Medicaid programs.
    b. Education. Assist Hospital in developing and implementing educational, training, and in-service programs for nonphysician personnel and provide or participate in educational or clinical programs for the medical staff as well as any medical students, interns, or residents in the Department.
    c. Technical advice. Advise Hospital's administration on operational and technical matters and make recommendations pertaining to the Department.
    d. Programs. Participate in professional organizations and programs and cooperate in the development of programs to enhance the Hospital's services.
    e. Consultation. Provide _____ hours per month of professional review and consultation services for Hospital personnel and physicians.
    f. Log of hours. Physician shall provide a detailed log of duty hours to the Hospital and submit it within ten (10) days following the end of each month describing all activities and services performed and certifying the number of hours and the days worked.
    g. Quality improvement. Participate in quality improvement meetings to review patient care, quality improvement, and operations pertaining to the Department.
    h. Legal compliance. Assist the Hospital and Department staff in complying with applicable state and federal laws and regulations

applying to the practice of medicine and maintenance of Hospital's Department.

2. Additional duties of physician

Physician shall have the following additional duties as the Director of the Department:

   a. Treatment policies. Physician shall abide by Hospital's policies and specifically agrees to provide services to employees, applicants for employment, and students of Hospital in accordance with the policies of Hospital and to provide all necessary services without regard to race, color, sex, age, disability, or other legally protected classification.

   b. Records. All medical records shall remain the property of the Hospital. Physician shall maintain medical records in accordance with the Hospital's policies and complete all records and reports in a timely fashion. Physician shall be entitled to access to medical records, as needed, in connection with responsibilities under this Agreement or as needed to reasonably conduct business or comply with state or federal law.

   c. Relationships. Physician shall establish and maintain positive working relationships with the patients within the Hospital, patient family members, or personal representatives, and with Hospital's employees, members of Hospital's medical staff, and outside referring practitioners and agencies.

   d. Hospital and medical staff policies. Physician shall comply with applicable bylaws, rules and regulations of the Medical Staff, and with the bylaws and policies of Hospital in delivering services under this Agreement.

   e. Risk management. Physician shall comply with the Hospital's risk management and malpractice prevention practices when performing services under this Agreement.

   f. Outside activities. The Hospital acknowledges that Physician maintains an outside medical practice. The Hospital acknowledges and consents to the continued conduct of Physician's outside medical practice provided that the outside medical practice or activities shall not have the effect of reducing services below required levels or of detracting from the prompt performance of services required under this Agreement.

   g. Independent medical judgment. Physician shall use his or her best professional judgment in determining when, how, where, and whether to render treatment to individual patients. The Hospital shall neither have nor exercise, nor attempt to exercise, any control over the professional judgment and decision making of Physician. Physician is free to accept and treat patients according to Physician's best judgment, or to transfer such patients for diagnosis or care to other practitioners or facilities in accordance with the patient's best interest, all without the loss of any benefits under this Agreement.

   h. Prohibited financial relationships. Neither Physician nor any member of Physician's immediate family may have a financial relationship (including an employment relationship) with the Hospital that is related to the provision of designated health services as defined at Section 1877 of the Social Security Act and commonly referred to as the "Stark Amendment" during the term of this Agreement unless Hospital provides express written consent in Hospital's sole discretion. Consent will be given or withheld based upon the perceived impact such a relationship (as perceived by the Hospital in its sole discretion) could have on this Agreement and the duties of Physician because of the application of Section 1877 of the Social Security Act (or similar state or federal legislation). If federal or corresponding state limitations are broadened to include other services, this paragraph shall be deemed to extend automatically to such broadened limitations. Physician certifies that, as of the effective date of this Agreement, no such prohibited financial relationship exists. Physician shall give Hospital written notice within five (5) business days following the creation of any such financial relationship during the term of this Agreement or any extension or renewal hereof. For purposes of this provision, immediate family is defined to mean the same as under the federal statute: spouse, natural or adoptive parent, child, sibling, stepparent, stepchild, stepbrother, stepsister, father-in-law, mother-in-law, daughter-in-law, son-in-law, brother-in-law, sister-in-law, grandparent, grandchild, and spouse of a grandparent or grandchild.

    i. Program default. Physician certifies that he or she is not now in default under, or upon execution and performance of this Agreement will be in default under, the National Health Service Corp Scholarship program, the Physician Shortage Area Scholarship program, the Health Education Assistance Loan program, or any other program that would permit offset of delinquent or defaulted obligations against payments due Physician under the Medicare Program now or during the terms of this Agreement.

3. Qualifications

   Physician must continuously meet each of the following qualifications:

    a. Membership on staff. At all times during the term of this Agreement, Physician shall maintain membership in good standing on the active professional staff of the Hospital and maintain admitting privileges and agree to abide by all Hospital and professional staff bylaws, rules, and regulations; provided, however, Physician shall not be prohibited from maintaining professional staff privileges at any other hospitals.

    b. License. Physician shall maintain an unrestricted license to practice medicine in the state during the term of this Agreement. Physician shall not permit his or her license to be revoked, surrendered, or suspended. Physician shall maintain current and unrestricted federal (DEA) and state narcotic registrations.

    c. Board certification. Physician shall become Board certified in his or her specialty within three years of the commencement date of this Agreement.

    d. Physical examination. Physician shall submit to a postoffer preemployment physical examination, and Hospital shall be entitled to inquire whether or not Physician is capable of performing the essential functions of the position with or without reasonable accommodation, and if accommodation is required, to inquire about the extent and nature of said accommodation.

e. Charity care; Medicare participation. Consistent with the Hospital charitable and nonprofit objectives, Physician shall see and treat patients regardless of their ability or inability to pay for services on the same basis as all other similarly situated patients of the Hospital. Physician shall also see and treat any Medicaid or Medicare patients coming to the Department and continually remain eligible for Medicare and Medicaid participation.

4. Physician to be employee of hospital

In performing the professional services and all duties described in this Agreement, Physician shall be a part-time employee of the Hospital, and Physician understands and agrees that Physician's salary shall be subject to tax withholding pursuant to state and federal tax laws, including federal income tax and taxes under the Federal Insurance Contributions Act (FICA) and Federal Unemployment Tax Act (FUTA). Physician, however, shall exercise his or her own independent professional judgment in the practice of medicine, and the Hospital shall in no way interfere with this independent professional judgment or direct Physician as to how to medically treat patients in any way except as set forth in this Agreement. Nothing in this paragraph, however, shall be deemed to prevent a review of Physician's professional competence by the appropriate physician peer review committees of the Hospital, as well as the duly licensed Director of Medical Education. Physician as a part-time employee shall not be entitled to any fringe benefits customarily afforded to full-time Hospital employees.

5. Salary

In exchange for the professional services to be performed under this Agreement, Physician shall receive an annual salary of _____ (_____) which shall be paid in equal installments at the same time as other Hospital employees are paid their salaries.

6. Professional liability coverage

Professional liability coverage shall be afforded by Hospital to Physician during the term of his or her employment, with coverage limits in the amount of Two Million Dollars ($2,000,000) for any one occurrence per year and Ten Million Dollars ($10,000,000) for all Hospital occurrences per year under the Hospital's Professional Liability Insurance policy. Following termination or expiration of this Agreement, the Hospital shall have no further obligation to furnish professional liability coverage; provided, however, all covered acts or omissions that occurred during the time Physician was an employee shall remain covered under the Hospital's Professional Liability Policy after Physician leaves the employment of the Hospital. If patients need to be admitted to a hospital other than the Hospital as a part of Physician's duties under this Agreement, Physician shall still be considered an employee of the Hospital and shall still have professional liability coverage under this paragraph while following those patients at other hospitals.

7. Term of agreement

This Agreement shall commence on the 1st day of July, 20__, and shall expire on June 30, 20__. If Physician has performed satisfactorily under this Agreement, and assuming the Hospital has a continuing need for Director of the Department, Hospital and Physician shall, at least one hundred twenty (120) days prior to the end of this Agreement, begin discussions regarding whether or not to extend this Agreement. If a mutual understanding cannot, for whatever reason, be reached regarding an extension, this Agreement shall expire according to its terms.

8. Default; termination

If Physician shall fail or refuse to perform any of his or her obligations or meet any of his or her duties under this Agreement, Hospital shall give Physician written notice specifying the nature of his or her default or breach. If Physician fails to cure the default or breach within ten (10) days after receipt of such notice, Hospital shall have the right, upon further written notice to Physician, to terminate this Agreement immediately; provided, however, that if Physician's license to practice medicine in the state is revoked, canceled, surrendered, or suspended, or Hospital medical staff privileges are limited, restricted, or revoked, or if he or she commits any illegal act in his or her practice or becomes involved in any immoral act or act involving moral turpitude regarding or adversely reflecting upon his or her medical practice or the Department, this Agreement may be summarily terminated by giving notice of such termination to Physician. Likewise, if Hospital shall fail or refuse to perform any of its obligations or meet any of its duties under this Agreement, Physician shall give Hospital written notice specifying the nature of the default. If Hospital fails to cure such default within ten (10) days after receipt of such notice, Physician shall have the right, upon further written notice to Hospital, to terminate this Agreement immediately. If at any time Physician is unable to perform his or her normal duties for a period of three (3) consecutive months by reason of illness, accident, disability, or similar causes, Hospital may, at its option, terminate this contract without further liability, except that the Hospital shall pay all salary due the Physician during the three- (3) month period of disability. Notwithstanding any provision of this Agreement to the contrary, however, Physician shall be entitled to all benefits of the Federal Family Leave Act without Hospital terminating this Agreement; provided, however, any leave under the Family Leave Act shall be without pay except for any accrued vacation or accrued sick days.

9. Assignment prohibited

Physician shall not assign any right nor delegate any duty under this Agreement. This Agreement shall be binding upon any of Hospital's successors in interest and may be assigned by Hospital without Physician consent.

10. Notices

Notices provided to be given pursuant to this Agreement shall be given either in writing in person, or in writing by certified mail, postage prepaid, return receipt requested, addressed as follows:

- **To Hospital:**

_____

_____

_____

_____

- **To Physician:**

_____

_____

_____

_____

11. Future legislation

In the event of future legislation, safe harbor regulations, government rule or regulation, policy, or governmental interpretation thereof that applies to this Agreement and prohibits or invalidates any of its provisions or causes the Hospital or Physician not to qualify under or otherwise be in violation (actual or potential) of any Medicare, Medicaid, or reimbursement regulations or other law or if the Hospital's continuing ability to qualify as a tax-exempt Section 501(c)(3) corporation is in jeopardy (actual or potential) at any time, as determined by the Hospital, then the parties hereto shall either forthwith cause to be made to this Agreement such amendments as may be reasonably required to bring its terms back into compliance or, in the alternative, the Hospital or Physician may summarily terminate this Agreement without penalty.

12. Confidentiality

To the extent permitted by law, neither Hospital nor Physician shall divulge the salary information contained in this Agreement to any other physicians. Both parties shall make a good-faith effort to keep the salary information confidential.

13. Miscellaneous conditions

The following conditions also apply to this Agreement:
  a. Recitals. The recitals at the beginning of this Agreement are intended to describe the intent of the parties and the circumstances under which this Agreement is executed and, consequently, shall be considered in the interpretation of this Agreement.
  b. Amendment. This Agreement may be amended only by the written consent of the parties.

c. Waiver. The failure or delay of either party to insist in any one or more instances upon performance of any terms or conditions of this Agreement shall not be construed as a waiver of past or future performance of any such terms, covenants, or condition, but the obligations of such party with respect thereto shall continue in full force and effect.

d. Severability. If one or more of the provisions contained in this Agreement are declared to be invalid, illegal, or unenforceable in any respect by a court of competent jurisdiction, the validity, legality, and enforceability of the remaining provisions of this Agreement shall not in any way be impaired thereby unless the effect of such declaration of the court would be to materially and substantially impair or diminish either party's rights and benefits hereunder.

e. Governing law. This Agreement shall be interpreted under and governed by the law of the State of _____, without regard to choice of law or conflict of law principles.

f. Entire agreement. This Agreement constitutes the entire agreement between the parties and replaces and supersedes all prior written and oral statements and understandings between the parties. Furthermore, there are no side deals, understandings, or other arrangements or agreements between the parties, either express or implied, pertaining to the subject matter of this Agreement.

PHYSICIAN   HOSPITAL

_____   By _____

                                            Title: _____

PROFESSIONAL SERVICES AGREEMENT—EMPLOYEE (FAMILY PRACTICE)

Director and Trainer for Family Practice Residency Program Agreement for Professional Services

This Agreement is entered into this ___ day of _____, 20__, effective the ___ day of _____, 20__, by and between _____, a nonprofit corporation ("Hospital") and _____, a physician specializing in family practice and who is duly licensed to practice medicine in the State of _____ ("Physician").

1. Statement of intent

The Hospital maintains an accredited family practice residency training program that includes training of residents at _____; the Hospital campus at _____; and continuity clinics affiliated with the Hospital's family practice residency training program (collectively "Clinics"). To continue meeting accreditation standards, the Hospital desires to designate Physician as a Director and one of its Trainers of the Hospital's family practice residency program in connection with the Clinics. Therefore, Hospital and Physician have agreed to enter into this Agreement for professional services.

2. Duties of physician

Physician, as a Director, shall assist in the training of Hospital family practice residents in the Clinics, consistent with applicable accreditation guidelines, and as directed by the Hospital, including seeing and treating patients as necessary in connection with such training. Physician shall be headquartered at _____. These duties shall be performed at the direction and under the supervision of the Hospital's Director of Medical Education; provided, however, that Physician shall exercise independent medical judgment, and the Hospital shall not exercise any dominion or control over Physician's professional services except as set forth in this Agreement. The duties of Physician shall include the following:
   A. Performing at least 40 hours of services at the Clinics per week. Physician shall also be the Trainer responsible for hands-on supervision of residents on a day-to-day basis. At other Clinic locations where there are already Trainers, Physician shall periodically visit the Clinics as requested by the Hospital's designee to verify the continuity of the clinic experience the residents are having and make recommendations to the residents, Trainers, and the Hospital.
   B. Supervising family practice residents who are training at the Clinics, including supervision of residents to ensure full compliance with the federal regulations that took effect July 1, 1996, in connection with residents and teaching hospitals, and where Part B is billed for patients who are Medicare beneficiaries as described in 60 Federal Register, Subpart D, Sections 415.170 through 415.174, including all interpretive regulations or amendments pertaining thereto. The Hospital shall furnish Physician with copies of applicable federal regulations so that

he can perform his duties under this subparagraph B. The Hospital's Legal Compliance Officer, as well as the Hospital's legal counsel, shall be available to Physician to help interpret any federal regulations.

C. Attending and contributing to the regular family practice residency meetings

D. Performing such other reasonable duties consistent with accreditation guidelines as may be required, including consultation or intervention with residents in conjunction with the Director of Medical Education and Chief of Staff of the Hospital.

Physician shall be a Hospital employee and shall receive employee benefits as provided below in this Agreement. Accordingly, the Hospital will withhold state and federal taxes regarding the fee paid to Physician under this Agreement, including federal income tax, FICA, and FUTA.

3. Responsibility to Hospital; compliance with law

Physician shall be loyal to the duties, goals, and objectives of the Hospital, all as expressed in the Articles of Incorporation and Bylaws and other policy statements of the Hospital. Physician shall carefully guard the Hospital's proprietary rights, and he shall not disclose any confidential information concerning the Hospital to third parties without the prior written consent of the Hospital. Physician represents to the Hospital that he is knowledgeable about the Hospital's family practice residency training program and also about federal regulations governing residents and teaching hospitals, specifically including the federal regulations effective July 1, 1996, applicable to freestanding family practice clinics and Part B billing for patients who are Medicare beneficiaries (60 Federal Register, Subpart D, Sections 415.170 through 415.174 and the interpretive regulations and all amendments thereto). Physician shall abide by all applicable state and federal laws in discharging his duties under this Agreement.

4. Professional standards

Physician, in addition to the duties described elsewhere in this Agreement, shall meet the following professional standards:

A. At all times during the term of this Agreement, Physician shall maintain membership in good standing on the professional staff of the Hospital, Active Staff Category, and abide by all applicable Hospital and Professional Staff bylaws, rules, and regulations as well as policies and procedures. Nothing in this Agreement shall in any way prohibit Physician from maintaining medical staff privileges at any other hospital.

B. Physician shall maintain an unrestricted license to practice medicine in the state during the term of this Agreement. He shall not permit his license to be revoked, surrendered, or suspended.

C. Physician shall be physically and mentally fully capable of competently and professionally discharging all duties under this Agreement subject to any reasonable accommodations required of the Hospital under the Americans with Disabilities Act (ADA) or any other federal, state, or local law.

D. Consistent with the Hospital's charitable and nonprofit objectives, Physician shall, if necessary, see and treat patients under this Agreement at the Clinics regardless of the patients' inability to pay for services.

5. Agreement fee

In exchange for the professional services to be performed by Physician under this Agreement, the Hospital shall pay Physician an annual salary of One Hundred Twenty Thousand Dollars ($120,000) per year, prorated and adjusted to the effective date and expiration date of this Agreement, with periodic payments being made at the same time as other Hospital employees are paid. The Hospital shall have the right to terminate this Agreement, without penalty, if, in the Hospital's opinion, a pattern is established by Physician where he is taking more vacation time or leave time than permitted under this Agreement and that pattern is having, in the opinion of the Hospital, a negative effect on the residency training program at the Clinics (subject to state and federal laws regarding disability and family emergency leaves, if applicable). In addition to the other payments by Hospital described in this Agreement, Physician shall be reimbursed for mileage and reasonable out-of-pocket expenses incurred for the benefit of the Hospital pursuant to Hospital policies and procedures. Requests for reimbursement shall be documented and shall be submitted in writing to the Hospital's Chief Financial Officer or designee.

6. Employee fringe benefits

In addition to the salary described above, Physician shall be entitled to receive the following benefits from the Hospital in connection with his employment:

A. Health and dental insurance. The Hospital shall make health insurance and dental insurance available to Physician and his immediate dependents pursuant to the Hospital's insurance plan for employees existing at the time of Physician's employment and as the insurance plan might be modified from time to time for all employees. The intent of this paragraph is that Physician shall be entitled to the same health insurance benefits during the term of his employment as are afforded to any other Hospital employee. Physician acknowledges that these health insurance benefits may be subject to change as to all Hospital employees from one Hospital fiscal year to another.

B. Continuing medical education. Physician shall be entitled to two (2) weeks of paid time off per year to attend continuing medical education courses within the United States and Canada. These courses must be approved in advance by the Hospital. Expenses eligible for reimbursement, but not to exceed Three Thousand Dollars ($3000) in any one year, shall including the following:

   i. Transportation to and from the meeting as well as local transportation to the meeting site

   ii. Tuition expenses

   iii. Lodging while at the meeting

iv. Direct reimbursement of reasonable food costs, excluding alcoholic beverages, gifts, or other nonessential expenses

v. Spousal expenses in connection with continuing medical education shall not be reimbursed.

C. Professional liability coverage. Professional liability coverage shall be afforded to Physician during the term of his employment, with coverage limits in the amount of One Million Dollars ($1,000,000) for any one occurrence per year and Five Million Dollars ($5,000,000) for all occurrences per year under the Hospital's Professional Liability Insurance policy together with an umbrella/excess coverage policy as may be deemed appropriate by the Hospital. Following termination or expiration of this Agreement, the Hospital shall have no further obligation to furnish professional liability coverage; provided, however, all covered acts or omissions that occurred during the time Physician was an employee shall remain covered under the Hospital's Professional Liability Insurance Policy after Physician leaves the employment of the Hospital. If patients desire or need to be admitted to a healthcare facility other than Hospital, Physician shall still be an employee of the Hospital while attending the patient, and he shall continue to have professional liability coverage under this paragraph subject to Physician providing an accounting to the Hospital regarding such patients so that the Hospital can monitor quality improvement issues and provide peer review of those activities pursuant to insurance underwriting requirements.

D. Vacation; sick leave. Beginning _____, 200__, Physician shall be entitled to three weeks of paid vacation per year (with the year measured from January 1) with the times being taken, if possible, in three one-week blocks or one two-week block and one one-week block and approved in advance by the Hospital. The vacation time shall not be carried over to the following year. These three weeks of vacation are in addition to the above-described paid time off to attend continuing medical education courses. Physician shall also be entitled to seven (7) days of paid sick leave per year (with the year measured from January 1), which may not be carried over to the following year.

E. Other benefits. In addition to the above-described fringe benefits, Physician shall be entitled to receive such other benefits as are received by other management-level Hospital employees that are not inconsistent with this Agreement. If there is a conflict between the Hospital's employee benefit plan and the terms of this Agreement, this Agreement shall control.

7. Term of agreement

This Agreement shall commence on _____, 20__, and shall extend through _____, 20__; provided, however, this Agreement may be terminated without cause and without penalty ("without cause" shall be defined as a termination not based on a material default as described below in paragraph 8) by either Physician or the Hospital for any reason prior to expiration by giving the other party at least one hundred eighty (180) days' prior written notice, assuming more than one hundred eighty (180) days remain before expiration.

8. Default; termination

If Physician shall fail or refuse to perform any of the obligations under this Agreement, Hospital shall have the right to give Physician written notice specifying the nature of the default or breach. If Physician fails to cure the default or breach within ten (10) days after receipt of such notice, Hospital shall have the right to declare that this Agreement is terminated immediately; provided, however, that if Physician has his license to practice medicine in the state materially changed to the detriment of the Hospital, revoked, canceled, surrendered, or suspended, or if he commits any illegal act or act of moral turpitude that could have an adverse effect on the Hospital, the Clinics, or the resident training program, this Agreement may be summarily terminated, without penalty, by giving notice of such termination to Physician. Likewise, if Hospital shall fail or refuse to perform any of its obligations or to meet all of the duties under this Agreement, Physician may give the Hospital written notice specifying the nature of the default. If Hospital fails to cure such default within ten (10) days after receipt of the notice, Physician shall have the right, without penalty, to terminate this Agreement immediately.

9. Notices

Notices provided to be given pursuant to this Agreement shall be sufficient if either given in writing in person or in writing by certified mail, postage prepaid, return receipt requested, addressed as follows:

- **To Hospital:**

_____

_____

_____

_____

- **To Physician:**

_____

_____

_____

_____

10. Future legislation

Physician and Hospital are of the opinion that this Agreement fully complies with all applicable state and federal laws in effect at the date this Agreement was signed. Either the Hospital or Physician, however, may immediately terminate this Agreement if any state or federal legislation, rule, or regulation is enacted after the execution of this Agreement or any governmental interpretation rendered or policy adopted that may prohibit or invalidate any provision of this Agreement or that might cause the Hospital or Physician to either not qualify under or be in violation of any Medicare, Medicaid, or other reimbursement regulations or other law or that might, in the Hospital's opinion, jeopardize the Hospital's tax-exempt status as a Section 501(c)(3) non-profit, educational, and charitable corporation.

11. Applicable law

This Agreement shall be governed by and construed under the laws of the State of _____.

12. Binding on successors

This Agreement is personal with Physician, and it shall not be assigned by Physician. This Agreement shall be binding upon and inure to the benefit of the Hospital as well as its successors in interest, grantees, or assigns.

13. Arbitration

The Hospital and Physician agree that any disputes that may arise between them under this Agreement shall be arbitrated in accordance with the following provisions:

   A. The parties desire to avoid and settle without litigation future disputes that may arise between them relative to this Agreement. Accordingly, the parties agree to engage in good-faith negotiations to resolve any such dispute. In the event they are unable to resolve any such dispute by negotiation, then such dispute concerning any matter whose arbitration is not prohibited by law at the time such dispute arises shall be submitted to arbitration in accordance with the arbitration rules of the American Arbitration Association (hereinafter "Rules"), then in effect, and the award rendered by the Arbitrator shall be binding as between the parties, and judgment on such award may be entered in any court having jurisdiction thereof.

   B. The parties shall be allowed to select one neutral Arbitrator from a list of five (5) nominees whose names will be provided by the American Arbitration Association, said Arbitrator shall be an Attorney at Law, and all decisions and awards shall be made by the Arbitrator except for decisions relating to discovery and disclosure as set forth herein.

   C. Notice of a demand for arbitration or of any dispute subject to arbitration by one party shall be filed in writing with the other party and with the American Arbitration Association's regional office. The parties agree that after any such notice has been filed, they shall, before the hearing thereof, make discovery and disclosure of all matters relevant to such dispute, to the extent and in the manner provided by the state rules of civil procedure. All questions that may arise with respect to the obligation of discovery and disclosure and the protection of the disclosed and discovered materials shall be referred to the Arbitrator so elected or may be brought before the state court where Hospital is located, in the event that the Arbitrator has not yet been selected or is otherwise not available to rule upon the matter within ten (10) days after the party seeks a ruling thereon. The state court may entertain such rulings in connection with an action to enforce the terms of this arbitration agreement, and the parties agree to expedite any such hearing or discovery motions or other matters relating to enforcement of this arbitration agreement by waiver of jury trial, waiver of right to remove to federal court, and by agreeing to take up any such matter within ten (10) days after the petition for enforcement is filed with the state court.

D.   Discovery and disclosure shall be completed no later than ninety (90) days after filing of such action for arbitration unless extended by the Arbitrator or by the court entertaining a petition to enforce this arbitration agreement, upon a showing of good cause by either party to said Arbitrator or court.

E.   The Arbitrator may consider any material that is relevant to the subject matter of such dispute even if such material might also be relevant to an issue or issues not subject to arbitration hereunder. A stenographic record shall be made of any arbitration proceeding by a court reporter to be mutually agreed upon.

F.   The Arbitrator's jurisdiction and authority to determine the dispute herein shall be limited to a determination of whether one party or the other has breached a material term or condition or promise in this Agreement, justifying the other party to terminate its further obligations hereunder, and to ordering specific performance by a party of its obligations and promises herein, but such Arbitrator shall not have the authority to enter a judgment for damages against either party to the extent that the party in whose favor the damages award was entered failed to exercise reasonable precaution to mitigate its damage.

G.   The parties shall be responsible for paying the fees and expenses of their respective attorneys, representatives, or advocates before the Arbitrator, but the parties shall share equally the fees of the neutral Arbitrator and of the American Arbitration Association and the costs of the original copy of the transcript prepared by the court reporter who makes the stenographic record, and of the attendance fee of that court reporter.

H.   The decision of the neutral Arbitrator shall be final and binding on the parties so long as rendered within the Arbitrator's authority as limited by this Agreement. Said Arbitrator shall be required to enter his or her decision in writing within fifteen (15) calendar days after the dispute is submitted to the Arbitrator at the conclusion of the hearing, unless the parties mutually agree to extend the date within which the Arbitrator's written decision and award shall be rendered and served on the parties.

14. Miscellaneous conditions
    The following conditions also apply to this Agreement:
    A.   Recitals. The recitals at the beginning of this Agreement are intended to describe the intent of the parties and the circumstances under

which this Agreement is executed and, consequently, shall be considered in the interpretation of this Agreement.

B. Amendment. This Agreement may be amended only by the written consent of the parties.

C. Waiver. The failure or delay of either party to insist in any one or more instances upon performance of any terms or conditions of this Agreement shall not be construed as a waiver of past or future performance of any such terms, covenants, or condition; but the obligations of such party with respect thereto shall continue in full force and effect.

D. Severability. If one or more of the provisions contained in this Agreement are declared to be invalid, illegal, or unenforceable in any respect by a court of competent jurisdiction, the validity, legality, and enforceability of the remaining provisions of this Agreement shall not in any way be impaired thereby unless the effect of such declaration of the court would be to materially and substantially impair or diminish either party's rights and benefits hereunder.

E. Entire Agreement. This Agreement constitutes the entire agreement between the parties and replaces and supersedes all prior written and oral statements and understandings between the parties. Furthermore, there are no side deals, understandings, or other arrangement or agreement between the parties, either express or implied, pertaining to the subject matter of this Agreement.

PHYSICIAN   HOSPITAL

_____   By _____

                                                          Title: _____

PROFESSIONAL SERVICES AGREEMENT—INDEPENDENT CONTRACTOR

Emergency Department Agreement for Professional Services (Independent Contractor)

THIS AGREEMENT is entered into this ___ day of _____, 200__, by and between _____ ("Hospital") and _____ ("P.C.").

Witnesseth:

WHEREAS, Hospital operates an Emergency Department providing emergency care and services to the public, and

WHEREAS, Hospital wishes to retain P.C. as an independent contractor to provide professional services in the Hospital's Emergency Department; and

WHEREAS, P.C. is a large entity with many physicians, and it would not be practical to employ some or all of said physicians individually;

NOW, THEREFORE, the Hospital and P.C. agree as follows:

1. General duties of P.C.
    A. P.C. furnish physician. P.C. shall furnish the services of its physicians as requested by Hospital who are capable of furnishing professional services hereunder (collectively "Physician").
    B. Treatment. P.C.'s Physician shall see and treat patients at the Emergency Department at the Hospital (hereinafter "ED"), and shall assist in performing those duties and responsibilities needed for the proper, efficient, and professional care and treatment of all patients presenting to the ED, and shall also perform all duties and responsibilities needed for the proper, efficient, and professional operation of the ED pursuant to the job description contained in Exhibit A attached to this Agreement. Hospital shall be responsible for all business management as well as scheduling, providing coverage, and formulating strategic plans.
    C. Scheduling. P.C.'s Physician shall perform services as scheduled by the Hospital with the mutual agreement of P.C. Physician at an hourly rate as specified in Exhibit B attached to this Agreement. Hospital shall attempt to arrange a schedule to reflect P.C.'s shift preference in recognition of any professional responsibilities elsewhere. The projected schedule is specified in Exhibit C attached to this Agreement.
    D. Revenue. P.C. and Physician hereby assign to the Hospital all rights they may now or hereafter possess to receive income, payment, and/or reimbursement for any and all professional medical services rendered by P.C. in the ED under this Agreement. P.C. shall have no right to bill patients under this Agreement. If requested by the Hospital, the P.C.'s Physician shall execute such documents as may be neces-

sary or desirable to implement said assignment with respect to public and private third-party reimbursement programs. The Hospital shall be responsible for all patient billings; however, P.C. shall do all things necessary for the Hospital to be able to generate patient billings, including patient diagnosis, treatment, and follow-up care.

E. Medical education. P.C.'s Physician shall also provide training and supervision for students, interns, and residents assigned to the ED as required by the Hospital's Director of Medical Education or the Chief of Staff, all consistent with applicable accreditation standards.

F. Other emergencies. While on duty and upon request, P.C.'s Physician shall be available for patient emergency situations needing backup or attention within the Hospital outside the ED, including Code Blue, for any house patient whether inpatient, outpatient, or otherwise.

G. Loyalty to Hospital. P.C. and its Physician shall be loyal to the duties, goals, and objectives of the Hospital, all as expressed in the Articles of Incorporation and Bylaws and other policy statements of the Hospital. P.C. and its Physician shall carefully guard the Hospital's proprietary rights, and P.C. and its Physician shall not disclose any confidential information concerning the Hospital to third parties without the prior written approval and consent of the Hospital.

2. Additional specific duties

P.C.'s Physician shall have the following additional specific duties and obligations at all times as an independent contractor of the Hospital:

A. Physician shall maintain membership in good standing on the professional staff of the Hospital (active staff category), maintain admitting privileges, and agree to abide by all Hospital and professional staff bylaws, rules, regulations, and policies in existence now and in the future.

B. Physician shall maintain an unrestricted license to practice medicine in the state. Physician shall remain in good standing with the Board of Medical Examiners and shall not be the subject of any Board of Medical Examiners sanctions, reprimands, or disciplinary actions. Physician shall not permit his or her license to practice medicine to be revoked, surrendered, or suspended. Physician shall maintain current and unrestricted federal (DEA) and state narcotics registrations.

C. Physician shall be board certified or board eligible in his or her specialty.

D. Physician shall actively participate on professional staff committees to which Physician is assigned and attend such committee meetings as may be required for quality improvement as well as accreditation. Physician shall maintain collegial relations with all other Physicians referring patients to the ED and shall provide services in a fashion that is not rude, curt, or unprofessional to patients, their families, or other Physicians.

E. Upon request, Physician shall help supervise any employees working with Physician.

F. Upon request, Physician shall advise the Hospital in expanding departmental services and formulating institutional long-range plans.

G. Upon request, Physician shall participate in marketing efforts in conjunction with the Hospital.

H. Physician shall assist in the education of students, interns, and residents as requested by the Hospital in the ED.

I. Consistent with the Hospital's charitable and nonprofit objectives as well as to ensure compliance with all federal and state laws and regulations, Physician shall see and treat patients regardless of their ability or inability to pay for services on the same basis as all other similarly situated patients of the ED or the Hospital. Physician shall also see and treat any Medicaid or Medicare patients presenting to Physician at the ED and will continually remain eligible for Medicare and Medicaid participation.

J. Physician shall fully and timely complete all patient charts and medical records regarding patients seen or treated by him in the ED in full compliance with the Hospital Medical Staff Bylaws and Hospital policies as well as accreditation standards. Records shall contain complete and accurate documentation of patient care via Hospital-provided documentation service (voice-activated system or dictation system).

K. Physician shall cooperate with the Hospital and other ED Physicians in preparing the schedule each month for coverage of the ED. Physician shall timely report for duty as required by the schedule so as to not have any gaps in coverage in the ED. Physician shall honor the schedule and shall be absent only in case of illness or personal or family emergency (in which event Physician shall provide the Hospital with adequate prior notice unless to do so would be an impossibility).

L. Physician shall be certified by the American Heart Association in advanced cardiac life support.

M. Physician shall be certified by the American College of Surgeons in advanced trauma life support.

N. Physician shall be certified in either PALS or APLS.

O. Physician shall maintain membership in the American College of Emergency Physicians (ACEP) and shall comply with CME requirements for ACEP Membership.

P. Physician shall abide by all applicable laws in the ED including, but not limited to, Medicare and Medicaid laws as well as the Emergency Medical Treatment and Active Labor Act.

3. Independent contractor

In performing the professional services under this Agreement, P.C. shall be an independent contractor and not an employee of the Hospital. As an independent contractor, P.C. and its Physician shall exercise their own independent professional judgment in seeing and treating patients, subject to the ordinary peer review of Hospital committees and subject to accreditation standards as well as the criteria of this Agreement. As an independent contractor, P.C. shall not be prohibited from furnishing professional services to other hospitals or from maintaining their own private practice. The Hospital shall not withhold any taxes from the payments made to P.C.; however, P.C. agrees that it shall be responsible to timely withhold any taxes owing regarding its employed Physician, including income taxes and taxes under the Federal Insurance Contributions Act (FICA) and Federal Unemployment Tax Act (FUTA). As an independent contractor, P.C. shall not be entitled to any fringe benefits that are customarily provided to Hospital employees. For example, P.C. and Physician acknowledge that they shall receive no health insurance, no vacation or sick time, nor any other benefits except as set forth in this Agreement.

4.   Contract fees

In exchange for professional services to be performed by P.C. through its Physician, P.C. shall be compensated as reflected in Exhibit B attached hereto and incorporated by this reference.

5.   Professional liability coverage

P.C. shall be responsible for providing professional liability insurance covering P.C. and its Physician with coverage in the minimum amount of One Million Dollars ($1,000,000) for any one (1) occurrence per year and Two Million Dollars ($2,000,000) for all occurrences per year. P.C. shall furnish a Certificate of Insurance to the Hospital prior to furnishing any professional services under this Agreement demonstrating the requisite professional liability insurance coverage. Upon expiration or termination of this Agreement, P.C. shall continue to maintain such professional liability insurance coverage for a period of at least two (2) years or, in the alternative, shall purchase extended reporting period coverage (tail coverage) at P.C.'s cost to make certain that there are no gaps in coverage concerning that period of time during which P.C. and its Physician provided professional services to the Hospital. All premiums and the costs of professional liability insurance coverage shall be borne by P.C. and not the Hospital.

6.   Term of this agreement

Subject to early termination as described below in this paragraph and as described below in paragraph 7 or elsewhere in this Agreement, this Agreement shall commence on the ___ day of _____, 200__, and shall expire on the ____ day of _____, 200__. At any time during the term of this Agreement either P.C. or Hospital shall have the right to terminate this Agreement without cause and without penalty by providing the other party with at least ninety (90) days' prior written notice after which this Agreement shall be null and void.

7.   Default; termination

If P.C. or its Physician shall fail or refuse to perform any of their obligations or meet any of the duties under this Agreement, Hospital shall give P.C. written notice specifying the nature of the default or breach. If P.C. fails to cure the default or breach within three (3) days after receipt of such notice, Hospital shall have the right, upon further written notice to P.C., to terminate this Agreement immediately; provided, however, that if P.C. Physician's license to practice medicine in the state is revoked, canceled, surrendered, or suspended, or Hospital medical staff privileges are limited, restricted, or revoked, or if P.C. commits any illegal act in P.C.'s practice or becomes involved in any immoral act or act involving moral turpitude regarding or adversely affecting the Hospital or any patients, this Agreement may be summarily terminated by giving notice of such termination to P.C. Likewise, if the Hospital shall fail or refuse to perform any of its obligations or meet any of its duties under this Agreement, P.C. shall give Hospital written notice specifying the nature of the default. If the Hospital fails to cure said default within three (3) days after receipt of such notice, P.C. shall have the right, upon further written notice to Hospital, to terminate this Agreement immediately.

8. Assignment

P.C's Physician shall personally perform the duties described in this Agreement and P.C. and Physician shall not assign any right nor delegate any duty under this Agreement.

9. Notices

Notices provided to be given pursuant to this Agreement shall be given by delivering the written notice in person or in writing by certified mail, postage prepaid, return receipt requested, addressed as follows:

- **To Hospital:**

_____

_____

_____

_____

- **To Physician:**

_____

_____

_____

_____

10. Future legislation

In the event of future legislation, safe harbor regulations, governmental rule or regulation, policy, or governmental interpretation thereof that applies to this Agreement and prohibits or invalidates any of its provisions or causes the Hospital or P.C. or its Physician not to qualify under or otherwise be in violation (actual or potential) of any Medicare, Medicaid, or IRS regulation, or if the Hospital's continuing ability to qualify as tax exempt Section 501(c)(3) corporation is in jeopardy (actual or potential) at any time, as determined by the Hospital, then the parties hereto shall either forthwith cause to be made to this Agreement such amendments as may be reasonably required to bring its terms back into compliance or, in the alternative, the Hospital or P.C. may summarily terminate this Agreement without penalty.

11. Confidentiality

To the extent permitted by law, Hospital, P.C., and Physician shall not divulge the fee information contained in this Agreement to any other P.C.s. Both parties shall make a good-faith effort to keep the fee information confidential.

12. Patient records

Upon expiration or termination of this Agreement, all patient records and charts shall remain in the possession of Hospital in its ED Department or its Medical Records Department.

13. Headings

Section headings in this Agreement are for convenience and reference purposes only and shall not be used to interpret or construe the provisions of this Agreement.

14. Disclosure

If requested, P.C. shall make a copy of this Agreement available to the U.S. Comptroller or designee in connection with any Medicare or governmental audit. This obligation shall continue for the duration of this Agreement and four (4) years thereafter, all pursuant to Section 1861 (V)(1)(L) of the Federal Social Security Act.

15. Miscellaneous conditions

The following conditions also apply to this Agreement:
  A. Recitals. The recitals at the beginning of this Agreement are intended to describe the intent of the parties and the circumstances under which this Agreement is executed and, consequently, shall be considered in the interpretation of this Agreement.
  B. Amendment. This Agreement may be amended only by the written consent of the parties.
  C. Waiver. The failure or delay of either party to insist in any one or more instances upon performance of any terms or conditions of this Agreement shall not be construed as a waiver of past or future performance of any such terms, covenants, or condition; but the obligations of such party with respect thereto shall continue in full force and effect.
  D. Severability. If one or more of the provisions contained in this Agreement are declared to be invalid, illegal, or unenforceable in any respect by a court of competent jurisdiction, the validity, legality, and enforceability of the remaining provisions of this Agreement shall not in any way be impaired thereby unless the effect of such declaration of the court would be to materially and substantially impair or diminish either party's rights and benefits hereunder.
  E. Governing law. This Agreement shall be interpreted under and governed by the law of the State of _____, without regard to choice of law or conflict of law principles.
  F. Entire agreement. This Agreement constitutes the entire agreement between the parties and replaces and supersedes all prior written and

oral statements and understandings between the parties. Furthermore, there are no side deals, understandings, or other arrangements or agreements between the parties, either express or implied, pertaining to the subject matter of this Agreement.

IN WITNESS WHEREOF, the parties have executed this Agreement as of the date set forth above.

P.C.   HOSPITAL

By _____   By _____

Title _____   Title: _____

Exhibit A—Independent Contractor Requirements

1. Provides efficient, high-quality patient care that reflects current professional practice norms
2. Practice management will be provided by the Hospital's ED Program Director.
3. Documents patient interactions in the patient's chart in a timely, comprehensive, and legible fashion via the Hospital-provided documentation service (voice-activated system or dictation system)
4. Attends all department staff meetings unless on duty in the ED or excused by the program Director
5. Presents himself or herself professionally and courteously to all patients, department staff, and all members of the Hospital community
6. Participates in appropriate medical staff committees as requested by Program Director, Chief of Staff, or Department Chairman
7. Participates in appropriate ED Quality Improvement and Utilization Review activities as requested
8. Participates in ED education activities, including but not limited to: nursing education programs, house staff educational programs, and paramedic educational programs
9. Responds to life-threatening situations in the Hospital when scheduled to be in the ED
10. Participates in relevant marketing and public relations activities on behalf of Hospital and the ED
11. Abides by ED's operations manual and policies and procedures.
12. Abides by the rules and regulations of Hospital and by its medical staff bylaws and credentialing requirements
13. Serves as a resource for local EMS services
14. Represents the Hospital in community affairs, both locally and regionally

Hospital Initials _____   Date: _____

Physician Initials _____   Date: _____

PROFESSIONAL SERVICES AGREEMENT—EMPLOYEE (EMERGENCY DEPARTMENT)

THIS AGREEMENT is entered into this ___ day of _____, 200__, by and between _____ ("Hospital") and _____ ("Physician").

Witnesseth:

WHEREAS, Hospital operates an Emergency Department providing emergency care and services to the public, and

WHEREAS, Hospital wishes to retain Physician as an employee to provide professional services in the Hospital's Emergency Department; and

NOW, THEREFORE, the Hospital and Physician agree as follows:

1. General duties
    A. Treatment. Physician shall see and treat patients at the Emergency Department at the Hospital (hereinafter "ED"), and shall assist in performing those duties and responsibilities needed for the proper, efficient, and professional care and treatment of all patients presenting to the ED, and shall also perform all duties and responsibilities needed for the proper, efficient, and professional operation of the ED pursuant to the job description contained in Exhibit A attached to this Agreement. Hospital shall be responsible for all business management as well as scheduling, providing coverage, and formulating strategic plans.
    B. Scheduling. Physician shall perform services as scheduled by the Hospital with the mutual agreement of Physician at an hourly rate as specified in Exhibit B attached to this Agreement. Hospital shall attempt to arrange a schedule to reflect Physician's shift preference in recognition of any professional responsibilities elsewhere. The projected schedule is specified in Exhibit C attached to this Agreement.
    C. Revenue. Physician hereby assigns to the Hospital all rights he or she may now or hereafter possess to receive income, payment, and/or reimbursement for any and all professional medical services rendered by Physician in the ED under this Agreement. Physician shall have no right to bill patients under this Agreement. If requested by the Hospital, Physician shall execute such documents as may be necessary or desirable to implement said assignment with respect to public and private third-party reimbursement programs. The Hospital shall be responsible for all patient billings; however, Physician shall do all things necessary for the Hospital to be able to generate patient billings, including patient diagnosis, treatment, and follow-up care.
    D. Medical education. Physician shall also provide training and supervision for students, interns, and residents assigned to the ED as required by the Hospital's Director of Medical Education or the Chief of Staff, all consistent with applicable accreditation standards.

E. Other emergencies. While on duty and upon request, Physician shall be available for patient emergency situations needing backup or attention within the Hospital outside the ED, including Code Blue, for any house patient whether inpatient, outpatient, or otherwise.

F. Loyalty to hospital. Physician shall be loyal to the duties, goals, and objectives of the Hospital, all as expressed in the Articles of Incorporation and Bylaws and other policy statements of the Hospital. Physician shall carefully guard the Hospital's proprietary rights, and its Physician shall not disclose any confidential information concerning the Hospital to third parties without the prior written approval and consent of the Hospital.

2. Additional specific duties

Physician shall have the following additional specific duties and obligations at all times as an employee of the Hospital:

A. Physician shall maintain membership in good standing on the professional staff of the Hospital (active staff category), and maintain admitting privileges, and agree to abide by all Hospital and professional staff bylaws, rules, regulations, and policies in existence now and in the future.

B. Physician shall maintain an unrestricted license to practice medicine in the state. Physician shall remain in good standing with the Board of Medical Examiners and shall not be the subject of any Board of Medical Examiners sanctions, reprimands, or disciplinary actions. Physician shall not permit his or her license to practice medicine to be revoked, surrendered, or suspended. Physician shall maintain current and unrestricted federal (DEA) and state narcotics registrations.

C. Physician shall be board certified or board eligible in his or her specialty.

D. Physician shall actively participate on professional staff committees to which Physician is assigned and attend such committee meetings as may be required for quality improvement as well as accreditation. Physician shall maintain collegial relations with all other Physicians referring patients to the ED and shall provide services in a fashion that is not rude, curt, or unprofessional to patients, their families, or other Physicians.

E. Upon request, Physician shall help supervise any employees working with Physician.

F. Upon request, Physician shall advise the Hospital in expanding departmental services and formulating institutional long-range plans.

G. Upon request, Physician shall participate in marketing efforts in conjunction with the Hospital.

H. Physician shall assist in the education of students, interns, and residents as requested by the Hospital in the ED.

I. Consistent with the Hospital's charitable and nonprofit objectives as well as to ensure compliance with all federal and state laws and regulations, Physician shall see and treat patients regardless of their ability or inability to pay for services on the same basis as all other similarly situated patients of the ED or the Hospital. Physician shall also see and treat any Medicaid or Medicare patients presenting to Physician at the ED and will continually remain eligible for Medicare and Medicaid participation.

J. Physician shall fully and timely complete all patient charts and medical records regarding patients seen or treated by him in the ED in full compliance with the Hospital Medical Staff Bylaws and Hospital policies as well as accreditation standards. Records shall contain complete and accurate documentation of patient care via Hospital-provided documentation service (voice-activated system or dictation system).

K. Physician shall cooperate with the Hospital and other ED Physicians in preparing the schedule each month for coverage of the ED. Physician shall timely report for duty as required by the schedule so as to not have any gaps in coverage in the ED. Physician shall honor the schedule and shall only be absent in case of illness or personal or family emergency (in which event Physician shall provide the Hospital with adequate prior notice unless to do so would be an impossibility).

L. Physician shall be certified by the American Heart Association in advanced cardiac life support.

M. Physician shall be certified by the American College of Surgeons in advanced trauma life support.

N. Physician shall be certified in either PALS or APLS.

O. Physician shall maintain membership in the American College of Emergency Physicians (ACEP) and shall comply with CME requirements for ACEP Membership.

P. Physician shall abide by all applicable laws in the ED including, but not limited to, Medicare and Medicaid laws as well as the Emergency Medical Treatment and Active Labor Act.

3. Employee

In performing the professional services under this Agreement, Physician shall be an employee of the Hospital. As an employee, however, Physician shall exercise his or her own independent professional judgment in seeing and treating patients, subject to the ordinary peer review of Hospital committees and subject to accreditation standards as well as the criteria of this Agreement. As an employee, Physician shall not be prohibited from furnishing professional services to other hospitals or from maintaining his or her own private practice. The Hospital shall withhold taxes from the payments made to Physician, including income taxes and taxes under the Federal Insurance Contributions Act (FICA) and Federal Unemployment Tax Act (FUTA). As an employee, Physician shall be entitled to fringe benefits that are customarily provided to Hospital employees.

4. Contract fees

In exchange for professional services to be performed by Physician, he or she shall be paid a salary as reflected in Exhibit B attached hereto and incorporated by this reference.

5. Professional liability coverage

Hospital shall be responsible for providing professional liability insurance covering Physician with coverage in the minimum amount of One Million Dollars ($1,000,000) for any one (1) occurrence per year and Two Million Dollars ($2,000,000) for all occurrences per year. Hospital shall furnish a Certificate of Insurance to the Physician prior to furnishing any professional services under this Agreement demonstrating the requisite professional liability insurance coverage. Upon expiration or termination of this Agreement, Hospital shall continue to maintain such professional liability insurance coverage for a period of at least two (2) years or, in the alternative, shall purchase extended reporting period coverage (tail coverage) at Hospital's cost to make certain that there are no gaps in coverage concerning that period of time during which Hospital and its Physician provided professional services to the Hospital. All premiums and the costs of professional liability insurance coverage shall be borne by the Hospital.

6. Term of this agreement

Subject to early termination as described below in this paragraph and as described below in paragraph 7 or elsewhere in this Agreement, this Agreement shall commence on the ___ day of _____, 20__, and shall expire on the ___ day of _____, 20__. At any time during the term of this Agreement, either Physician or Hospital shall have the right to terminate this Agreement without cause and without penalty by providing the other party with at least ninety (90) days prior written notice after which this Agreement shall be null and void.

7. Default; termination

If Physician shall fail or refuse to perform any of his or her obligations or meet any of the duties under this Agreement, Hospital shall give Physician written notice specifying the nature of the default or breach. If Physician fails to cure the default or breach within three (3) days after receipt of such notice, Hospital shall have the right, upon further written notice to Physician, to terminate this Agreement immediately; provided, however, that if Physician's license to practice medicine in the state is revoked, canceled, surrendered, or suspended, or Hospital medical staff privileges are limited, restricted, or revoked, or if Physician commits any illegal act in Physician's practice or becomes involved in any immoral act or act involving moral turpitude regarding or adversely affecting the Hospital or any patients, this Agreement may be summarily terminated by giving notice of such termination to Physician. Likewise, if the Hospital shall fail or refuse to perform any of its obligations or meet any of its duties under this Agreement, Physician shall give Hospital written notice specifying the nature of the default. If the Hospital fails to cure said default within three (3) days after receipt of such notice, Physician shall have the right, upon further written notice to Hospital, to terminate this Agreement immediately.

8. Assignment

Physician shall personally perform the duties described in this Agreement, and Physician shall not assign any right nor delegate any duty under this Agreement.

9. Notices

Notices provided to be given pursuant to this Agreement shall be given by delivering the written notice in person or in writing by certified mail, postage prepaid, return receipt requested, addressed as follows:

- **To Hospital:**

_____

_____

_____

_____

- **To Physician:**

_____

_____

_____

_____

10. Future legislation

In the event of future legislation, safe harbor regulations, governmental rule or regulation, policy, or governmental interpretation thereof that applies to this Agreement and prohibits or invalidates any of its provisions or causes the Hospital or Physician not to qualify under or otherwise be in violation (actual or potential) of any Medicare, Medicaid, or IRS regulation, or if the Hospital's continuing ability to qualify as a tax-exempt Section 501(c)(3) Corporation is in jeopardy (actual or potential) at any time, as determined by the Hospital, then the parties hereto shall either forthwith cause to be made to this Agreement such amendments as may be reasonably required to bring its terms back into compliance or, in the alternative, the Hospital or Physician may summarily terminate this Agreement without penalty.

11. Confidentiality

To the extent permitted by law, Hospital and Physician shall not divulge the fee information contained in this Agreement to any other persons. Both parties shall make a good-faith effort to keep the fee information confidential.

12. Patient records

Upon expiration or termination of this Agreement, all patient records and charts shall remain in the possession of Hospital in its ED Department or its Medical Records Department.

13. Headings

Section headings in this Agreement are for convenience and reference purposes only and shall not be used to interpret or construe the provisions of this Agreement.

14. Severability

If any part of this Agreement is found to be invalid, all remaining portions of the Agreement shall remain in full force and effect, notwithstanding any invalidity.

15. Applicable law

This Agreement shall be interpreted and construed in accordance with the laws of the State of _____.

16. Disclosure

If requested, Physician shall make a copy of this Agreement available to the U.S. Comptroller or designee in connection with any Medicare or governmental audit. This obligation shall continue for the duration of this Agreement and four (4) years thereafter, all pursuant to Section 1861(V)(1)(L) of the Federal Social Security Act.

17. Miscellaneous conditions

The following conditions also apply to this Agreement:

A. Recitals. The recitals at the beginning of this Agreement are intended to describe the intent of the parties and the circumstances under which this Agreement is executed and, consequently, shall be considered in the interpretation of this Agreement.

B. Amendment. This Agreement may be amended only by the written consent of the parties.

C. Waiver. The failure or delay of either party to insist in any one or more instances upon performance of any terms or conditions of this Agreement shall not be construed as a waiver of past or future performance of any such terms, covenants, or conditions; but the obligations of such party with respect thereto shall continue in full force and effect.

D. Severability. If one or more of the provisions contained in this Agreement are declared to be invalid, illegal, or unenforceable in any respect by a court of competent jurisdiction, the validity, legality, and enforceability of the remaining provisions of this Agreement shall not in any way be impaired thereby unless the effect of such declaration of the court would be to materially and substantially impair or diminish either party's rights and benefits hereunder.

E. Governing law. This Agreement shall be interpreted under and governed by the law of the State of _____, without regard to choice of law or conflict of law principles.

F. Entire agreement. This Agreement constitutes the entire agreement between the parties and replaces and supersedes all prior written and oral statements and understandings between the parties. Furthermore, there are no side deals, understandings, or other arrangements or agreements between the parties, either express or implied, pertaining to the subject matter of this Agreement.

IN WITNESS WHEREOF, the parties have executed this Agreement as of the date set forth above.

PHYSICIAN   HOSPITAL

By _____   By _____

                                             Title: _____

Exhibit A—Employment Requirements

1. Provides efficient, high-quality patient care that reflects current professional practice norms
2. Practice management will be provided by the Hospital's ED Program Director.
3. Documents patient interactions in the patient's chart in a timely, comprehensive, and legible fashion via the Hospital-provided documentation service (voice-activated system or dictation system)
4. Attends all department staff meetings unless on duty in the ED or excused by the program Director
5. Presents himself or herself professionally and courteously to all patients, department staff, and all members of the Hospital community
6. Participates in appropriate medical staff committees as requested by Program Director, Chief of Staff, or Department Chairman.
7. Participates in appropriate ED quality improvement and utilization review activities as requested
8. Participates in ED education activities, including but not limited to: nursing education programs, house staff educational programs, and paramedic educational programs
9. Responds to life-threatening situations in the Hospital when scheduled to be in the ED
10. Participates in relevant marketing and public relations activities on behalf of Hospital and the ED
11. Abides by ED's operations manual and policies and procedures
12. Abides by the rules and regulations of Hospital and by its medical staff bylaws and credentialing requirements
13. Serves as a resource for local EMS services
14. Represents the Hospital in community affairs, both locally and regionally

Hospital Initials _____   Date: _____

Physician Initials _____   Date: _____

PHYSICIAN RECRUITMENT AGREEMENT—INDEPENDENT CONTRACTOR

THIS AGREEMENT dated as of _____, 20___ ("Effective Date"), by and among ___[name]___ HOSPITAL, INC., a ___[state]___ not-for-profit corporation (referred to herein as "Hospital"), _____, a ___[state]___ professional association (referred to herein as "Group"), and [_____], M.D. (referred to herein as "Physician").

Recitals

1. Hospital is an organization exempt from federal income tax under Sections 501(a) and 501(c)(3) of the Internal Revenue Code of 1986, as amended ("Code"), and, in furtherance of its charitable and other exempt purposes, Hospital owns and operates two licensed hospitals where medical services are made available to the community of [name] County, [state], and surrounding areas, which includes rural or economically disadvantaged areas.

2. In implementing its patient service role, Hospital strives to maintain a medical setting that attracts and retains qualified physicians and enables them to use and strengthen their skills in furtherance of the promotion of quality medical care in the community. Hospital is further committed to ensuring the availability of physicians for patients within the community.

3. Hospital has determined that [name of specialty] physicians are needed to meet the present and future needs of the residents of [region] [name] County [description of service area] (hereinafter referred to as the "Service Area") and other communities served by Hospital, and that there is a current shortage and continued anticipated shortage of [specialty] in the Service Area as evidenced by the physician demand and community need assessment prepared by the [consulting firm].

4. Physician has recently completed training in, has never practiced [specialty] in [city/state], and has agreed to locate his or her practice in the Service Area, and Group has agreed to employ Physician and open a second practice location in [name] County and the Service Area on the basis of an offer of recruitment assistance made by Hospital.

5. Hospital has determined that to persuade Group to employ Physician and Physician to locate his or her practice to the Service Area, it is necessary to provide a certain level of support as specified herein to ensure that Physician's practice will be financially viable during his or her first year of practice.

6. Group is an existing medical practice in [name] County that has agreed to expand its services and has extended an offer of employment to Physician.

7. To accomplish the foregoing, Hospital provided assurance in early [year] that it would support the recruitment of a physician to the Service Area and on that basis Group employed Physician in [month/date], subsequently entered a contract for the development of property in the Service Area, and thereafter in [month/date] began occupancy of the developed property.

NOW THEREFORE, to ensure the provision of additional quality medical [name of specialty] services to the Service Area, Hospital has determined that the benefit of assisting with recruiting Physician to practice in the Service Area in the form of a net income guarantee for Physician as hereinafter set out is appropriate. In consideration thereof, Physician and Group agree to the terms, conditions, covenants, agreements, and obligations herein stated. It is now mutually agreed by and among the parties hereto as follows:

1. Physician Responsibilities. During and throughout the term of this Agreement, Physician agrees to the following:

   1.1 Physician represents that he or she currently holds and will maintain in good standing and without interruption, restriction or sanction: (a) board certification or eligibility by the American Board of Medical Specialties in the specialty of [name]; (b) licensure by the State of [name] to practice medicine; (c) status as a Medicare and Medicaid participating provider physician, and further represents that he or she has not been excluded from participating in or sanctioned by any state or federal healthcare program; (d) registration by the Federal Drug Enforcement Administration to dispense and administer controlled substances; (e) medical staff membership and [name of specialty] privileges at Hospital and other hospitals in the community that service the Service Area.

   1.2 Accept the offer of employment by Group and engage in the full-time practice of (specialty) medicine at an office within a reasonable distance from Hospital (consistent with Hospital's time/distance policy) that is located within the Service Area (referred to herein as the "[name of area] Office") for a period of not less than ____ (_) years, unless terminated due to cause. It is understood and agreed that reasonable distance shall mean not more than ____ (_) minutes drive time as established by the Hospital drive time map prepared by the [name] County Metropolitan Planning Organization (the "Map") and located in the Hospital's Medical Staff office.

   1.3 Upon the opening of Group's practice location in the Service Area, maintain customary office hours of at least five (5) days a week and devote at least forty (40) hours a week at the [name of area] Office or in surgery to direct care, diagnosis, and treatment of patients.

It is recognized that Physician will have reasonable periods of absence for continuing medical education, vacations, and similar purposes, for which periods Physician will arrange adequate coverage.

1.4 Attend and participate in division, section, and appropriate committee meetings of the Hospital's Medical Staff, maintain medical record completion as required, assist, if requested to do so, in quality review activities of Hospital, and otherwise abide by the obligations placed on Medical Staff members under the Bylaws, Rules and Regulations, and Policies of the Medical Staff.

1.5 Accept and provide consultations for hospitalized patients at both [name] Medical Center and [name] – [name of area] Office upon physician request.

1.6 Be a participating provider in the federal Medicare and [state] Medicaid programs. Physician shall accept and treat Medicare and Medicaid patients at Hospital as well as at the [name of area] Office and other patients regardless of their ability to pay. Physician's obligation with respect to providing uncompensated care shall be to provide a reasonable amount of uncompensated care in relation to the total practice.

1.7 Physician agrees to refrain from signing any other document, contract, or agreement containing provisions that may conflict with any provision in this Agreement. If Physician signs a conflicting document the terms of this Agreement shall govern.

2. Group Responsibilities. During and throughout the term of this Agreement, Group agrees to:

2.1 Employ and assign Physician or another practitioner of Group to the [name of area] Office, assure his or her availability for the provision of [name of specialty] patient services as required by this Agreement, and pay Physician compensation at not less than the Compensation rate specified in Section 3.1.

2.2 Ensure that Physician and any other physicians employed by Group maintain in good standing and without interruption, restriction, or sanction: (i) board certification in the specialty of [name of specialty]; (ii) licensure by the State of [name of state] to practice medicine; (iii) status as a Medicare and Medicaid participating provider physician, and represent that none have been excluded from participation in or sanctioned by any federal or state healthcare program; (iv) registration by the Federal Drug Enforcement Administration to dispense and administer controlled substances; and (v) medical staff membership and [name of specialty] privileges at Hospital.

2.3 Maintain an office for the practice of medicine in the specialty of [name of specialty] in the Service Area staffed by Physician with customary office hours five (5) days per week, with evening or weekend hours if warranted by patient demand, forty (40) hours per week, throughout the term of this Agreement, and for a period of ___ ( ) years thereafter from and after the commencement date.

2.4 Repay the amounts of financial incentives advanced for Physician hereunder, with interest, in the manner specified in Section 3.2.1 and the Promissory Note executed pursuant hereto, unless the service repayment provisions of Section 3.2.1 apply.

2.5 Group agrees that its employment agreement and any other agreements with physician will not contain any provisions that conflict with the provisions of this Agreement.

2.6 Ensure that Physician and all physicians affiliated with or employed by Group who provide medical services at Hospital provide such services in a manner consistent with the standards of practice of the American Board of [Specialty Society] and in accordance with all applicable laws and regulations, accreditation standards, and the Bylaws, Rules and Regulations, and the Policies of the Medical Staff of Hospital.

3. Recruiting Incentives. In consideration for services to be rendered by Physician and Group pursuant to this Agreement and to facilitate Group's employment of Physician and establishment of a new office practice in the Service Area for the purposes herein stated, Hospital will assist Group with certain costs associated solely with Physician beginning practice, as follows:

3.1 Group has agreed to employ Physician and compensate Physician at an annual compensation level (including salary and benefits) for the first twelve (12) months of Physician's employment of _____ ($_____) ("Compensation"). Hospital will provide a guarantee against net practice income up to fifty percent (50%) of the Compensation amount or a maximum of _____ ($_____) for the first twelve- (12) month period of Physician's employment, as further set out below.

3.2 Hospital's guarantee payments will begin upon the date Physician begins practice in accordance with Section 1.4 at the [name of area] Office (referred to herein as commencement date) which is _____, 20__. The guarantee payments will thereafter be made monthly for a period of up to twelve (12) months and shall be based on the amount by which reasonable practice expenses (as hereinafter defined) attributable to Physician exceed Physician's gross collections, as further described below.

3.2.1 Hospital will pay Group each month one half (1/2) of the negative Net Practice Income, if any, related to Physician's practice, up to _____ ($_____) during the twelve- (12) month term. After the close of each month, Group will provide to Hospital (Attn: [name] , Vice President Finance) a monthly billing report detailing Physician's gross collections and practice expenses, as defined below, attributable solely to Physician, for the month. Within ten (10) days of receipt thereof, Hospital will issue payment to Group in an amount equal to one half (1/2) of the amount by which the reasonable practice expenses exceed gross collections attributable to Physician at the [name of area] office. In the event Physician's gross collections in any month in the twelve-(12) month period exceed reasonable practice expenses attributable to Physician for the month, Group and Physician are obligated to pay the difference to Hospital, until the guarantee amounts previously advanced by Hospital are repaid. This reconciliation may occur at the end of each quarter or within thirty (30) days after the end of the twelve- (12) month term of this Agreement. Any Hospital guarantee advances that are not repaid after the final reconciliation shall constitute an interest-bearing obligation of Group that shall be paid back with interest over a thirty-six- (36) month period beginning the first day of the first month after the expiration of the twelve- (12) month term or any termination of this Agreement that gives rise to the repayment obligation, whichever first occurs (hereinafter referred to as the "Debt Commencement Date"), and in accordance with the attached promissory notes. However, Hospital will allow Physician and Group to earn service payback of Hospital guarantee advances less the amounts repaid provided that Physician or another recruit acceptable to Hospital and Group remain in active practice at the [name of area] Office or another medical office in the Service Area for an additional thirty-six (36) months subsequent to the Debt Commencement Date with one thirty-sixth (1/36) of the balance to be considered repaid for each month that the Physician remains in practice at the [name of area] Office or in the Service Area.

3.2.2   "Net Practice Income" is defined as gross collections from all payer sources minus reasonable practice expenses ("practice expenses") relating to Physician that the Internal Revenue Service considers as deductible business expenses for federal income tax purposes. Examples of practice expenses that may be included are in Attachment A, and shall include only those expenses as they incrementally relate to Physician. Practice expenses shall not include: (a) any bonuses drawn by Physician, including personal income taxes and deferred compensation plans; (b) any wages, salaries, or other compensation paid to any member of Physician's immediate family who works in the practice (any such compensation shall be deemed compensation to Physician); (c) any wages, salaries, or other compensation paid to employees of the practice that exceeds compensation for comparable positions in the local market place; (d) any automobile expenses for Physician or other practice employees; (e) any charitable contributions made on behalf of Physician or the Group. Net practice income will be computed on a cash basis.

    3.2.3 In the event of Physician's death, disability, or incapacity rendering him or her unable to practice medicine for a period of thirty (30) days or more, this Agreement shall terminate.

    3.2.4 In the event Physician separates from Group for any reason, this Agreement shall terminate. The repayment obligation specified in Section 3.2.1 shall commence, capped at the guarantee amount previously paid by Hospital.

4. Independent Contractor Status. Nothing in this Agreement is intended to or shall be construed as creating an agency, partnership, employment, joint venture, or other relationship between Physician, Hospital, Group, and the Partners thereof. Accordingly, Physician understands and agrees that he or she shall not be entitled to any of the rights and privileges established for employees of Hospital.

   It is further expressly agreed that Hospital shall neither have nor exercise any control over the professional medical judgment or methods used by Physician or partners or employees of Group in the delivery of physician services to patients. However, Physician and Partners agree that they shall observe the requirements set forth in this Agreement, in Hospital's Medical Staff's Bylaws, Rules, Regulations, and Policies, the accreditation standards of the Joint Commission for Accreditation of Healthcare Organizations (JCAHO), applicable laws and regulations, and that Physician and Group shall perform their duties and functions in conformance with currently approved practices in the field of [name of specialty] and in a competent and professional manner.

5. Insurance. Group, for the benefit of itself, Physician, its employees, and each Partner of Group, shall maintain and provide Hospital with a certificate or certificates of insurance evidencing the continuation of professional liability coverage (by insurance companies acceptable to Hospital) covering each practitioner in an amount of not less than $250,000 per occurrence/$750,000 aggregate for any liability of Group and its employees and staff throughout the term of this Agreement. Group shall obtain an endorsement requiring that if said policy is canceled for any reason, notice of cancellation shall be provided by insurance company to the Administrator of Hospital.

6. Billing for Services. Group shall bill for all professional services rendered in the practice, whether to inpatients or outpatients. Billing and collection by Group shall be in a manner consistent with all laws, rules, and regulations applicable to billing and collections, and Group shall use best efforts to collect all billings promptly. Group shall receive and deposit in a Group bank account all fees for Physician's professional services.

7. Access to Books and Records. The following clause is included because of the possible application of Section 1395x(v)(1)(I) of Title 42 of the United States Code to this Agreement; but if that section be found inapplicable to this Agreement, then this clause shall be deemed not to be a part of this Agreement and shall be null and void:

   Until the expiration of four (4) years after the furnishing of services under this Agreement, Physician shall make available, upon written request of the Secretary of Health and Human Services, or the Comptroller General of the United States, or any of their duly authorized representatives, this Agreement and such books, documents, and records of Physician as are necessary to certify the nature and extent of any costs incurred by Physician with respect to this Agreement. Physician agrees to notify Hospital in writing within five (5) days of receipt of any such request. If Physician or Group carries out any duties under this Agreement through a subcontract for the value or cost of $10,000 or more over a twelve- (12) month period, with a related organization, such subcontract shall contain a clause placing the same duty on the subcontractor as this contract places on Physician. This clause shall survive the termination of this Agreement according to terms.

In the event the law or regulations are effectively amended to increase or decrease the annual amount necessary to require this clause, the amount set forth herein shall be deemed amended retroactively without the necessity of any action by the parties hereto, to include the terms of any rules, regulations, or judicial or administrative interpretations or decisions promulgated or made under Section 1395x(v)(1)(I) of Title 42 of the United States Code, to the extent that the terms of such rules, regulations, interpretations, or decisions differ herefrom. Notwithstanding the presence of this clause in this Agreement, this clause shall only be applicable if the actual dollar amount paid in any twelve- (12) month period equals or exceeds the above stated threshold amount.

8. Assignment. Hospital may assign or transfer its rights and responsibilities pursuant to this Agreement to an affiliate of Hospital without prior written approval of or notice to Physician or Group. This Agreement is personal to Physician and Group and may not be assigned to any person. This Agreement and all provisions shall inure to the benefit of, and be binding upon, the parties hereto and their respective successors and assigns. The obligation to reimburse Hospital for any money advanced to Group to guarantee the income of Physician shall be binding upon the heirs, personal representatives, estate, successors, and assigns of Physician and Group.

9. Term of Agreement. The term of this Agreement shall commence on the Commencement Date and continue for a period of twelve (12) months. Notwithstanding the stated term, certain obligations set forth in this Agreement, such as the repayment provision evidenced by the Promissory Notes, shall continue after the termination or expiration of this Agreement until the respective obligations of the parties hereto, one to the other, are satisfied in full.

10. Termination.

    10.1 Upon any material violation of the terms of this Agreement by Physician or Group, Hospital shall give written notice thereof to Physician and Group giving Physician and/or Group ten (10) days to cure the same; failure of Physician or Group to cure such violation(s) within ten (10) days after notice is given shall be grounds for Hospital to terminate this Agreement.

10.2 Either Hospital, Group, or Physician may terminate this agreement with ten (10) days' prior written notice, upon receipt of notification from third-party payers, governmental agencies, or other agencies that may have authority relative to Hospital/Physician Group contracts or over any part of this Agreement or receipt of other information, which either party in good faith believes requires that this Agreement must be renegotiated or revised to conform with rules or standards of any third-party payers or agencies referred to above.

10.3 Hospital may terminate this Agreement without prior notice upon Physician's loss, suspension, reduction, restriction, or probation of medical licensure, Drug Enforcement Administration certification, medical staff membership or clinical privileges at any hospital, or upon failure to obtain or cancellation of professional liability insurance coverage.

10.4 In the event that Physician or Group institutes any suit in a court or any proceeding before regulatory or governmental body in a position adverse to Hospital (excepting only when such action is explicitly protected by law); or upon the indictment of Physician or any partner or employee of Group for a felony offense; or upon any conduct by Physician or any partner or employee of Group that jeopardizes, as determined in the reasonable good-faith judgment of Hospital, the reputation of Hospital, interferes with Hospital operations, or puts any licensure, accreditation, or tax-exempt status of Hospital at risk of loss (excepting only when such conduct is explicitly protected by law), Hospital may terminate this Agreement effective on the date so specified in written notice of such action provided by Hospital.

10.5 Should this Agreement be terminated by Physician or Group without cause, as a result of the death or disability of Physician as specified in Section 3.2.3, or by Hospital with cause, the repayment provisions specified in Section 3.2.1 shall become effective upon the termination date without the opportunity for service payback. The determination by Hospital to terminate this Agreement for any reason stated in Sections 10.1 through Section 10.4 shall be considered termination for cause giving rise to the repayment provision.

11. Compliance with Laws and Regulations.

11.1 Physician, Group, and Hospital acknowledge and agree that the performance of this Agreement is subject to compliance with all applicable federal and state laws including but not limited to federal statutes and regulations pertaining to Medicare and Medicaid and to Hospital's tax-exempt status under Section 501(c)(3) of the Code. This includes laws and regulations that may be enacted in the future, as well as those now in effect.

Accordingly, all parties agree to do whatever may be necessary or appropriate and also to cooperate with the other so that legal compliance will be ensured, including cooperation by Group and

Physician with Hospital's Corporate Integrity Program. In addition, it is specifically provided that Hospital may terminate this Agreement and recover from Physician or Group, pursuant to Section 3.2.1, any payment that is determined by a court or government agency to be improper or inconsistent with Hospital's tax-exempt status under Section 501(c)(3) of the Code, or any other federal or state law, rule, or regulation.

Group and Physician enter into this Agreement with the intent of conducting their relationship and all business activities in full compliance with applicable [state], local, and federal law, including the laws known as the Stark law, the Medicare and Medicaid Anti-Fraud and Abuse law, and the [state] Patient Self-Referral Act. Notwithstanding any unanticipated effect of any of the provisions herein, no party will intentionally or with indifference conduct itself under the terms of this Agreement in a manner to constitute a violation of the Stark law, Medicare and Medicaid Anti-Fraud and Abuse law, the [state] Patient Self-Referral Act, or any other applicable laws.

12. Amendment. This Agreement may be amended only by written agreement of Hospital, Group, and Physician.

13. Interpretation. This Agreement shall be governed by and construed in accordance with the laws of the State of [name] and, in the event of any litigation or other action with respect to the Agreement or any of its terms, venue shall lie exclusively in [name] County. The paragraph headings are for convenience only and shall not be construed to explain or interpret any provision.

14. Physician Discretion and Community Benefit Covenant. The parties to this Agreement acknowledge and agree that Group provides essential healthcare services that are in short supply in the community served by Hospital. Hospital desires through this Agreement to make these services more readily available and accessible to the community. Hospital, Group, and Physician expressly acknowledge and agree that this Agreement is not entered into for the purpose of requiring or inducing referrals or patient admissions to Hospital. Accordingly, Group and Physician shall have complete discretion according to their own medical judgment for selecting the site for inpatient or outpatient hospital and diagnostic services for all patients. Also, neither Physician, Partners, nor Group is barred from establishing staff privileges at, providing services in, or making referrals to any other facility of their discretion. The objectives of Hospital in this Agreement are to encourage Physician to practice medicine and to provide professional services to patients in the Service Area. The parties expressly agree that, at all times, the needs of the patients shall take priority, and Physician and Partners shall solely decide with their patients to which hospital facility to admit any particular patient. Physician, and Group acknowledge, and the parties agree, that neither Physician nor Partners are under any obligation whatsoever, either express or implied, to admit, treat, and/or refer any patients to [name] Hospital.

15. Confidentiality. It is understood and agreed that the details of this Agreement shall be held in strict confidence, except as may otherwise be required to carry out other provisions of this Agreement.

16. Complete Agreement. This Recruitment Agreement, the associated promissory notes, and the security agreement constitute the Complete Agreement by and among the parties; there are no other agreements or arrangements written or verbal between or among them relating to the subject matter hereof.

17. Waiver. Any waiver of enforcement of a provision or provisions or waiver of a breach or breaches of this Agreement, whether or not recurring, shall not be construed as a waiver of any subsequent enforcement or breach.

18. Notices. All notices required to be sent hereunder shall be deemed sufficient if in writing and if personally delivered, delivered by commercial courier service, or if mailed by United States mail, certified or registered mail, postage prepaid, to, in the case of Hospital:

[Name of] Hospital
[Street Address]
[City/State/Zip]
Attn: Chief Executive Officer

and in case of Physician or Group:

Attn: _____

IN WITNESS WHEREOF, the parties have executed this Agreement the day and year first written above.

PHYSICIAN   [Name of] HOSPITAL

By _____   By _____
          PHYSICIAN   Vice President

Date: _____   Date: _____

[Name of Group]

A [state] professional association

By: _____

Name: _____

Its: _____

Date: _____

Attachment A

A. Group expenses related specifically to Physician: Health insurance premium, dental insurance premium, life insurance premium, Professional program membership dues, and CME not to exceed $2500/year

B. Group overhead expenses attributable to Physician that may be included on a pro rata basis: Wages and benefits of employees hired specifically to support Physician, medical supplies, office supplies, billing services, fees, biohazardous waste removal, long-distance telephone, and transcription costs.

NURSE PRACTITIONER RECRUITMENT AGREEMENT—
FORGIVABLE LOAN

This Nurse Practitioner Recruitment Agreement is entered into this ____ day of _____, 200__, by and among _____, a not-for-profit corporation ("Hospital"); _____ ("P.C."); and _____ ("Practitioner").

Recitals

A. The Hospital is a not-for-profit corporation as described under Section 501(c)(3) of the Internal Revenue Code. The Hospital is organized and operated for the purposes of promoting and providing healthcare services to the public and is also organized for charitable, scientific, and educational purposes.

B. The Hospital through its Board of Trustees has determined that it is consistent with the Hospital's charitable, scientific, and educational purposes to encourage and assist physicians as well as nurse practitioners to practice in the Hospital's community, including rural communities of the state.

C. Practitioner is presently in an educational program to become a nurse practitioner and upon completion of her education is willing to devote her services to the rural community of _____, _____, and to make her professional services available in that community on a full-time basis provided that certain financial incentives are made available to her so that she can start her practice.

D. P.C. is willing to bring Practitioner into P.C.'s existing practice in the rural community of _____, _____, and to assist her in the start-up of practice.

E. The Board of Trustees of the Hospital has determined that a Nurse Practitioner Recruitment Agreement should be entered into that will be in the best interest of the rural community of _____, _____. Furthermore, the Board of Trustees of the Hospital on _____, 200__, reviewed and approved the terms of the proposed Nurse Practitioner Recruitment Agreement, and all parties wish to set forth their agreement in writing.

NOW, THEREFORE, the Hospital, P.C., and Practitioner agree as follows:

1. Loan to practitioner (income guarantee)

In exchange for Practitioner's commitment to devote her services as a Nurse Practitioner in the rural community of _____, _____, as described in this Agreement, the Hospital hereby agrees and commits to lend her sums of money as described below in this paragraph over a one- (1) year period of time, which loan commitment shall commence on July 1, 20__, and end on June 30, 20__. The loan shall be in the form of an income guarantee for Practitioner for a one- (1) year period of time, but only if she devotes her services as a Nurse Practitioner in the rural community of _____, _____, in the office of P.C. on a full-time basis.

If in the one- (1) year period of time during the loan commitment period revenues from Practitioner's services as a Nurse Practitioner in _____, _____, net of reasonable and customary overhead expenses as determined by the Hospital, do not reach Forty Thousand Dollars ($40,000) (as annualized and projected on a monthly basis), the Hospital, upon the request of Practitioner, shall lend a sum of money to her to bring her income, net of overhead expenses, to the level of Forty Thousand Dollars ($40,000) per year. Practitioner may draw on the loan during the one- (1) year loan commitment period of time on a monthly basis or such other periodic basis as may be mutually agreeable between Hospital and Practitioner. P.C. and Practitioner, upon request of the Hospital, shall make business and financial records available to the Hospital to verify the income level of Practitioner and the overhead expenses attributable to her, which records shall be kept confidential by the Hospital to the extent allowed by law.

2.   Repayment

Any sums advanced under the loan commitments described above to Practitioner shall accrue interest at the fixed rate of two (2) percentage points over the Prime Rate as published in the *Wall Street Journal* as of the first date when any sums are advanced under the loan commitment. No payments of either interest or principal shall be required during the first year if Practitioner is otherwise in compliance with this Agreement; provided, however, accrued interest at the end of the first year shall be added to the unpaid principal. Beginning on July 1, 200__, and for a period of three (3) years thereafter, payment of principal and interest shall be made in equal monthly installments until all sums are paid in full; provided, however, Practitioner shall not be deemed to be in default in the repayment of the loan if the alternative repayment provisions of paragraph 4 below are being fully met.

3.   Promissory note and security

Practitioner shall execute a Promissory Note for each draw under the loan commitment in a form to be prescribed by the Hospital. If she neglects to execute a Promissory Note, however, this Agreement shall constitute a Promissory Note and shall be evidence of her promise to pay all sums advanced by the Hospital pursuant to the terms of this Agreement. Implementation of the loan, as well as the obligation for obtaining necessary Promissory Notes and security for the loan, including a mortgage on real estate owned by Practitioner, if any, shall be the responsibility of the Chief Financial Officer of the Hospital.

4.   Alternative repayment of loan

As an alternative means of repayment of the loans described in paragraph 1 of this Agreement, the Hospital shall acknowledge that one third (1/3) of the principal balance and accrued interest on loans already made under paragraph 1 of this Agreement has been paid beginning on July 1, 20__, and on July 1 of each year thereafter for a total of three (3) years (with a proration being made on a monthly basis) if Practitioner has met all of the following community service requirements:

    A. Practitioner shall devote her services on a full-time basis as described in this Agreement as a Nurse Practitioner in the rural community of

       _____, _____.

    B. Practitioner shall not restrict or limit the number of Medicare or Medicaid patients who are seen or treated by her within the scope of her license and certification and shall remain eligible to participate in the Medicare and Medicaid programs and shall observe all applicable rules and regulations pertaining to those programs.

    C. Practitioner shall accept patients referred by the Hospital's referral services regardless of the patient's ability to pay so long as the treatment shall be within the scope of her license and certification.

    D. Practitioner shall not limit the number of indigent or charitable patients seen or treated by her within the scope of her license and certification. She shall keep a record of all such patients and make those records available to the Hospital; provided, however, such report shall not reveal a patient's name and shall not violate physician-patient confidentiality requirements.

If all the above described community service requirements are met, at the end of three (3) years all of the principal balance and accrued interest on the loans made by the Hospital to Practitioner under paragraph 1 of this Agreement shall be acknowledged by the Hospital as paid in full. Practitioner acknowledges that for each year the above-described loan is repaid by community service, the Hospital will be obligated under federal law to issue IRS Form 1099, and Practitioner shall be responsible for all income tax consequences flowing from loan forgiveness.

5. Obligations of P.C.

    P.C. agrees to bring Practitioner into its medical practice in _____,_____, and to provide her with staff, office space, furniture, examination rooms, equipment, and other amenities necessary to provide Nurse Practitioner services. If Practitioner or P.C. ever terminates their arrangement, for whatever reason, P.C. shall have no obligations or liability to the Hospital under this Agreement, and Practitioner solely shall be liable to repay any sums under this Agreement to the Hospital.

6. Freedom in referrals

    Hospital, P.C., and Practitioner understand and agree that nothing contained in this Agreement shall in any way require or suggest that P.C. or any other physicians associated with P.C. refer or admit patients to the Hospital at any time whatsoever. They shall be absolutely free to refer or admit patients to any hospital or other healthcare facility that they, in consultation with their patients, deem appropriate, in their sole discretion, all without loss of any benefits whatsoever under this Agreement.

7. Third-party reporting

P.C. and Practitioner recognize that the Hospital is a participant in various third-party payment programs including, without limitation, Medicare and Medicaid. P.C. and Practitioner agree to cooperate fully with the Hospital and provide assistance to the Hospital for participation in such programs, including furnishing, upon request, financial information or other books, records, and documentation concerning this Agreement for a period of up to four (4) years after the termination or expiration of this Agreement to the United States Comptroller General, or designee, pursuant to Section 1861(v)(1)(L) of the Federal Social Security Act.

8. Default

If any party fails or refuses to perform the obligations under this Agreement, the affected party shall give the defaulting party written notice specifying the nature of the default. If the default is not substantially cured within ten (10) days after personal delivery or receipt of the mailed notice, the affected party shall have the right to terminate this Agreement immediately. If Practitioner's license and certification as a Nurse Practitioner in the State is restricted, revoked, canceled, surrendered, or suspended so that Practitioner does not maintain her license and certification in a full and unrestricted manner, and such condition continues for more than thirty (30) continuous days, this Agreement may, at the option of the Hospital, be summarily terminated by giving notice of the termination to the other parties to this Agreement; provided, however, such a termination shall not eliminate the duty to repay any sums of money owed by Practitioner to the Hospital pursuant to the above-described loan commitment.

9. Entire agreement

This Agreement constitutes the entire understanding among the parties, except for the agreement between P.C. and Practitioner, and all prior negotiations and understandings among the parties have been merged into this Agreement. There are no understandings, representations, or side agreements, either oral, written, or implied, among the parties other than those set forth in this Agreement and in the agreement between P.C. and Practitioner.

10. Future legislation and interpretations

The parties to this Agreement are of the opinion that all of the terms of this Agreement comply with present law; however, the parties are mindful of the potential for possible healthcare legislation in the future at the federal and state levels. Furthermore, the parties are aware that federal and state regulations are subject to periodic interpretations and court decisions that could affect this Agreement. In the event of future legislation, court decision, governmental regulation, policy, or governmental interpretation thereof that applies to this Agreement and prohibits or invalidates any of its provisions, or causes the Hospital, P.C., or Practitioner not to qualify under or otherwise be in violation of any Medicare or Medicaid reimbursement regulations, or other laws, or if the Hospital's continuing ability to qualify as a tax-exempt Section 501(c)(3) corporation is in jeopardy at any time because of this Agreement, as determined by the Hospital, then the parties shall either forthwith cause to be made to this Agreement such amendments as may be reasonably required to bring its terms back into compliance with the law or, in the alternative, terminate this Agreement. In the event of such termination, no party shall have any further duties or obligations under this Agreement except that Practitioner shall be required to pay back all loans advanced by the Hospital, including interest, and said loans shall be repaid in full within ninety (90) days of termination unless other acceptable means of repayment are approved by the Hospital in its reasonable discretion consistent with federal and state law.

11. Notices

Written notices required to be given under this Agreement shall be deemed served when personally received or in lieu of personal service when deposited in the United States Mail, by certified mail, postage prepaid, return receipt requested, and addressed as follows:

- **To Hospital:**

_____

_____

_____

_____

- **To P.C.:**

_____

_____

_____

_____

- **To Practitioner:**

_____

_____

_____

_____

12. Condition

This Agreement is subject to Practitioner successfully completing her education and obtaining her license and certification in the state by July 1, 20__, to lawfully furnish services as a Nurse Practitioner, including the ability to see and treat patients outside the presence of a licensed physician within the scope of her license and as allowed by state law regarding qualified rural and medically underserved areas. If Practitioner does not so obtain her license and certification in the state by _____, 20__, the Hospital, P.C., or Practitioner may terminate this Agreement without penalty.

13. Miscellaneous conditions
   The following conditions also apply to this Agreement:
   A. Recitals. The recitals at the beginning of this Agreement are intended to describe the intent of the parties and the circumstances under which this Agreement is executed and, consequently, shall be considered in the interpretation of this Agreement.
   B. Amendment. This Agreement may be amended only by the written consent of the parties.
   C. Waiver. The failure or delay of either party to insist in any one or more instances upon performance of any terms or conditions of this Agreement shall not be construed as a waiver of past or future performance of any such terms, covenants, or condition; but the obligations of such party with respect thereto shall continue in full force and effect.
   D. Severability. If one or more of the provisions contained in this Agreement are declared to be invalid, illegal, or unenforceable in any respect by a court of competent jurisdiction, the validity, legality, and enforceability of the remaining provisions of this Agreement shall not in any way be impaired thereby unless the effect of such declaration of the court would be to materially and substantially impair or diminish either party's rights and benefits hereunder, subject to the rights of the parties to otherwise terminate this Agreement as provided elsewhere in this Agreement.
   E. Governing law. This Agreement shall be interpreted under and governed by the law of the State of _____, without regard to choice of law or conflict of law principles.

IN WITNESS WHEREOF, the parties have caused this Agreement to be duly executed and delivered as of the date and year first above written.

HOSPITAL

By _____

Title:_____

PRACTITIONER

By _____

Title: _____

P.C.

By: _____

MEDICAL OFFICE LEASE AGREEMENT—HOSPITAL AND PHYSICIAN

Medical Office Lease Agreement Hospital-Owned Space

1. Parties
   This Medical Office Lease Agreement is entered into this ____ day of _____, 200__, effective as of the date set forth below in paragraph 3, by and between _____, a nonprofit corporation ("Landlord") and _____, a duly licensed physician ("Tenant").

2. Premises
   In consideration of the rents and agreements set forth herein, Landlord leases to Tenant and Tenant leases from Landlord the following described premises situated at _____ in the City of _____:

   > Approximately _____ gross square feet of
   > space as shown on the attached floor plan marked
   > Exhibit A within the building known as
   > _____ and operated by the
   > Landlord at _____ in the City of _____,
   > State of _____ ("Premises"),

   with the improvements thereon and all rights, easements, and appurtenances belonging thereto, including a nonexclusive right of use, in common with others, of the parking areas, driveways, means of ingress and egress regarding the property known as "_____" at _____ in the City of _____. Furthermore, Landlord grants to Tenant a nonexclusive right of use, in common with others, of all common areas within the building known as "_____." All uses of the Premises, common area, the parking areas, driveways, and means of ingress and egress shall be subject to reasonable rules and regulations of the Landlord.

3. Term
   Subject to earlier termination as provided in this Lease, Landlord and Tenant agree that the commencement and termination dates of this Lease Agreement are as follows:
   Lease commencement: _____, 20____
   Lease termination: _____, 20____

3A. Option
   So long as Tenant is not in default under this Lease Agreement, he shall have the right and option to extend this Lease Agreement after the expiration thereof for an additional five (5) years on the same terms and conditions except that rent shall be adjusted to a level mutually agreeable to Landlord and Tenant; provided, however, that rent in any one year of the option period shall not exceed the prior year's rent by more than five

percent (5%). If agreement cannot be reached regarding rent for the option period, neither Landlord nor Tenant shall have any further rights or duties concerning the option beyond the expiration date of this Lease Agreement. If Tenant wishes to exercise his option under this paragraph, he shall give written notice to Landlord at least 120 days prior to the lease termination date described above in paragraph 3.

4. Rent

In consideration of the leasing of the Premises, Tenant agrees to pay Landlord rent due on the 1st day of each month of this Lease, as set forth in Exhibit B; provided, however, that for each day or partial day the improvements to the Premises described in the attached Exhibit C are not completed after _____, 20__, Tenant shall have one (1) week's rent credited unless the delay on the part of Landlord is caused by an act of God or some other major force beyond Landlord's control.

5. Possession

Tenant shall be entitled to possession on the 1st day of the term of this Lease and shall yield possession back to the Landlord at the time and date of the expiration or termination of this Lease.

6. Use of premises

Tenant agrees during the term of this Lease to use the Premises only for a medical office.

7. Quiet enjoyment

Landlord covenants that the Tenant, on performing all of the Agreements by the Tenant to be performed in this Lease, shall and may peaceably have, hold, and enjoy the Premises for the term of this Lease free from eviction or disturbance by the Landlord.

8. Care and maintenance of premises

Except as set forth below in this paragraph or elsewhere (including Exhibit C), Tenant shall be responsible for making all necessary renovations, repairs, and improvements to the Premises in order that Tenant may operate the Premises as a medical office. All such renovations, repairs, and improvements that are or become affixed to the Premises and are not movable shall become the property of the Landlord upon expiration or termination of this Lease. Landlord shall keep the roof, structural parts of the floor, walls, and other structural parts of the Premises, and the building in good repair. Tenant shall, after taking possession of the Premises, and until termination of this Lease, at its own expense, care for and maintain the Premises in a reasonably safe and serviceable condition, except for structural parts of the Premises that shall be Landlord's responsibility. Tenant shall furnish its own interior decorating. Tenant shall not knowingly permit or allow the Premises to be damaged or depreciated in value by any act or negligence of the Tenant, its agents, or employees. Landlord shall maintain and make necessary repairs to the sanitary sewer system, plumbing, water pipes, and electrical wiring as well as the heating, ventilating, and air-conditioning equipment. Landlord shall maintain adequate heat for the Premises and shall be responsible for the plate glass in the windows of the Premises, except for any negligence or act of Tenant. Tenant shall make no structural alterations or improvements to the Premises without the prior written consent of the Landlord after submitting plans and specifications. Landlord shall be responsible for removing snow and ice from the parking lot, driveways, and sidewalks serving the Premises.

9. Utilities and services

Landlord shall provide all water, sewer facilities, gas, heat, electricity, power, air-conditioning, and other similar services and utilities for the Premises, including repairs. Janitorial and cleaning services shall be furnished by Tenant for the Premises.

10. Surrender of premises

Tenant agrees that upon the termination of this Lease, it will surrender, yield up, and deliver the Premises in good and clean condition, except for ordinary wear and tear and depreciation arising from the lapse of time, or damage without fault or liability of the Tenant. Tenant may, at the expiration of this Lease, provided that Tenant is not in default hereunder, remove any movable equipment that Tenant has placed in the Leased Premises, including wall-hung microscopes and Tenant-owned nurses' counters, provided that Tenant repairs any and all damages caused by the removal. Nothing in this paragraph shall be construed as allowing Tenant to remove any attached cabinets, sinks, counters, doors, shelving, built-in equipment, or other equipment or improvements affixed or attached to the Premises.

11. Hazardous substances

Except as provided below, Tenant shall not maintain or store on or about the premises any hazardous substances as defined by any environmental laws of the United States or state or local law or regulation. Notwithstanding the general prohibition contained herein, however, Tenant shall be permitted to maintain and store the usual and customary substances found in a medical office so long as Tenant complies with all applicable laws.

12. Real estate taxes

Tenant shall not be responsible for paying any real estate taxes and special assessments.

13. Insurance

Landlord and Tenant shall each keep their respective property interests in the Premises and their liability in regard thereto and the use thereof as well as the personal property on the Premises, reasonably insured against hazards and casualties, including fire, theft, vandalism, and those casualty items usually covered by an extended coverage insurance policy. Tenant shall procure and deliver to the Landlord a certificate of insurance from an acceptable insurance company describing the required coverage with limits of liability reasonably acceptable to Landlord. The certificate shall name the Landlord as an additional insured party and shall provide that it may not be materially changed or canceled without at least fifteen (15) days' prior written notice. The insurance proceeds shall be made payable to the parties hereto as their interests may appear, except that the Tenant's share of such insurance proceeds is hereby assigned and made payable to the Landlord to secure any rent and other obligations then due, delinquent, and owing Landlord by Tenant. Tenant shall not do or knowingly permit the doing of any act that would violate any insurance policy or increase the insurance rates in force upon the Premises. Landlord and Tenant, for good and valuable consideration, hereby mutually waive their respective rights of recovery against each other for any loss incurred by fire or any casualty if there shall be extended coverage and other property insurance or liability policies existing for the benefit of the respective parties in amounts sufficient to repair or restore the Premises and damages caused by such casualty and, if necessary, each party shall apply to its insurer to obtain waivers of subrogation.

14. Destruction
    A. Partial destruction of premises or common areas. If the improvements to the Premises or if the common areas shall be partially destroyed by fire, or other casualty, whereby the Premises or common areas shall be rendered unusable only in part, Landlord shall cause the damage to be repaired (due allowance being made for settlement of insurance claims and delays resulting from governmental restrictions or controls, or other causes beyond Landlord's control) and the Lease shall remain in full force and effect except that the rent payable by Tenant shall be abated in proportion to that portion of the Premises or common areas rendered unusable, until such portion of the Premises or common areas is restored.

    B. Total destruction of premises or common areas. If by reason of fire or other casualty the Premises or common areas shall be rendered wholly unusable, or if the damage results from a cause not covered by fire and extended coverage insurance, or if the casualty occurs during the last year of the term of this Lease, Landlord shall have the option either to: (a) cause such damage to be repaired, in which event this Lease shall remain in full force and effect except that the rent shall be abated in proportion to that part of the Premises or common areas rendered unusable until said Premises or common areas are restored; or (b) terminate this Lease by providing Tenant with written notice thereof within sixty (60) days after the casualty, in which event this Lease shall cease as of the date of said damage or destruction, and the rent shall be adjusted equitably as of such date.

    C. Partial destruction of building. In the event that twenty-five percent (25%) or more of the building known as "_____" is damaged or destroyed by fire or other casualty, notwithstanding the fact that the Premises may be unaffected, Landlord may terminate this Lease by providing Tenant with written notice within sixty (60) days after the occurrence of the damage or destruction. Landlord's obligation to repair any damage hereunder shall be limited to the proceeds actually received by Landlord from insurance coverage and shall be limited to the basic building, roof, and structural parts thereof, including those items for which Landlord is responsible under paragraph 8 of this Lease, and in no event shall it include any repairs or replacement of tenant improvements, betterments, fixtures, or contents made or placed by Tenant in or about the Premises.

D. Tenant's duties regarding destruction. Tenant, after the occurrence of any fire or other casualty, shall, at its own cost and expense (unless Landlord or Tenant elects to terminate the Lease as described in this paragraph 14), promptly repair and restore Tenant's equipment, personal belongings, and furnishings, but not any fixtures or non-moveable items. Tenant shall not be entitled to any abatement of rent in the event of a casualty if the damage is due to the negligence of Tenant or its employees.

E. Tenant's rights of termination. Wherever in this paragraph 14 Landlord is given the right to terminate this Lease due to casualty or destruction, Tenant shall likewise have the same right of termination with the same notice requirements.

15. Condemnation

If all or a sufficient portion of the building, Premises, or common areas shall be condemned by any public authority or acquired under threat of condemnation, so as to render the building, Premises, or common areas unsuitable for the Tenant's business and intended purposes, or unsuitable for the Landlord's intended purposes, either Tenant or Landlord may terminate this Lease by serving upon the other party a written notice of its intention to do so within sixty (60) days after the condemnation award shall be entered or payment made by the governmental authority.

16. Tenant's fixtures

All furniture, trade fixtures, and movable equipment owned by Tenant and installed in the Premises by Tenant (unless such fixtures or equipment were installed as a replacement for furniture, fixtures, or equipment owned by Landlord in the Premises as of the date the Premises were first occupied by Tenant) shall remain the property of Tenant and shall be removable from time to time or upon the expiration or earlier termination of this Lease; provided, however, such removal shall be done without causing damage to the Premises and provided that Tenant is not in default hereunder. Prior to termination of the Lease, Tenant shall repair, at Tenant's expense, any damage to the Premises caused by the removal of any furniture, fixtures, or equipment.

17. Holding over

If Tenant remains in possession of the Premises after the expiration or earlier termination of this Lease, and Landlord thereafter accepts rent from Tenant, Tenant shall be deemed to be occupying the Premises as a tenant from month to month, subject to all of the conditions and obligations of this Lease insofar as the same are applicable to a month-to-month tenancy.

18. Subordination

Tenant agrees that this Lease and all interests of Tenant in the Premises shall be subordinate to any mortgages or other security instruments that may now exist or hereafter be placed upon the Premises by Landlord. Tenant hereby agrees to recognize any future purchaser of the Premises or any party taking title to the Premises by virtue of foreclosure, deed in lieu of foreclosure, or other conveyance as the new Landlord ("Attornment"), provided that Tenant's right to quiet possession of the Premises is not disturbed and the terms and conditions of this Lease continue in full force and effect. The subordination by Tenant is self-operative; however, Tenant agrees to execute, upon thirty (30) days' prior written request, such instruments as Landlord may reasonably request confirming such subordination and Attornment. In the event any lender requires as a condition of a loan secured by the Premises that any amendments be made to this Lease that shall not require Tenant to make any additional payments or otherwise materially change the rights or obligations of the Tenant hereunder, Tenant shall, upon Landlord's request, execute and deliver appropriate amendments.

19. Assignment and sublease

Tenant shall not assign this Lease nor sublet the Premises, or any portion thereof, without first obtaining the prior written consent of Landlord, which consent shall not be unreasonably withheld. Any rent charged to a subtenant in excess of the rent under this Lease shall be paid to Landlord. Landlord shall not be obligated to consent to any sublease or assignment if not consistent with the use of the Premises as a medical office. Any assignment or subletting approved by Landlord shall release or discharge any obligation of Tenant under this Lease if Landlord approves the credit rating of the subtenant or assignee demonstrating its ability to fully assume the financial obligations under this Lease, which approval shall not be unreasonably withheld. The term "Assignment" includes any transfer by operation of law or otherwise of this Lease, any transfer of effective control or ownership of Tenant if Tenant is a professional corporation or partnership and any sale of all or substantially all of the assets owned or used by Tenant in the operation of the medical office on the Premises. Tenant shall not, either voluntarily or by operation of law, mortgage, pledge, or encumber the Premises.

20. Indemnification

Landlord and Tenant hereby mutually agree to indemnify and hold harmless each other against and from any and all costs, claims, penalties, fines, damages, or liability arising, directly or indirectly, from: (a) use by Landlord or Tenant of the Premises, adjacent sidewalks, parking lot, common areas, or anything else within the building; (b) the conduct of Tenant's medical practice or Landlord's business or anything else done or permitted by Landlord or Tenant to be done on or about the Premises or the building; (c) any breach or default in the performance of Landlord's or Tenant's obligations under this Lease; (d) other acts or omissions of Landlord or Tenant, their employees, contractors, agents, patients, or invitees.

20A.   Termination by tenant

In addition to any other rights that Tenant might have to terminate this Lease as described elsewhere, Tenant may terminate this Lease, without penalty, for the following reasons, or upon the following events, and according to the following notice provisions:

A.   Upon the death of Tenant, or if Tenant is a professional corporation, upon the death of the primary shareholder.

B.   Upon the disability of Tenant, or if Tenant is a professional corporation, upon the disability of the primary shareholder. For the purposes of this section, the term "disability" shall mean the physical or mental incapacity or inability to practice medicine, all as determined by Tenant's disability insurance carrier.

C.   Upon the retirement of Tenant from the practice of medicine, or if Tenant is a professional corporation, upon the retirement of the primary shareholder.

D.   If this Lease is terminated for any of the reasons set forth above in subparagraphs A., B., or C., the termination shall take effect on the first day of the next month following written notice to Landlord of such termination, and Tenant shall vacate the Premises as of that date. A failure to vacate the Premises shall be treated as a holdover tenancy on a month-to-month basis under this Lease, and Tenant shall pay rent during any holdover tenancy as described in this Lease.

21. Mechanic's lien

Notice is hereby given that no contractor, subcontractor, supplier, or anyone else who may furnish any material, service, or labor for any improvement, alteration, or repair to the Premises shall at any time be entitled to any lien on the Premises. For the further security of the Landlord, the Tenant agrees to give actual notice in advance to the Landlord concerning any contractors, subcontractors, and suppliers who may furnish or agree to furnish any such material, services, or labor regarding the Premises. In the event a Mechanic's Lien shall at any time be filed against the Premises by reason of work, labor, services, or material performed or furnished at Tenant's request or direction, then Tenant shall forthwith cause the same to be promptly discharged. If Tenant shall fail to cause such lien to be discharged within thirty (30) days after notification of the filing thereof, Landlord may, but shall not be obligated to, discharge the same by paying the amount claimed to be due and the amount so paid by Landlord, and all costs and expenses, including reasonable attorney fees incurred by Landlord, shall be due and payable by Tenant to Landlord immediately upon receipt by Tenant of Landlord's demand therefore in the form of additional rent; provided, however, the mechanic's lien need not be paid in full and released if the Tenant, in good faith, is diligently contesting the mechanic's lien. If, however, the existence of the mechanic's lien constitutes a default or breach of any mortgage or loan agreement regarding the Landlord, Landlord shall have the right to require Tenant to either pay the mechanic's lien and cause it to be released or to post a bond pursuant to applicable law.

22. Access

Landlord or Landlord's agents or employees may enter the Premises during normal business hours (or at other times in the case of an emergency) to examine the Premises; to make necessary repairs required of Landlord under this Lease; to show the Premises to potential buyers, lessees, or lenders; and to make such alterations as Landlord deems necessary to meet its obligations under this Lease so long as such access does not unreasonably affect Tenant's use of the Premises. Landlord shall make every reasonable effort always to give Tenant advance notice of Landlord's desire to obtain access.

23. Tenant default

Tenant shall be in default under this Lease (i) if Tenant abandons or vacates the Premises, (ii) if Tenant fails to make a payment of rent in a timely fashion, (iii) if Tenant shall violate any requirement of this Lease and fail to cure the default within the required grace period, or (iv) if Tenant shall make an assignment for the benefit of creditors or be adjudicated a bankruptcy or file any petition in bankruptcy. Upon default, Landlord shall have the option to declare this Lease terminated and to reenter the Premises. In the event of any default by Tenant under this Lease, Landlord shall be entitled to terminate this Lease upon giving Tenant thirty (30) days' prior written notice of the default and an opportunity to cure the default within thirty (30) days; provided, however, that if more than thirty (30) days are reasonably required to cure the default, Tenant shall not be deemed in default if Tenant commences such cure within the thirty- (30) day period and thereafter diligently prosecutes such cure to completion.

24. Landlord's default

Landlord shall be in default under this Lease if Landlord fails to perform any of its obligations hereunder without cure for a period of thirty (30) days after written notice thereof is provided to Landlord; provided, however, that if more than thirty (30) days are reasonably required to cure the default, Landlord shall not be deemed in default if Landlord commences such cure within the thirty- (30) day period and thereafter diligently prosecutes such cure to completion. In the event of any sale of the Premises, Landlord shall be entirely freed and relieved of all liability under any and all of the covenants and obligations contained in or derived from this Lease. The purchaser, at such sale or any subsequent sale of the Premises, shall be deemed to have assumed and agreed to carry out any and all of the covenants and obligations of the Landlord under this Lease. Should Landlord or its successor in interest or assignee fail to continuously exist and operate primarily as it presently is doing and such failure would in the reasonable opinion of Tenant materially alter his medical practice, Tenant may terminate this Lease by giving Landlord sixty (60) days' prior written notice.

25. Equipment

Included in the leasehold interest being leased to Tenant shall be all fixtures and improvements that will be installed by Landlord on the Premises immediately prior to the commencement of this Lease. Tenant shall be responsible for maintaining said fixtures and improvements and at the end of the Lease Term shall return said items to Landlord in good working condition, ordinary wear and tear excepted.

26. Future legislation or interpretation.

Landlord and Tenant are of the opinion that this Lease complies with all laws presently in effect as they apply to hospitals and physicians. In the event of future legislation, safe harbor regulations, governmental rule or regulation, policy, or governmental interpretation thereof which applies to this Lease and prohibits or invalidates any of its provisions or causes Landlord or Tenant not to qualify under or otherwise be in violation of any Medicare, Medicaid or other reimbursement regulations or other laws or if the Landlord's continuing ability to qualify as a tax-exempt Section 501(c)(3) corporation is in jeopardy at any time, as determined by the Landlord, because of the terms of this Lease, then Landlord and Tenant shall forthwith cause to be made to this Lease such amendments as may be reasonably required, and which shall be mutually agreeable, to bring the terms of this Lease back into compliance with law. If this Lease cannot be so amended by mutual consent, either the Landlord or the Tenant shall have the right to terminate this Lease without penalty by giving sixty (60) days' prior written notice.

27. Notices

Any notice permitted or required to be given under this Lease shall be adequate if either delivered in person or delivered by certified United States Mail, postage prepaid, return receipt requested, or delivered by overnight courier such as Federal Express and addressed as follows:

- **To Landlord:**

_____

_____

_____

_____

- **To Tennant:**

_____

_____

_____

_____

28. Freedom in referrals

Landlord and Tenant understand and agree that nothing contained in this Lease shall in any way require or suggest that Tenant, or any persons affiliated or associated with Tenant, refer or admit patients to the hospital or healthcare facility owned or operated by Landlord at any time whatsoever.

Tenant shall be absolutely free to refer to admit patients to any hospital or healthcare facility that Tenant deems appropriate, in Tenant's sole discretion, all without loss of any rights or benefits whatsoever under this Lease.

IN WITNESS WHEREOF, the parties hereto have executed this Lease on the day and year first written above.

LANDLORD: TENANT:

By _____   By _____

Title:_____

PHYSICIAN RECRUITMENT GUIDELINES

A. Legal Parameters

The recruitment activities of ABC are guided by laws governing tax-exempt organizations as well as the federal Medicare regulatory structures. These include prohibitions against (i) substantial benefits to private individuals that are not supported by demonstrated hospital or community need, (ii) any remuneration (whether cash or in kind) to any physicians for the purpose or with the intent of increasing referrals to or the business activity at ABC, and (iii) referrals to ABC for designated health services (including hospital services) by physicians with financial relationships with the hospital, unless a legal exception is satisfied. Therefore, there are certain guiding principles that must be adhered to, and all recruitment arrangements must receive the advance approval of ABC legal counsel and the Board of Trustees.

Safe harbor legal protection under the federal anti-kickback statutes and Stark laws is limited. Recruitment incentives paid, even in part, to induce or in exchange for referrals, could be considered a violation of the anti-kickback statutes. Recruitment incentives also create financial relationships under the Stark law between the hospital and physician(s) recipients of the incentive. Therefore, unless an exception applies, the physician(s) would be prohibited from referring to the hospital for designated health services (including hospital services) and the hospital prohibited from billing for such services. An exception to the Stark law permits recruitment incentives paid to a recruited physician who relocates to the area provided certain conditions are met. The Internal Revenue Service prohibits transactions by tax-exempt organizations that result in an excess benefit to private individuals without commensurate supporting hospital or community need. If these private individuals are considered "disqualified persons" under the IRS "intermediate sanctions" law, those involved in the excess benefit transactions are subject to personal fines. This includes management personnel.

Physician recruitment guidelines were developed by the legal services department and finalized in early 1999. The ABC Board of Trustees Executive Committee approved the guidelines on February 24, 1999. However, these guidelines may not keep pace with the rapid regulatory changes. Therefore, while a copy of the approved guidelines is attached, consultation with legal counsel should occur before discussions begin.

B. Guiding Principles

1. Recruitment activity may only be pursued in support of demonstrated community or hospital need. The specific needs/requirements must be addressed in the contract and monitored over the life of the agreement.
2. Remuneration:
   a. Any incentives or remuneration provided must be commercially reasonable, consistent with fair market value, and may not take into account or be based upon the volume or value of

any referrals or business otherwise generated or anticipated by the physician(s) involved.

   b. The remuneration must be stated in the agreement, must cover all promises and agreements (no other payments or side deals), and may not be modified.

3. Recruits must be from outside of the geographic area and agree to relocate to our community, or be graduating from a training program.

4. The physician involved may not be requested or required, expressly or implicitly, to refer any patient to the hospital and may not be prohibited from obtaining medical staff privileges at any other facility in the community.

5. The preferred structure is a direct recruiting arrangement between the hospital and the recruit. Recruitment to an existing practice may occur provided: (i) the hospital first identifies and documents a specific hospital or community need for the particular specialty; (ii) establishes the terms and conditions of the recruitment package; (iii) identifies an acceptable recruit (or recruits) (e.g., Level I, bilingual, female obstetrician); (iv) offers the opportunity to expand a practice to all medical staff members within the specialty equally; and (v) a tripartite agreement is signed.

C. Recruitment Guidelines

1. Recruitment must be consistent with demonstrable community and/or Hospital need.
   a. If there is not a community or Hospital need supported by objective evidence, do not proceed.
   b. Terms of recruitment agreement must support demonstrated need. That is, the recruitment activity should bear a reasonable relationship to the identified need, which should relate to the promotion and protection of health in the community or the Hospital's exempt purpose.
   c. Recruitment should also be consistent with Hospital plan, mission, and policy.

2. Recruitment incentive or compensation may not be tied to the anticipated value or volume of referrals or business to be generated between the parties. The recruit may not be required expressly or implicitly to refer to the Hospital.

3. Recruit from *out* of market area (i.e., physician must relocate residence *and* practice, and develop new patient base in area); or physician may be recruited directly from training.
   a. The recruit must establish practice in Hospital service area of identified need.
   b. With very limited exception, "cross-town" recruiting is not acceptable.

4. The entire recruitment package must be commensurate with the identified need and be reflected in a written, signed agreement.
   a. The terms of the agreement must be commercially reasonable and consistent with fair market value.

      i. The agreement must be negotiated at arm's length.

      ii. The recruitment package must be reviewed and approved by the Board Executive Committee for this purpose.

      iii. Comparability data must be obtained, reviewed, and considered by negotiators and Board Executive Committee in determining reasonableness and fair market value.

    b. If intent is to bring into a current practice, then: (i) the hospital first identifies and documents a specific hospital or community need for the particular specialty, (ii) establishes the terms and conditions of the recruitment package, (iii) identifies an acceptable recruit (or recruits), (iv) offers the opportunity to expand practice to all medical staff members within the specialty equally, and (v) a tripartite agreement is signed. Furthermore, if recruit joins existing group, incentives will be limited, per paragraph 11 below.

    c. There may *not* be any side agreements; all issues and payments (i.e., recruitment incentives, relocation expenses, etc.) must be reflected in the written agreement.

5. Any person with a conflict of interest must refrain from participating in negotiating, acting, or voting regarding the transaction.

6. A 1099 form must be issued to the recruit and/or practice, depending on agreement, to reflect the value of *all* benefits received.

7. File documentation to reflect the following is essential and must be submitted to the Board Executive Committee for review and to legal services *prior* to approval of the transaction:

    a. Community and/or Hospital benefit or need (e.g., need analysis, medical staff patterns, medical staff retirement, documented lack of Medicaid/indigent care providers/bilingual providers, emergency room call coverage, etc.)

    b. Fair market value (e.g., salary surveys)

    c. Commercial reasonableness of entire package

    d. Notes, or other documentation reflecting arm's-length negotiation (e.g., RFP, correspondence) and adherence to guidelines

8. Recruitment packages and these guidelines will be reviewed periodically to ensure activities of Hospital do not substantially benefit private interests.

9. Selection of permissible incentives (identified below) and combinations that may be offered must be made on a case-by-case basis on the basis of all relevant facts and with the advice of legal counsel.

10. If recruit joins an existing group, 11a, 11b, or 11c below may be selected. Relocation expenses in accordance with hospital policy, capped at 50% of actual expenses, may be provided directly to the recruit and must be reflected in the agreement and included in the loan amount.

11. Permissible recruitment incentives include the following:

    a. Income guarantees

      i. Hospital may guarantee up to 100% of fair market value income for first year of practice. Guarantee may be provided up to two (2) years in special circumstances with documented reasons therefore. When recruit is joining an existing practice, hospital may guarantee up to 50% of fair market value income for first year of practice.

   ii. If guarantee is based upon net income, a reasonable fixed cap on expenses must be established by accounting and stated in agreement.

   iii. In most circumstances, guarantee must be structured as a secured loan with promissory note and security agreement with accounts receivable and/or equipment as security.

   iv. Agreement must require continued presence and practice by recruit/group for entire guarantee period, and four (4) years thereafter, forgiveness ratable (25% per year) over four- (4) year period. [The four- (4) year period is subject to reduction based upon specific benefit to the hospital with approval of legal counsel.]

   v. Hospital must periodically inspect books and records of practice regarding income and expenses of recruit.

b. Loans, loan guarantees

   i. Loan rate must be reasonable and reflect market rates [prime plus one percent (1%) or two percent (2%)]. Loan must have reasonable repayment period and be evidenced by promissory note with security agreement, per above.

   ii. Loan repayment may be deferred for a reasonable period of time; interest continues to accrue.

c. Office expansion or renovation assistance may be provided to an existing practice when necessary to accommodate a new recruit. Assistance may not exceed fifty percent (50%) of commercially reasonable cost of the expansion necessary to accommodate the new recruit. It must be structured as a secured loan, and the loan may be forgiven ratably (25% per year) over a four- (4) year period provided practice conditions are satisfied.

d. Relocation expenses

   i. Only those that relate to moving household goods and family members from old residence to first new residence are reimbursable. Meal and lodging reimbursement must be consistent with Hospital policy.

   ii. Must have a reasonable cap.

e. Reasonable interview travel expenses consistent with hospital policy.

f. Lease/sublease. Hospital may lease space to a new recruit or practice that is accepting a recruit and provide commercially reasonable build-out assistance. This must be structured as a secured loan that is forgiven ratably over four (4) years (25% per year) provided the practice conditions are satisfied.

   i. There may be no other incentive.

   ii. May not include: start-up costs, nonphysician salary subsidy, sign-on bonuses.

g. Search firm fees must be paid directly to search firm.

12. All recruitment packages/agreements, incentives, payments must be:
    a. Approved by legal services
    b. Consistent with these guidelines unless approved otherwise by the Executive Committee of the Board of Trustees and Legal Services.
13. Hospital will not recruit or assist with the recruitment of a Level III practitioner (as defined by Medical Staff policy).

POSITION POSTINGS

XYZ Health System

[Date]
Contact: [Name of Recruiter]
Tel: (555) 555-1212 | Fax: (555) 555-1214
Current Physician Needs For:
XYZ [name of campus]
XYZ [name of campus]
XYZ [name of campus]

General Demographic Information:

- Located in upper Northwest [name of state] and recently selected as an All-American City
- Convenient distance from major metropolitan areas in [state], [state], and [state]
- Population for [name of service area] is 400,000; service area is 1.3 million
- None of these positions qualifies for a waiver.
- Physicians must be willing to work full-time; no part-time positions available.
- Nationally ranked public and private schools
- Numerous festivals, sporting, and cultural events

Gastroenterology (1):

New Information
Position Available: Immediate

Facility: XYZ [name of campus], [city, state]

Requirements: Fellow or practicing physician

Practice: To join private SSG of 4. Rotate through 5 facilities. Must be able to perform ERCPs as well as other invasive procedures, or willing to learn (Group willing to train on ERCPs). All invasive procedures performed in hospitals. Full rotational basis for new consults and patients. Averaging 25 procedures a month. Averaging 10 patients each in office and 5 inpatients. Approximately 300 referring physicians. Four and a half day workweek. Zero capitated managed care.

Call: 1:4

Compensation and Benefits: Salary of $200,000 with quarterly bonus for 1st and 2nd years. After 2 years, there is option for buying into the partnership. Overhead approximately 30%. Two weeks vacation for 1st year, 3 weeks the 2nd year, and 1 week of CME. Practice potential $500K. Paid relocation and interview expenses. Sign-on bonus available for this position.

Hematology/Oncology (1):

Position Available: Immediate

Facility: XYZ [name of campus], [city, state]

Requirements: Would prefer practicing physician but will consider fellow.

Practice: Join 3 other hematology/oncologists in single specialty group at XYZ Cancer Treatment Center. Averaging 20–25 patients in clinic and 5 inpatients. Ninety percent of practice is physician referral. Approximately 9,000 hem/onc visits and 9,000 chemo visits per year.

Call: 1:5

Compensation and Benefits: Salary of $250,000 and incentive bonuses based upon percentage of total production and clinic expenses, paid malpractice, 5 CME days with generous allowance, vacation, health and life insurance, and relocation up to $10,000.

*Internist/Endocrinologist (1):

New Position
Position Available: Immediate

Facility: XYZ [name of campus], [city, state]

Requirements: Completion of accredited residency program. Must be willing to take boards within 2 years.

Practice: General Internal Medicine and Endocrinology practice. Both inpatient and outpatient services. Average 5 inpatients and 20–25 outpatients.

Call: Possibly 1:4 (Hospitalist services available)

Neonatologist (1):

New Position
Position Available: Immediate

Facility: XYZ [name of campus], [city, state]

Requirements: Fellowship trained in Neonatology. Board certified or board eligible with imminent plans to sit for the boards. Warm and compassionate, outgoing personality to work with families. Would prefer practicing physician but will consider fellow.

Practice: Join 1 other Neonatologist and 1 NP; 150+ referring physicians; 17+ referring hospitals; Level III nursery with 26–30 beds; average daily census: 15–18; approximately 350 admission/year; active air and ground transport team; 24-hour in-house respiratory therapy; no ECMO or complicated heart surgery; high-frequency oscillation and nitric oxide; pediatric subspecialties: cardiology, genetics, hematology, infectious disease, neurology, and surgery.

Call: Favorable schedule: one week on/one week off

Compensation and Benefits: Generous base salary of $250K plus incentive; sign-on bonus and/or stipend available to qualified candidates; paid interview, relocation, and malpractice insurance expenses; partnership after one year with practice potential of $400K; generous pension plan; CME stipend.

Orthopedics, General (1):   **Position Available: Immediate**
Facility: XYZ [name of campus], [city, state]
Requirements: Practicing physician or fellow.
Practice: Join large SSG of 10 Orthopedists. Average 20–40 patients daily. 10% Pediatrics.
Call: 1:7
Compensation and Benefits: $250–$275K, depending on experience; paid malpractice, full health insurance plan, life insurance, disability, retirement/401K, annual CME and relocation. Stipend and/or sign-on *bonus available to qualified candidates.*

Orthopedics, Foot & Ankle (1):   **Position Available: Immediate**
Facility: XYZ [name of campus], [city, state]
Requirements: Must have Foot & Ankle Fellowship. *Practicing physician or fellow.*
Practice: Join large SSG of 10 orthopedists. Average 20–40 patients daily. 5% Pediatrics. Must be willing to do general orthopedics while building practice.
Call: 1:7
Compensation and Benefits: $250–$275K, depending on experience; paid malpractice, full health insurance plan, life insurance, disability, retirement/401K, annual CME and relocation. Stipend and/or sign-on bonus available to qualified candidates.

Orthopedics, Hand (1):   **Position Available: Immediate**
Facility: XYZ [name of campus], [city, state]
Requirements: Must have Hand Fellowship. *Practicing physician or fellow.*
Practice: Join large SSG of 10 Orthopedists. Average 20–40 patients daily. 5% Pediatrics. Existing Hand Surgeon is available to mentor and train.
Call: 1:7
Compensation and Benefits: $250–$275K, depending on experience; paid malpractice, full health insurance plan, life in-

surance, disability, retirement/401K, annual CME and relocation. *Stipend and/or sign-on bonus available to qualified candidates.*

Psychiatry, Geriatric

New Position
PositionAvailable: Immediate

Facility: XYZ [name of campus], [city, state]

Requirements: Must have completed accredited residency program. *Practicing physician or fellow.*

Practice: Join SSG of 2 general psychiatrists. Will forward additional information as soon as possible.

Call:

Compensation and Benefits: $150–$175K, depending on experience; paid malpractice, full health insurance plan, life insurance, disability, retirement/401K, annual CME and relocation. Stipend and/or sign-on bonus available to qualified candidates.

Vascular Surgeon (1)

New Position
Position Available: Immediate

Facility: XYZ [name of campus], [city, state]

Requirements: Must have Vascular Fellowship. *Practicing physician or fellow.*

Practice: *Replacing retiring physician.* Ready-made practice to walk into. Physician is willing to stay for 6 months to train new physician in arteriograms, abdominal aortic aneurysms, and endovascular procedures, transfer patient load, and will help build relationships with greater than 80 referring physicians. Operate AM/clinics PM. Average 180 patients/month in office; 50–70 surgical cases/month. Four-day work week. 3 FT; 1 PT personnel—one is a certified vascular tech, RN and Certified RN First Assist. Performs endovascular and general vascular procedures with a specially trained OR Team. No access work. In-office noninvasive vascular lab.

Compensation and Benefits: 100% Guarantee of Collections. Up to $300K, depending on experience and qualifications. Practice Potential is $500K annually. *Stipend and/or sign-on bonus available to qualified candidates.*

Source: Christus Schumpert Health System, Shreveport, Louisiana. Used with permission.

CONTINGENCY SEARCH AGREEMENT—PRIMARY CARE

This Agreement is between _____ (hereinafter referred to as "ABC") and [NAME OF RECRUITMENT FIRM] (hereinafter referred to as "Recruiter").

A. Responsibilities

The following sets forth the responsibilities the parties have mutually agreed to regarding the recruitment of physician as specified by ABC. In performing the services specified in this Agreement, Recruiter shall act at all times and in all respects as an independent contractor. Nothing herein shall be construed to create an employer–employee relationship between Recruiter and ABC.

Recruiter agrees to:

1. Search, screen, and prequalify potential physician candidates who meet the specifications of ABC.
2. Interview potential physician candidates by telephone to ascertain compatibility with ABC's specifications.
3. Present in writing to ABC only those candidates who have been verbally presented and accepted by ABC.
4. Present only those candidates who have expressed a desire for continued interest regarding the position(s) available.
5. Assist in planning, coordination, and follow-up of all physician site visits.
6. Keep ABC updated and current on contacts with all candidates.

ABC health system agrees to:

1. Provide Recruiter with recruitment specifications and general contract terms.
2. Assume financial responsibility for the travel and recruitment expense for all physician visits as preauthorized by ABC.
3. Provide feedback to Recruiter regarding physician on-site visits and the status of contract negotiations.

B. Placement Fee

ABC agrees to pay a placement fee of $10,000 when a candidate is "placed," which means the candidate referred by Recruiter becomes employed by or independently contracted with ABC or any other physician group for which ABC is recruiting, whether by written Employment Agreement or Independent Practice Agreement, and Recruiter has fulfilled all responsibilities set for this section A (1-6) of this Agreement.

The placement fee shall be due and payable if a placement occurs as described in this paragraph anytime within one (1) year of acceptance of candidate by ABC. Fifty (50) percent of the placement fee ($5,000.00) shall be due and payable within ten (10) working days upon full execution of candidate's Employment Agreement or Independent Practice Agreement; with the remaining fifty (50) percent ($5,000.00) due within ten (10) working days of the actual start date of the candidate.

C. Guarantee

In the event that a candidate recruited by Recruiter fails to appear on his or her start date or fails to remain in his or her position for any reason for a period of ninety (90) days after his or her actual start date, Recruiter shall conduct a search for a minimum of six (6) months in an effort to provide a replacement candidate who satisfies the specifications of ABC at no additional charge to the above agreed fee for each physician.

In the event Recruiter fails to locate and recruit a replacement who satisfies all the terms of this Agreement, including but not limited to the requirement that such candidate remain in the position for at least ninety (90) days, Recruiter shall refund 100% of the fee paid for that position, and this Agreement shall otherwise remain in effect until the end of the term.

D. Term

This Agreement shall have an initial term of one (1) year from the date given below, although either party has the right to terminate this Agreement for any reason prior to the expiration of such term with ten (10) days' advance written notice.

E. Confidentiality

All information, whether written or oral, that is requested from or voluntarily furnished by ABC shall be in the strictest of confidence and used only for the purposes specified in this Agreement.

F. Contract Conditions

All claims and requests, pursuant to or in addition to this contract, are to be only in writing. All understandings or modifications are to be only with mutual written consent. In the event that legal fees are incurred by either party pursuant to enforcing the terms of this contract, or to enforce an arbitration decision reached pursuant to the terms of this contract, the nonprevailing party will be responsible for such legal fees.

G. Miscellaneous

This Agreement shall be governed by the laws of the State of [_____].

This Agreement constitutes the entire agreement of the parties and contains all of the agreements between the parties and may not be modified except in writing and signed by both parties.

If any portion of this Agreement for any reason shall be determined by a court of competent jurisdiction to be invalid or unenforceable, the remaining portion or portions shall be valid, enforceable, and carried into effect when to do so would accomplish the present legal and valid intentions of the parties.

IN WITNESS THEREOF, the parties have caused this Agreement to be executed by their authorized representatives on the day and date first below written.

For ABC,   For Recruiter,

_____   _____

Date: _____   Date: _____

Source: Elliot Health System, Manchester, New Hampshire.
Used with permission.

CONTINGENCY SEARCH AGREEMENT—SPECIALTY AND SUBSPECIALTY

This Agreement is between _____(hereinafter referred to as "ABC") and [NAME OF RECRUITMENT FIRM] (hereinafter referred to as "Recruiter").

A. Responsibilities

The following sets forth the responsibilities to which the parties have mutually agreed regarding the recruitment of physician as specified by ABC. In performing the services specified in this Agreement, Recruiter shall act at all times and in all respects as an independent contractor. Nothing herein shall be construed to create an employer–employee relationship between Recruiter and ABC.

Recruiter agrees to:

1. Search, screen, and prequalify potential physician candidates who meet the specifications of ABC.
2. Interview potential physician candidates by telephone to ascertain compatibility with ABC's specifications.
3. Present in writing to ABC only those candidates who have been verbally presented and accepted by ABC.
4. Present only those candidates who have expressed a desire for continued interest regarding the position(s) available.
5. Assist in planning, coordination, and follow-up of all physician site visits.
6. Keep ABC updated and current on contacts with all candidates.

ABC health system agrees to:

1. Provide Recruiter with recruitment specifications and general contract terms.
2. Assume financial responsibility for the travel and recruitment expense for all physician visits as preauthorized by ABC.
3. Provide feedback to Recruiter regarding physician on-site visits and the status of contract negotiations.

B. Placement Fee

ABC agrees to pay a placement fee of $15,000.00 when a candidate is "placed," which means the candidate referred by Recruiter becomes employed by or independently contracted with ABC or any other physician group for which ABC is recruiting, whether by written Employment Agreement or Independent Practice Agreement, and Recruiter has fulfilled all responsibilities set for this section A (1-6) of this Agreement.

The placement fee shall be due and payable if a placement occurs as described in this paragraph anytime within one (1) year of acceptance of candidate by ABC. Fifty (50) percent of the placement fee ($7,500.00) shall be due and payable within ten (10) working days upon full execution of candidate's Employment Agreement or Independent Practice Agreement;

with the remaining fifty (50) percent ($7,500.00) due within ten (10) working days of the actual start date of the candidate.

C. Guarantee

In the event that a candidate recruited by Recruiter fails to appear on his or her start date or fails to remain in his or her position for any reason for a period of ninety (90) days after his or her actual start date, Recruiter shall conduct a search for a minimum of six (6) months in an effort to provide a replacement candidate who satisfies the specifications of ABC at no additional charge to the above agreed fee for each physician.

In the event Recruiter fails to locate and recruit a replacement who satisfies all the terms of this Agreement, including but not limited to the requirement that such candidate remain in the position for at least ninety (90) days, Recruiter shall refund 100% of the fee paid for that position, and this Agreement shall otherwise remain in effect until the end of the term.

D. Term

This Agreement shall have an initial term of one (1) year from the date given below, although either party has the right to terminate this Agreement for any reason prior to the expiration of such term with ten (10) days' advance written notice.

E. Confidentiality

All information, whether written or oral, that is requested from or voluntarily furnished by ABC shall be in the strictest of confidence and used only for the purposes specified in this Agreement.

F. Contract Conditions

All claims and requests, pursuant to or in addition to this contract, are to be only in writing. All understandings or modifications are to be only with mutual written consent. In the event that legal fees are incurred by either party pursuant to enforcing the terms of this contract, or to enforce an arbitration decision reached pursuant to the terms of this contract, the non-prevailing party will be responsible for such legal fees.

G. Miscellaneous

1. This Agreement shall be governed by the laws of the State of _____.
2. This Agreement constitutes the entire agreement of the parties and contains all of the agreements between the parties and may not be modified except in writing and signed by both parties.
3. If any portion of this Agreement for any reason shall be determined by a court of competent jurisdiction to be invalid or unenforceable, the remaining portion or portions shall be valid, enforceable, and carried into effect when to do so would accomplish the present legal and valid intentions of the parties.

IN WITNESS THEREOF, the parties have caused this Agreement to be executed by their authorized representatives on the day and date first below written.

For ABC,   For Recruiter,

_____   _____

Date: _____   Date: _____

Source: Elliot Health System, Manchester, New Hampshire.
Used with permission.

**PHYSICIAN RECRUITMENT QUESTIONNAIRE—PREINTERVIEW
PHYSICIAN QUESTIONNAIRE**

Thank you for your interest in ABC Urgent Care. Please complete all areas and answer all questions.

Name _____

Address _____

SSN _____ DOB _____

Place of Birth _____

Telephone: Home _____ Work _____

Pager _____

*(State) License No. _____ Date of Issue _____

*(State) Registration _____ Exp. Date _____

*Other Licensed States and Numbers _____

*DEA Registration _____ Exp. Date _____

*BCBS Number _____ UPIN _____

*Medicare Number(s) _____

If you had Medicare numbers in other states, please list these as well.

Board Certified _____ Specialty _____

If not certified, when do you plan to take the Boards? _____

Please list below any Malpractice insurance policy(s) coverage and *attach at least 10 years of claim history and coverage.*

Malpractice Insurance Co. _____

Period of policy _____

Please attach additional page if necessary. We *must* have 10 years for verification of coverage with no gaps.

*Please provide the following medical education information. (Please include **name, city, state, month,** and **year of graduation**).

Undergraduate _____ From _____ to _____

Graduate School _____ From _____ to _____

Medical School _____ From _____ to _____

Internship _____ From _____ to _____

Residency _____ From _____ to _____

Fellowship _____ From _____ to _____

PROVIDER REFERENCES (Must be Board Certified in your Specialty). Please include complete address and phone number.

1._____

2._____

3._____

Please send copies of your [State] License, [State] Registration, DEA, and Board Certifications or Residency Certificates and Emergency Care Foreign Medical Graduate (ECFMG) certificates (if applicable). These certificates are required for employment. If you do not have copies, please request them from the appropriate sources. I have a listing of sources on file, if you need assistance.

Source: Doctor's Urgent Care Centre, Fayetteville, North Carolina.
Used with permission.

PROFESSIONAL QUESTIONS AND ATTESTATION

During the past 5 years:

1. Has your license to practice in this state or any other state been denied, restricted, limited, suspended, or revoked, or are any of these actions ending with respect to your license? Have you been reprimanded by a state licensing agency? ☐ Yes ☐ No

2. Has your DEA (state or federal) license been restricted, limited, suspended, or revoked, or are any of these actions pending with respect to your DEA registration? ☐ Yes ☐ No

3. Have your hospital admitting privileges been revoked, suspended, reduced, or not renewed? Have disciplinary proceedings been instituted against you? Are any of these actions pending with respect to your hospital admitting privileges? ☐ Yes ☐ No

4. Have you voluntarily relinquished hospital privileges, DEA registration, academic appointments, or any professional status while an investigation was being conducted? ☐ Yes ☐ No

5. Has your participation in Medicare, Medicaid, or other government programs been denied, suspended, or revoked? Have any monetary penalties been levied against you? Have you been or are you under investigation by a regulatory agency? ☐ Yes ☐ No

6. Have any complaints been filed against you with a medical society? ☐ Yes ☐ No

7. Have any professional liability judgments been entered against you, including arbitration, or are there suits pending? ☐ Yes ☐ No

8. Have any professional liability claims settlements, not involving litigation or arbitration, been paid by you or on your behalf? ☐ Yes ☐ No

9. Has your professional liability insurance been canceled, denied, or premiums increased or surcharged based on claims history? ☐ Yes ☐ No

10. Have you been convicted of a crime (other than a traffic offense), or do you have any felony or misdemeanor charges pending, other than traffic offenses? ☐ Yes ☐ No

11. Do you presently have any condition that affects, or is reasonably likely to affect, your ability to perform professional or medical practice duties appropriately? ☐ Yes ☐ No

12. Do you presently have any condition that would require any accommodations to perform medical practice duties safely and effectively?
☐ Yes ☐ No

13. Do you have a chemical dependency problem that is not currently in remission?
☐ Yes ☐ No

Please provide an explanation for any questions to which you responded yes. Use a separate page if necessary.

_____

_____

_____

_____

_____

_____

_____

_____

_____

_____

_____

_____

_____

_____

_____

_____

_____

I certify that the information contained in this document is complete and accurate to the best of my knowledge. I agree to provide information as required to support this document. I specifically authorize and release ABC Urgent Care Center and/or its representatives to consult with any third party who may have information bearing on my professional qualifications, credentials, competence, character, mental or emotional stability, physical condition, ethics, behavior, financial condition, or any other matter, as well as to inspect or obtain any and all communications, reports (including but not limited to credit reports), records, statements, documents, recommendations, or disclosure of said third parties that may be material to such questions. I also specifically authorize said third parties to release said information to ABC Urgent Care Center and/or its authorized representatives upon request. I hereby release them from any liability any and all individuals and institutions or organizations who in good faith and without malice concerning my professional competence, ethics, character, education, training, licensing, and other qualifications, provide information to ABC Urgent Care Center.

Signature _____

Degree _____ Date _____

Please return to:

Name
Title
Address
Phone
Fax
Facility/Campus

Source: Doctor's Urgent Care Centre, Fayetteville, North Carolina.
Used with permission.

DEFINING THE POSITION—GETTING A FEEL FOR THE OPPORTUNITY (PHYSICIAN RECRUITMENT QUESTIONNAIRE)

Practice Specifics

Name of Practice _____

Principal Contact _____

E-mail Address _____

Phone _____ Fax _____

Private Line _____

Location _____

Position _____

Compensation $ _____

Call Schedule _____

Partnership Track? _____ If yes, then when? _____

Benefits

Incentive/Bonus? _____

Malpractice Paid? _____

Loan Repayment? _____

Vacation/Holiday _____

CME Time off? _____ If yes, any stipend amount _____

Life Insurance? _____

Insurance Benefits?
Health? _____ Disability? _____ For Dr. Only? _____ For Dr. & Family? _____

Tax Shelter? _____

Pension Plan? _____

Relocation Expense? _____

Other Benefits? (e.g., professional dues, licensing fees, or publications paid)

_____

Preferences		**Circle One**		
Fellowship	Yes	No		
Years of Experience	< 3	3 to 10 >		< 10
American Trained	Yes	No		

Preferred Medical Schools (please list) _____

Special Requests or Skills _____

Best Time/Day to Meet with Candidates _____

Prefer Phone Interview First? _____

Return to:

Name
Title
Phone
Fax
Facility/Campus

Source: Sarah S. Foster, Health Quest, Poughkeepsie, New York.
Used with permission.

CANDIDATE SCREENING—INITIAL INTERVIEW (PHYSICIAN INTERVIEW QUESTIONNAIRE)

Candidate: _____ Date: _____

1. What are you seeking in a practice setting? _____

2. Do you prefer an _____ employed position or a _____ guarantee of collections arrangement? Why? _____

3. What are you looking for in group size? _____

4. Why are you considering leaving your current position? Residency completion _____ Fellowship completion _____ Other _____

5. What would you like to have in the practice that you do not currently have? _____

6. Availability? _____

7. By when do you want to have made your decision? _____

8. What type of procedures are you currently performing? _____

9. For what type of procedures will you be requesting privileges? _____

10. What is your current call schedule?

    1:_____ Weekends _____ and ER _____

    What would you prefer?

    1:_____ Weekends _____ and ER _____

11. How many patients are you currently seeing? _____

    Inpatients _____ Clinic _____

12. How many patients are you comfortable seeing? _____

    Inpatients _____ Clinic _____

13. What is your current payer mix? _____

    What is preferred? _____

14. What is your current financial and benefit package? _____

15. What are you looking for in terms of compensation and benefits? ____

16. Do you have any student loans? _____ Yes _____ No

    If yes, how much? _____

17. Is loan forgiveness a requirement for your acceptance of a position? _____ Yes _____ No

18. Does your current contract include a noncompete clause? _____ Yes _____ No

    If so, is that why you want to relocate? _____ Yes _____ No

19. If you accept another position, will you be financially obligated to your current facility/group? _____ Yes _____ No

20. Have your hospital privileges ever been restricted? _____

21. Have your hospital privileges ever been suspended due to incomplete medical records? _____

    How many times in the last two years? _____

22. Have you been the subject of any disciplinary action? _____

    Have you been considered for any disciplinary action? _____

23. Do you know of any written complaints about you by patients, hospital staff, or members of the medical staff? _____

24. Why would you consider moving to _____ (any ties)?

25. What are your community needs? _____

26. Are you looking at other opportunities? _____ Yes _____ No

    If yes, are you willing to share any of the details with me? _____

Additional information _____

Follow up: _____

Source: Christus Schumpert Health System, Shreveport, Louisiana.
Used with permission.

CANDIDATE INTERVIEW CHECKLIST

Candidate Name: _____

Specialty: _____

Date(s) of Interview/Stay: _____

Interview #: _____

Practices to Visit: _____

To Do		Comments/Arrangements
Book flight		
Car rental		
Hotel reservation		
Meeting scheduled w/Medical Director		
Contact physicians and office managers in practices you will be visiting re: availability to meet candidate; lunch/dinner also		
Meeting scheduled w/Practice Administrator		
Verify/arrange someone to give tour of hospital to candidate		
Verify/arrange someone to give tour of practices to candidate		
Contact realtor to schedule real estate tour		
Make dinner reservation		
Complete written itinerary		
Put together packet for candidate and mail		
If married, include extra copies of itinerary for spouse		
Additional Information		

Source: Elliot Health System, Manchester, New Hampshire. Used with permission.

CANDIDATE INTERVIEW QUESTIONNAIRE

Conducting the Candidate Interview

Name: _____

Specialty: _____

Date: _____

Home Address: _____

City: _____ State: _____ Zip: _____

Phone: _____ E-mail: _____

Practice Opportunity

1. What specialized equipment will you need? _____

2. What are you looking for in a practice opportunity? _____

Personal

3. Spouse/Significant other's name: _____

   His/her career: _____

   Impact on your decision: _____

4. What led you into the medical field? _____

Licensure/Certification

5. Licensed in what states: _____

6. License applications pending in what states? _____

7. Board certified: _____ Specialty _____ Date: _____

8. Board eligible: _____ Specialty _____ Date: _____

Professional Accomplishments

  9. Honors/Awards: _____

10. Publications: _____

11. Military Service? _____ Branch: _____ Rank: _____

    Base/Hospital: _____ Dates: _____

    Duties: _____

Practice Style

12. What work/call schedule do you hope to establish? _____

13. Share three things from your residency and/or work experience of which you are particularly proud:

    a. _____

    b. _____

    c. _____

14. For what have you been criticized during the past four years or so (with respect to your medical practice)? _____

    Do you agree? _____ Why or why not? _____

    _____

15. What aspects of your specialty do you like the best? _____

    _____

    _____

16. What aspects of your specialty do you like the least? _____

17. What do you consider your three greatest strengths?

    a. _____

    b. _____

    c. _____

18. Everyone has weaknesses, and good physicians are aware of theirs. What would you identify as your weaknesses?

a. _____

b. _____

c. _____

19. What do your subordinates (nurses, support staff) say about you?

_____

_____

20. What would they like to have you do differently? _____

_____

_____

21. How do you criticize/correct your subordinates? _____

_____

_____

22. What do your colleagues say about you? _____

_____

_____

23. What is the most difficult thing you have had to do in your medical experience?

_____

_____

Miscellaneous

24. What are the factors you will take into consideration when choosing a practice opportunity?

_____

25. Is there anything else you would like me to know about you or your qualifications?

_____

_____

Source: Sitka Community Hospital, Sitka, Alaska. Used with permission.

CANDIDATE PEER INTERVIEW EVALUATION
(GRID CANDIDATE EVALUATION)

Name of Candidate: _____

Please rate this candidate according to the following criteria and return this

form to _____, or fax to (____) ____-_____.

Criteria This Candidate	Strongly Agree	Agree	Disagree	Cannot Evaluate
1. Will work well with a multidisciplinary team				
2. Has extensive knowledge of current therapies and treatments.				
3. Has knowledge of recent advances in surgical techniques and procedures				
4. Will develop a referral network outside our primary service area				
5. Can plan a well-executed implementation plan for the unit				
6. Can articulate quality indicators that he/she will review to ensure good outcomes				
7. Has a vision and plan to grow a quality program				
8. Is customer-service driven				
9. Will be a good fit with our medical and hospital staff				
10. Has the experience we need to develop a quality program				

Comments:

I would ____ strongly recommend ____ recommend ____ not recommend this candidate.

Source: Sitka Community Hospital, Sitka, Alaska. Used with permission.

CANDIDATE EVALUATION CHECKLIST—INTERVIEWER'S EVALUATION GRID

Candidate: _____   Position: _____

Reviewer: _____   Date: _____

Rating Scale:
Excellent: Above established standards
Satisfactory: Meets established standards
Unsatisfactory: Falls below established standards

Professional Requirements and Attributes	Excellent	Satisfactory	Unsatisfactory
Training and experience			
Medical staff rapport—how well will he/she relates			
Patient rapport—how well will he/she relates			
General medical knowledge			
Knowledge of position			
Personal Attributes			
Congenial personality			
Articulation			
Enthusiasm			
Confidence			
Personal rapport with interviewer			
Opportunity Match	**Yes**	**No**	**Do not know**
Can we meet the candidate's needs?			
Professional			
Financial			
Personal			
Spouse and family			

If not, why? _____

Recommendations:

Pursue without reservation _____

Pursue with the following reservations: _____

Do not pursue because: _____

Additional comments: _____

Source: Sitka Community Hospital, Sitka, Alaska. Used with permission.

LETTER TO REVIEWERS

Date

Dr. _____
ABC Medical Center
Street Address
City, State, Zip Code

Dear Dr. _____ :

Thank you for taking the time to meet with Dr. _____
during his/her visit on (date) . I would appreciate your input and evaluation of this candidate as an addition to the medical staff.

Please answer the questions below and return the letter to my office. If you
prefer to send it by fax rather than coming by the office within the next
day or so, please send it to my attention at (____) ____-_____.

Thank you for your timely response.

1. What was your overall impression of the candidate?

   Professional:

   Personal:

2. What key points about the area or hospital do you feel we should emphasize with this physician and/or significant other that seemed to be of
   interest to him or her?

3. On a scale of 1–10, how confident are you that Dr. _____
   would be willing to relocate and make a long-term commitment?

4. In your opinion, what were the negative factors, if any, that would present hurdles to relocation?

5. In your observations, what are other areas of notable interest that we
   should address?

Thank you again for your participation.

Sincerely,

Name,
CEO/Administrator

Source: Sitka Community Hospital, Sitka, Alaska. Used with permission.

PHYSICIAN ORIENTATION AND DEVELOPMENT

Physician Name: _____   **Practice Location:** _____

Start Date: _____   **Practice Administrator:** _____

New Physician Orientation (to be completed within first two weeks):

Orientation	Completed	Date
• MSO Orientation • Billing Director • MSO VP • Practice Administrator • Director of Finance		
Hospital Orientation		
Clinical Liaison		
Coding Specialist		
Medical Director Mtg.		
Office Orientation (w/OM)		

30-Day Visit: (with Medical Director)

30-Day Visit Due	Productivity	Schedules	Communication	Other Issues	Date Completed	Minutes Distributed

Comments/Summary:

Quarterly Review (with Medical Director, VP MSO, and Practice Administrator)

Quarterly Visit Due	Productivity	Schedules	Communication	Other Issues	Date Completed	Minutes Distributed

Comments/Summary:

Quarterly Visit Due	Productivity	Schedules	Communication	Other Issues	Date Completed	Minutes Distributed

Comments/Summary:

Annual Visit: (with Medical Director, VP MSO, and Practice Administrator)

Annual Visit Due	Productivity	Schedules	Communication	Other Issues	Date Completed	Minutes Distributed

Comments/Summary:

Source: Elliot Health System, Manchester, New Hampshire. Used with permission.

PHYSICIAN RETENTION PLAN

There are six general reasons why physicians leave a practice:

- Lack of professional interaction, support, call coverage, camaraderie
- Spousal and/or family dissatisfaction
- Economic dissatisfaction and lack of hope for improvement
- Management that does not seek or use input
- Facility, equipment, support personnel, and quality issues
- Fear or loss of professional skills

Recognizing these factors and implementing a plan to address them will ensure physician retention. The retention process begins with recruiting the physician. The first step is identifying and qualifying the candidate. Qualifying a candidate occurs through an in-depth screening to identify a match—who would be a candidate who meets all of the criteria outlined by the recruitment team to the recruitment agency. Once the candidate is qualified and scheduled for a visit, the retention process begins. Below is a detailed outline of the process for year 1:

1. Candidate qualified
2. Recruiter/Recruitment Coordinator does analysis of family needs
   - Employment of spouse
   - Day care needs
   - Schooling (special ed, higher ed)
   - Cultural needs
   - Spiritual needs
   - Recreational
3. Visit is scheduled.
   - Recruitment Coordinator contacts candidate for dates, handles all travel arrangement, and sends a relocation packet to the candidate that includes the interview itinerary, maps, directions, guidebooks, and any other pertinent information needed based on the family assessment. Recruitment Coordinator provides contact information for the candidate/family (i.e., cell phone, pager number, etc.)
4. The unforgettable family visit
   - Present practice opportunity positively and honestly.
   - Arrange for ample ABC affiliates to meet candidate.
   - Arrange appropriate appointments (or assist with such) based on family analysis (i.e., school contacts, day care information, employment needs of spouse, etc.).
   - Make them feel welcome (i.e., welcome basket in hotel room).
   - Make visit stress free. Provide excellent maps/directions to places family will visit. Offer to make appointments for them. Drive them if possible. Suggest sites for them to see while they visit, and assist with arrangements.

   Make sure the visit provides them with all the information they need about the practice opportunity, but also make sure they have a good time.

5. Contract offered by Medical Director. When the contract is extended, the following items should be discussed/reviewed with the candidate: salary guarantee, retirement plan, insurance benefits, vacation time, CME, and any other benefits offered. A realistic start date should be agreed upon taking into consideration the following:
   - Contract review
   - State licensure and hospital credentialing process
   - Third-party insurance company credentialing
   - House hunting and relocation

6. Once the contract is extended, a follow-up call from the Recruiter, Recruitment Coordinator, or Medical Director should occur within 48 hours. If the contract has not been signed within 10 business days, a second follow-up phone call should occur. If the contract has not been signed within 15 days, a second (or third, whichever applies) visit should be suggested.

7. Upon receipt of signed contract a phone call from the Recruitment Coordinator should occur, reviewing the house-hunting and relocation portion of the contract. Recruiter should offer assistance with this process to ensure a smooth transition to the area for the new physician and his or her family.

8. Upon receipt of signed contract, the credentialing process begins. (Credentialing process diagram attached).

9. Once a local address is established for the new physician, the Recruitment Coordinator should provide new physician and his/her family with access to community resources (i.e., town office information, dry cleaners, grocery stores, etc.)

10. Once the family arrives to their new home, a welcome basket should be sent.

11. Recruitment Coordinator should provide a community tour for the new physician and family and act as a resource while family is transitioning to new area. The Recruitment Coordinator should provide a forum for social integration within the first 30 days of the arrival of the new physician and his/her family to help ensure that they feel part of the community (e.g., arrange for a luncheon or a dinner with other physicians and family in the network with similar interests, etc.)

12. A physician mentor should be assigned to the new physician. The mentor will act as a resource for the new physician during his/her first six months of employment. A comprehensive orientation to the health system should be given, to include orientation to the MSO, the Hospital, the physician's practice, the hospitalist program, key administrators, and the medical community. (Outline of orientations to hospital and MSO are attached.)

13. Medical Director should visit physician at his or her practice after first 30 days. Three quarterly visits should occur with Medical Director, VP MSO, and Practice Administrator for first year of employment.

14. Provide a comprehensive marketing initiative for the new physician through media venues.

15. Medical Director should maintain an open-door policy for new physicians. A forum should be held once a month for the first six months for

new physicians to go and discuss any problems or concerns, hosted either by the medical director or a long-time physician. These sessions can be hosted at the hospital during lunch time.

The following are retention strategies that should continue during the early years (years 1–3). Typically, if a physician stays for three years, he or she is most likely to remain.

1. Facilitate ability of practitioners to use most/all of their medical expertise/skills. Provide avenues for those physicians who want to learn new skills to be able to do so. For example, if you have a physician who is trained to do endoscopic procedures, you should do your best to arrange for him or her to be able to do them. If there are practitioners who wish to learn to do such a procedure, you should have a process in place so this can happen. Encourage practitioners to develop new professional interests.
2. Recognize the varying needs of individual practitioners to achieve professional satisfaction and support activities toward achieving such satisfaction (i.e., teaching opportunities, research interests, lecturing at medical meetings, etc.).
3. Minimize administrative hassles. Maintain an overall reasonable workload/schedule, including days worked per week and on-call schedule.
4. Have a recognition plan in place.
5. Provide a forum for the new physicians and their families to meet other physicians and their families through scheduled social events or personal introductions. Try to find other physicians and their families in the health system who share common interests and arrange for introductions. Assist the new practitioner and his or her family in making a smooth transition to the community. The Recruitment Coordinator should facilitate such functions and meetings.

Once a physician has remained for three years, the risk of him or her leaving is much less. Most of the strategies for retention in the early years apply to retention in the later years. Some additional strategies for retention in the later years are as follows:

1. Encourage physicians to develop new professional skills and interests that can be incorporated into their practices.
2. Seek input from senior physicians during key decision-making processes.
3. Consider a years-of-service recognition plan in which call coverage is reduced, benefits improve, awards given, and so forth.

Source: Elliot Health System, Manchester, New Hampshire.
Used with permission.

CHECKLIST FOR INITIATING HOSPITAL-EMPLOYED PHYSICIAN PRACTICE

Physician Practice: _____   **Date:** _____

A. Preagreement Activities

Task	Department(s)	Date	Status

1. Obtain independent appraisal of practice:
  • Include list of assets to be acquired.
  • Include list of liabilities to be assumed.
	Planning		

2. Fair market value salary survey	Planning		
3. Confirm community and hospital need.	Planning		
4. Establish range of compensation package.	CEO/Legal		
5. Review practice agreements to determine assignability/termination.	Planning/Legal		

B. Physician Employment

Task	Department(s)	Date	Status
1. Contract negotiations	CEO/Legal Project VP		
2. Develop salary structure.	CEO/Legal Project VP		
3. Develop benefits structure.	CEO/Legal Project VP		
4. Determine start date and contract term.	CEO/Legal Project VP		
5. Credentialing process	Med Staff		

C. Acquisition Activities

Task	Department(s)	Date	Status
1. UCC search, certificates of good standing, liens, civil filings, etc.	Legal Project VP		
2. Prepare related legal documents, such as assignments, estoppel agreements, etc.	Legal Project VP		
3. Seller board approval	CEO/Legal Project VP		
4. Buyer board approval	CEO/Legal Project VP		

D. Financial

Task	Department(s)	Date	Status
1. Review managed care contracts: • Obtain assignments? • Negotiate new contracts. • Place under existing contracts.	Mgd Care/ Pt. Bus Srvc		
2. Obtain Medicare provider numbers.	Pt. Bus Service		
3. Review tax considerations.	Fiscal Services		
4. Create cost centers.	Fiscal Services		
5. Review current revenue/expenses and develop operating budget.	Fiscal Services Project VP		
6. Develop financial reporting procedures.	Fiscal Services		
7. Review office current billing policies and procedures.	Fiscal Services Compliance		
8. Fee schedule review	Fiscal Services Compliance		

E. Information Systems/Communications

Task	Department(s)	Date	Status
1. Review billing system: • Add to UCH physician billing. • Continue independent billing.	Pt. Bus Service Compliance MIS		
2. Transcription system • Add to UCH transcription. • Continue independent transcription.	HIM/MIS		
3. Review equipment and software functionality: • Add to UCH inventory. • Terminate agreements.	MIS		
4. Determine system support requirement.	MIS		
5. Office telephone, pager, cellular, and long-distance access	Communications		
6. Computer access	MIS		

F. Medical Records

Task	Department(s)	Date	Status
1. Review medical records procedures.	HIM Compliance		
2. Perform coding audit.	HIM Compliance		
3. Establish process for medical records management.	HIM		

G. Insurance

Task	Department(s)	Date	Status
1. Professional liability	VP (Insurance)		
2. Property	VP (Insurance)		
3. Business/office liability	VP (Insurance)		

H. Contract Review/Management

Task	Department(s)	Date	Status
1. Property leases	Planning/Legal		
2. Equipment leases	Material Mgmt., Fiscal Services		
3. Software license agreements	MIS/Legal Fiscal Services		
4. Services	Fiscal Services Legal		
5. Consulting	Fiscal Services Legal		

I. Human Resources

Task	Department(s)	Date	Status
1. Determine whether support staff will be employed.	Project VP/HR		
2. Develop job descriptions.	Project VP/HR		
3. Complete applications.	HR		
4. Health screening	Employee Health HR		

	Department(s)	Date	Status
5. Background screening, including OIG	HR Compliance		
6. Salary negotiations/hiring	Project VP/HR		
7. Orientation	Education/HR		
8. Other			

J. Marketing/Public Relations

Task	Department(s)	Date	Status
1. Notification letter to patients	Project VP/Legal Public Relations		
2. Notices in newspaper	Public Relations		
3. Letterhead/stationary/business cards	Public Relations		
4. Telephone book/Yellow Pages	Public Relations		
5. Review current practice brochures.	Public Relations		
6. Review current advertisement.	Public Relations		
7. Building signage	Public Relations		

K. Office Operations

Task	Department(s)	Date	Status
1. Purchasing/obtaining medical supplies	Materials Mgmt., Fiscal Services		
2. Employee time accounting	HR/Payroll		
3. Accounting and A/P procedures	Fiscal Services		

Task	Department(s)		
4. Interoffice mail	Mail Room		
5. E-mail	MIS		
6. Purchasing/obtaining medications	Materials Mgmt. Pharmacy		
7. Purchasing/obtaining office supplies	Materials Mgmt.		
8. Cash collection procedures	Fiscal Services Pt. Bus. Services		
9. A/R management	Pt. Bus. Services		

L. Construction/Relocation

Task	Department(s)	Date	Status
1. Identify space requirements.	Project VP Construction		
2. Identify space availability/alternatives.	Project VP Construction Prop. Mgmt.		
3. Develop layout/plans.	Project VP Construction		
4. Identify medical equipment requirements.	Project VP/ Materials Mgmt./ Construction		
5. Identify office equipment requirements.	Project VP/ Materials Mgmt./ Construction		

6. Identify furniture requirements.	Project VP/ Materials Mgmt./ Construction		
7. Identify computer and communications equipment requirements.	Project VP, MIS Construction		
8. Prepare capital budget.	Project VP		
9. Prepare project budget.	Project VP Construction		
10. Construct or remodel space.	Project VP Construction		
11. Relocate office.	Project VP Construction		

Index

Notes

Notes

Notes

Notes

Notes

Notes

Notes

Notes

Notes

Notes